D0523339

# Ratio & Proportion WITHDRAWN Dosage Calculations

**Anthony Patrick Giangrasso, Ph.D.**
Professor of Mathematics
LaGuardia Community College
Long Island City, NY

**Dolores M. Shrimpton, M.A., R.N.**
Professor of Nursing
Kingsborough Community College
Brooklyn, NY

**DATE DUE**

| | |
|---|---|
| SEP 0 8 2010 | |
| SEP 0 8 2010 | |
| JUN 2 0 2011 | |
| MAR 0 5 2012 | |
| | |
| | |
| | |
| | |
| | |
| | |
| | |
| | |
| | |

BRODART, CO.      Cat. No. 23-221

**PEARSON**

Upper Saddle River, New Jersey, 07458

Library of Congress Cataloging-in-Publication Data
Giangrasso, Anthony Patrick.
    Ratio & proportion dosage calculations / Anthony Patrick Giangrasso, Dolores M. Shrimpton.
       p. ; cm.
    Includes index.
    ISBN-13: 978-0-13-513596-9
    ISBN-10: 0-13-513596-6
1.  Pharmaceutical arithmetic  I. Shrimpton, Dolores M. II. Title. III. Title: Ratio and proportion dosage
calculations.
    [DNLM: 1.  Drug Dosage Calculations—Problems and Exercises.  QV 18.2 G433r 2010]
    RS57.G53 2010
    615'.1401513—dc22

                                                              2008046839

**Publisher:** Julie Levin Alexander
**Publisher's Assistant:** Regina Bruno
**Editor-in-Chief:** Maura Connor
**Senior Acquisitions Editor:** Kelly Trakalo
**Editorial Assistant:** Lauren Sweeney
**Director of Development:** Stephanie Klein
**Development Editor:** Michael Giacobbe
**Media Project Manager:** Lorena Cerisano
**Director of Marketing:** Karen Allman
**Senior Marketing Manager:** Francisco Del Castillo
**Marketing Coordinator:** Michael Sirinides

**Marketing Assistant:** Crystal Gonzalez
**Managing Editor, Production:** Patrick Walsh
**Production Editor:** Leo Kelly, Macmillan Publishing Solutions
**Production Liason:** Yagnesh Jani
**Manufacturing Manager/Buyer:** Ilene Sanford
**Senior Design Coordinator:** Christopher Weigand
**Interior and Cover Designer:** Wanda Espana
**Composition:** Macmillan Publishing Solutions
**Printer/Binder:** Webcrafters. Inc.
**Cover Printer:** Phoenix Color

Notice: Care has been taken to confirm the accuracy of information presented in this book.  The authors, editors, and the publisher,
however, cannot accept any responsibility for errors or omissions or for consequences from application of the information in this book
and make no warranty, express or implied, with respect to its contents. The authors and publisher have exerted every effort to ensure
that drug selections and dosages set forth in this text are in accord with current recommendations and practice at time of publication.
However, in view of ongoing research, changes in government regulations, and the constant flow of information relating to drug therapy
and drug reactions, the reader is urged to check the package inserts of all drugs for any change in indications of dosage and for added
warnings and precautions.  This is particularly important when the recommended agent is a new and/or infrequently employed drug.

Copyright © 2010 by Pearson Education, Inc., Upper Saddle River, New Jersey 07458. Pearson. All rights reserved. Printed in the
United States of America. This publication is protected by Copyright and permission should be obtained from the publisher prior to
any prohibited reproduction, storage in a retrieval system, or transmission in any form or by any means, electronic, mechanical,
photocopying, recording, or likewise. For information regarding permission(s), write to: Rights and Permissions Department.

Pearson® is a registered trademark of Pearson plc

Pearson Education Ltd.
Pearson Education Singapore Pte. Ltd.
Pearson Education Canada, Ltd.
Pearson Education—Japan
Pearson Education Australia Pty. Limited

Pearson Education North Asia Ltd., Hong Kong
Pearson Educación de Mexico, S.A. de C.V.
Pearson Education Malaysia Pte. Ltd.
Pearson Education Inc., Upper Saddle River, New Jersey

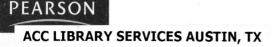

ACC LIBRARY SERVICES AUSTIN, TX

10 9 8 7 6 5 4 3 2
ISBN 10:        0-13-513596-6
ISBN 13:    978-0-13-513596-9

# Dedications

To Anthony J. Calio, MD, who has used his skill to keep me healthy enough to continue working and enjoying life well beyond "retirement age." The etymology of the word "doctor" is "teacher," and Dr. Calio is a wonderful instructor who is generous with his time, both with his patients and with the young physicians he oversees. Dr. Calio exemplifies the words of Hippocrates, "With purity and holiness I will pass my life and practice my art."

**—Anthony Giangrasso**


In loving memory of my beautiful redheaded niece, Tara Ann Donahue, Tara's mother Mary Ann Donahue, aunt Cheryl Donahue, and her grandparents, my mom and dad, Mary and Francis X. Donahue. You are all loved and missed very much.

A huge thank you to my co-author, Dr. Anthony Giangrasso, a wonderful mathematician, tremendous tennis player, and all around great guy. Tony, it has been a lot of work, but great fun as well.

**—Dolores Shrimpton**

# About the Authors

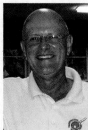 **ANTHONY GIANGRASSO** was born and raised in Maspeth, NY. He attended Rice High School on a scholarship and in his senior year was named in a citywide contest by the *New York Journal-American* newspaper as New York City's most outstanding high school scholar-athlete. He was also awarded a full-tuition scholarship to Iona College, from which he obtained a BA in mathematics, magna cum laude, with a ranking of sixth in his graduating class.

Anthony began his teaching career as a fifth-grade teacher in Manhattan as a member of the Christian Brothers of Ireland, and taught high school mathematics and physics in Harlem and Newark, NJ. He possesses an MS and Ph.D. from New York University, and has taught at all levels from elementary school through graduate school. He is currently teaching at Adelphi University and LaGuardia Community College, where he was chairman of the mathematics department. He has authored eight college textbooks through twenty-one editions.

Anthony's community service has included membership on the Boards of Directors of the Polish-American Museum Foundation, Catholic Adoptive Parents Association, and Family Focus Adoptive Services. He was the president of the Italian-American Faculty Association of the City University of New York, and the founding Chairman of the Board of the Italian-American Legal Defense and Higher Education Fund, Inc. He and his wife, Susan, are proud parents of three children Anthony, Michael, and Jennifer. He enjoys tennis, and in 2007 for the second time was ranked #1 for his age group in the Eastern Section by the United States Tennis Association.

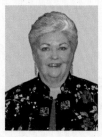 **DOLORES SHRIMPTON** is the immediate past president of the New York State Associate Degree Nursing Council, where she also served as the vice president and member of its Board of Directors. She was the co-chair of the CUNY Nursing Discipline Council for more than ten years, an active member of the Nurses Association of the Counties of Long Island (NACLI), D14 of the New York State Nurses Association, an active member of the Nursing Capacity Team, which founded the Brooklyn Nursing Partnership (BNP). She has served on the Board of Directors and as the first co-vice president of the BNP. She was also the project co-director of the New York State Coalition for Nursing Educational Mobility (NYSCNEM). She serves on a number of Advisory Boards of LPN, associate degree, and baccalaureate degree nursing programs.

Dolores has received many awards for her achievements in nursing. In 2008 she was honored for her commitment to nursing by the Brooklyn Nursing Partnership (BNP). She is the recipient of the Presidential Award in Nursing Leadership from NACLI, the Mu Upsilon award for Excellence in Nursing Education, and the 2006 Mu Upsilon award for Excellence in Nursing Leadership. Dolores has taught a wide variety of courses in practical nursing, diploma, and associate degree nursing programs. Her area of clinical practice is maternity, with a focus on labor and delivery.

# Preface

In 1995, the Institute of Medication issued its landmark report, "To Err Is Human: Building a Safer Health System," which claimed that nearly 100,000 people died annually due to medical errors. Since that report, greater emphasis has been placed on improving "safety" in medication administration. One aspect of that safety is accuracy in drug calculations. *Ratio & Proportion Dosage Calculations* is not merely a textbook about math skills; it is also an introduction to the professional context of safe drug administration. Calculation skills and the rationales behind them are emphasized throughout.

This book uses the Ratio and Proportion method for dosage calculations, a time-tested approach based on simple mathematical concepts. It helps the student develop a "number sense," and largely frees the student from the need to memorize formulas. Once the technique is mastered, students will be able to calculate drug dosages quickly and safely.

Because of the growing use and acceptance of handheld calculators, the first chapter of this textbook includes **keystroke sequences** to enable checking of calculations on the calculator. Illustrative examples proceed in small increments from the simple to the more complex. The text uses examples of realistic drug orders containing both the trade and generic names of the medications prescribed.

Because of safety considerations, the apothecary system should no longer be used in drug orders. Therefore, a discussion of the apothecary system is not included in the body of the textbook, but has been placed in Appendix B for those who would like to study it.

*Ratio & Proportion Dosage Calculations* is a combined text and workbook. Its consistent focus on safety, accuracy, and professionalism make it a valuable part of a course for nursing or allied health programs. It is also highly effective for independent study and may be used as a refresher for dosage-calculation skills and as a professional reference.

*Ratio & Proportion Dosage Calculations* is arranged into four basic learning units:

**Unit 1: Basic Calculation Skills and Introduction to Medication Administration**
Chapter 1 includes a diagnostic test of arithmetic and reviews the necessary basic mathematics skills. Chapter 2 introduces the student to the essentials of the medication administration process. Chapter 3 introduces the Ratio and Proportion method in small increments using a simple, step-by-step, common sense approach.

**Unit 2: Systems of Measurement**
Chapters 4 and 5 present the metric and household systems of measurement that nurses and other allied health professionals must understand in order to interpret medication orders and calculate dosages. Students learn to convert measurements between and within measurement systems.

**Unit 3: Oral and Parenteral Medications**
Chapters 6, 7, 8, and 9 prepare students to calculate oral and parenteral dosages and introduce them to the essential equipment needed for administration and preparation of solutions.

**Unit 4: Infusions and Pediatric Dosages**
Chapters 10 and 11 provide a solid foundation for calculating intravenous and enteral dosage rates and flow rates and include titrating IV medications. Pediatric dosages and daily fluid maintenance needs are discussed in Chapter 12.

In addition to these topics, this edition includes a substantial amount of information about safety in medication administration and follows the *National Patient Safety Goals of the Joint Commission*. Readers will learn how to interpret actual drug labels, package inserts, and various forms of medication orders, as well as how to select the appropriate equipment to administer the prescribed dose.

# Benefits of Using *Ratio & Proportion Dosage Calculations*

- Constant skill reinforcement through frequent practice opportunities.
- More than 1,000 problems for students to solve.
- Actual drug labels, syringes, drug package inserts, prescriptions, and medication administration records (MARs) are illustrated throughout the text.
- Ample work space on every page for note taking and problem solving.
- Worked out solutions to practice exercises are found in the textbook in Appendix A.

# Acknowledgments

Our special thanks to the nursing and mathematics faculty and the students at LaGuardia Community College and Kingsborough Community College. Also, a special thank you to our editor, Kelly Trakalo, and development editor, Michael Giacobbe, and to the production and marketing teams at Pearson.

Thank you also to the following manufacturers for supplying labels and art for this textbook:

Abbott Laboratories; American Pharmaceutical Partners; Amgen, Inc.; Astra Zeneca; Baxter; Bayer Pharmaceutical Corporation; Eisai, Inc.; Eli Lilly and Company; Forrest Pharmaceuticals, Inc.; GlaxoSmithKline; Merck and Company, Inc.; Novartis Pharmaceuticals; Pfizer, Inc.; Purdue Pharma; Roxane Laboratories; Teva Pharmaceutical Industries Ltd.

**Reviewers for *Ratio & Proportion Dosage Calculations***
*Eileen Costello, RN, MSN*
Dean, School of Health Sciences
Mount Wachusett Community College
Gardner, MA

*Pamela Fowler, MS, RNC*
Assistant Professor
Rogers State University
Claremore, OK

*Jim Hodge, Ed.D.*
Professor of Mathematics
Mountain State University
Beckley, WV

*Janet Lile, RN, MSN, Ph.D.*
Nursing Instructor
College of the Sequoias
Visalia, CA

*Vincent J. Maltese, Jr., MA*
Dean of Science/Mathematics
Monroe County Community College
Monroe, MI

*Mandyam A. Tirumalachar, MD, FRCP*
Adjunct Professor
Austin Community College
Austin, TX

# Contents

**CHAPTER 3**  **Ratio and Proportion    73**

**Unit 2**  **Systems of Measurement    105**

**CHAPTER 4**  **The Metric and Household Systems    106**

# Learn to Calculate Dosages Safely and Accurately!

## The Ease of Learning with Ratio & Proportion

**Ratio & Proportion Dosage Calculations** provides the ease of learning the ratio and proportion method of calculation with a building block approach of the basics.

Name: _____     Date: _____

### Diagnostic Test of Arithmetic

The following Diagnostic Test illustrates all the arithmetic skills needed to do the computations in this textbook. Take the test and compare your answers with the answers found in Appendix A. If you discover areas of weakness, carefully review the relevant review materials in Chapter 1 so that you will be mathematically prepared for the rest of the textbook.

1. Write 0.375 as a fraction in lowest terms. _____

2. Write $\frac{28,500}{100,000}$ as a decimal number. _____

3. Round off 6.492 to the nearest tenth. _____

4. Write $\frac{5}{6}$ as a decimal number rounded off to the nearest hundredth. _____

5. Simplify $\frac{0.63}{0.2}$ to a decimal number rounded off to the nearest tenth. _____

6. $0.038 \times 100 =$ _____

7. $4.26 \times 0.015 =$ _____

8. $55 \div 0.11 =$ _____

9. $90 \times \frac{1}{300} \times \frac{20}{3} =$ _____

10. Write $5\frac{3}{4} \div 23$ as a fraction and as a decimal number. _____

11. Write $\frac{7}{100} \div \frac{3}{100}$ as a mixed number. _____

12. Write $\frac{\frac{4}{5}}{20}$ as a simple fraction in lowest terms. _____

**The Diagnostic Test of Arithmetic** helps students rediscover their understanding of basic math concepts and guides them in identifying areas for review.

---

### EXAMPLE 3.6

Is $\frac{30}{120} = \frac{6}{18}$ a true portion?

To determine if this proportion is true, cross multiply. If the products obtained are equal, then the proportion is true.

Cross multiply

$$\frac{30}{120} = \frac{6}{18}$$

$$(6)(120) = (30)(18)$$
$$720 \neq 540$$

Because the products are not equal, $\frac{30}{120} = \frac{6}{18}$ is not a true proportion.

---

**Learn by Example.** Each chapter unfolds basic concepts and skills through completely worked out questions with solutions.

### EXAMPLE 6.1

The order reads *Cymbalta (duloxetine HCl) 120 mg PO daily.*

Read the drug label shown in ● Figure 6.1. How many capsules of this antidepressant drug will you administer to the patient?

**NDC 0002-3240-30**
**30 capsules          PU3240**

**Cymbalta®** *DELAYED RELEASE CAPSULES*
duloxetine HCl

**30 mg**

Each capsule contains 33.7 mg of duloxetine hydrochloride equivalent to 30 mg duloxetine.

**Rx only**

www.Cymbalta.com     *Lilly*

Dispense in a tightly closed container. Keep out of the reach of children.
Eli Lilly and Company
Indianapolis, IN 46285, USA
Expiration Date/Control No.
WW 8931 AMX

See accompanying literature for dosage. Store at 25°C (77°F); excursions permitted to 15-30°C (59-86°F).

Medication Guide is to be dispensed to patients.

3 0002-3240-30 9

● Figure 6.1
**Drug label for Cymbalta.**
*(Copyright Eli Lilly and Company. Used with permission.)*

# Safe and Accurate Dosage Calculation

Safe and accurate dosage calculation comes from practice and critical thinking.

**Try These for Practice, Exercises,** and **Additional Exercises,** found in every chapter, tests your comprehension of material.

Workspace

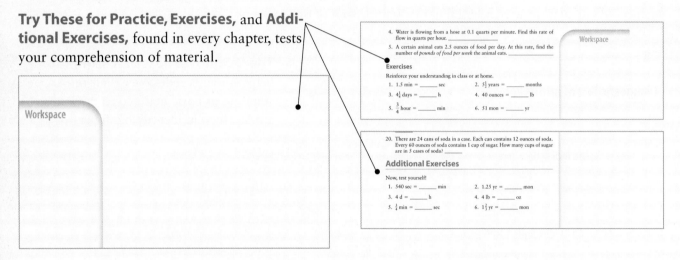

4. Water is flowing from a hose at 0.1 quarts per minute. Find this rate of flow in quarts per hour. _____

5. A certain animal eats 2.5 ounces of food per day. At this rate, find the number of *pounds of food per week* the animal eats. _____

Workspace

**Exercises**

Reinforce your understanding in class or at home.

1. 1.5 min = _____ sec      2. $5\frac{1}{2}$ years = _____ months

3. $4\frac{1}{4}$ days = _____ h      4. 40 ounces = _____ lb

5. $\frac{3}{4}$ hour = _____ min      6. 51 mon = _____ yr

20. There are 24 cans of soda in a case. Each can contains 12 ounces of soda. Every 60 ounces of soda contains 1 cup of sugar. How many cups of sugar are in 5 cases of soda? _____

**Additional Exercises**

Now, test yourself!

1. 540 sec = _____ min      2. 1.25 yr = _____ mon

3. 4 d = _____ h      4. 4 lb = _____ oz

5. $\frac{3}{4}$ min = _____ sec      6. $1\frac{2}{3}$ yr = _____ mon

**Cumulative Review Exercises** begin in Chapter 4 and review mastery of earlier chapters.

**Case Studies.** Clinical case scenarios allow the student opportunities for critical thinking as they apply concepts and techniques presented in the text.

Workspace

**Cumulative Review Exercises**

Review your mastery of earlier chapters.

1. 7.8 g = _____ mg      2. 0.25 mg = _____ mcg

3. 4.5 L = _____ mL      4. 12 T = _____ oz

5. 1,200 mL = _____ L      6. 7.6 kg = _____ g

7. Convert 750 mL to liters.

8. How many teaspoons are contained in 5 T?

9. The order reads Carafate 1 g PO q.i.d. Convert this dose to milligrams.

10. The patient must receive 250 mg of Cloxacillin PO q6h. Change to grams.

11. Change 0.65 mg to micrograms.

12. The physician ordered 2 T of Mylanta PO q2h. How many teaspoons of this antacid would you prepare?

13. The order is Colace 150 mg PO t.i.d. the label reads 150 mg/15 mL. How many milliliters would you prepare?

14. Change 250 mL to liters.

15. Change 0.032 g to milligrams.

**Case Study 6.1**

Mr. M. is a 68-year-old male patient with a past medical history of diabetes mellitus Type II and severe ischemic cardiomyopathy. He reported that for 6 weeks he had been experiencing shortness of breath and fatigue with moderate activity, difficulty sleeping at night, and has a weight gain of 5 lbs, even though he described his appetite as poor. There is no evidence of smoking or illegal drug use. Upon examination, the practitioner noted periorbital edema and bilateral 4+ pitting edema in both lower extremities. His present weight is 154 lb and his vital signs are BP 160/100, T 98.4, P 104, and R 28. Mr. M. was admitted for intravenous support and aggressive diuresis.
His orders are as follows:

■ Complete CBC and SMA18

2. At 8 P.M., Mr. M.'s v
ganic brand of chicken broth, w
390 mg salt in each 1 cup serving.
(a) How many mL of chicken
patient receive?
(b) How many grams of salt did
(c) How much more salt should
sume for the remainder of th

3. The diuretic drug Lasix (furoser
able in 20 mg tablets.
(a) How many tablets will you a
the stat dose?
(b) How many tablets will the
received within the first 20 h

4. How many milliequivalents of t
supplement micro-K will the

**Notes** and **Alerts** highlight concepts and principles for safe medication calculation and administration.

## ALERT

Because the volume of ordinary household spoons, cups, and glasses may vary, medications should not be administered using ordinary household utensils.

## NOTE

Whenever you set up a proportion, both fractions should have the units of measurement in corresponding positions. That is, the numerators should have matching units (*oz* in this case), and the denominator units (*glasses* in this case) should also match.

**Realistic Illustrations.** Real drug labels and realistic syringes aid in identifying and practicing with what you will encounter in actual clinical settings.

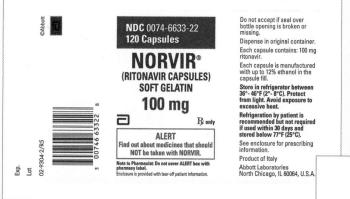

NDC 0074-6633-22
**120 Capsules**

**NORVIR®**
(RITONAVIR CAPSULES)
SOFT GELATIN

**100 mg**

℞ only

**ALERT**
Find out about medicines that should
NOT be taken with NORVIR.

Note to Pharmacist: Do not cover ALERT box with pharmacy label.
Enclosure is provided with tear-off patient information.

Do not accept if seal over bottle opening is broken or missing.

Dispense in original container.

Each capsule contains: 100 mg ritonavir.

Each capsule is manufactured with up to 12% ethanol in the capsule fill.

**Store in refrigerator between 36°- 46°F (2°- 8°C). Protect from light. Avoid exposure to excessive heat.**

**Refrigeration by patient is recommended but not required if used within 30 days and stored below 77°F (25°C).**

See enclosure for prescribing information.

Product of Italy

Abbott Laboratories
North Chicago, IL 60064, U.S.A.

©Abbott

Exp.
Lot

02-9304-2/R5

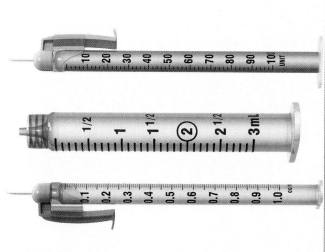

# Additional Student Resources

**Pearson's Dosage Calculation Tutor.** This CD-ROM comes packaged with every textbook. A unique interface guides the user through animated examples of chapter topics, provides practice questions, chapter challenge test, and a comprehensive final test.

**Companion website.** Go to www.prenhall.com/giangrasso for an online study guide. The companion website provides even more review and practice questions.

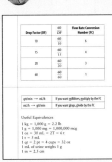

**Pocket Reminder Card.** Use this handy reference for examples and equivalency charts to accurately calculate medical dosages wherever and whenever you need to.

# Additional Instructor Resources

**Instructor's Manual.** The instructor's manual that accompanies this book provides extra test questions and answers, answers to the additional exercises that are found in the book, a list of key terms, possible teaching approaches relevant to each chapter, an overview of learning outcomes for each chapter, and comprehensive examinations with answers. This instructor's manual helps instructors prepare lectures and examinations quickly.

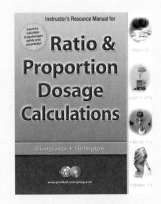

**Instructor' Resource CD-ROM.** This CD-ROM resource contains a computerized test generator, plus PowerPoint slides to help guide lectures and a link to the Instructor's Manual.

**Online Course Management.** Pearson's online course management solutions feature all of the instructor resources and companion website materials in a flexible, easy-to-use format. Course management tools allow customization of course content, online testing, gradebook functionality, and robust communication tools. Please contact your Pearson sales representative for Pearson's course management options, or if you require customization to a different course-management platform.

# Unit

# Basic Calculation Skills and Introduction to Medication Administration

**Chapter 1**

## Review of Arithmetic for Medical Dosage Calculations

**Chapter 2**

## Safe and Accurate Drug Administration

**Chapter 3**

## Ratio and Proportion

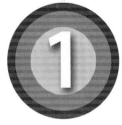

**Chapter**

# Review of Arithmetic for Medical Dosage Calculations

## Learning Outcomes

$$5\frac{3}{4} \div 23$$

After completing this chapter, you will be able to

1. Reduce and build fractions.
2. Add, subtract, multiply, and divide fractions.
3. Simplify complex fractions.
4. Convert between decimal numbers and fractions.
5. Add, subtract, multiply, and divide decimal numbers.
6. Round decimal numbers to a desired number of decimal places.
7. Write percentages as decimal numbers and fractions.
8. Find a percent of a number and the percent of change.
9. Estimate answers.
10. Use a calculator to verify answers.

Medical dosage calculations can involve whole numbers, fractions, decimal numbers, and percentages. Your results on the *Diagnostic Test of Arithmetic*, found on the next page, will identify your areas of strength and weakness. You can use Chapter 1 to improve your math skills or simply to review the kinds of calculations you will encounter in this text.

# Diagnostic Test of Arithmetic

The following Diagnostic Test illustrates all the arithmetic skills needed to do the computations in this textbook. Take the test and compare your answers with the answers found in Appendix A. If you discover areas of weakness, carefully review the relevant review materials in Chapter 1 so that you will be mathematically prepared for the rest of the textbook.

1. Write 0.375 as a fraction in lowest terms. _____

2. Write $\frac{28,500}{100,000}$ as a decimal number. _____

3. Round off 6.492 to the nearest tenth. _____

4. Write $\frac{5}{6}$ as a decimal number rounded off to the nearest hundredth. _____

5. Simplify $\frac{0.63}{0.2}$ to a decimal number rounded off to the nearest tenth. _____

6. $0.038 \times 100 =$ _____

7. $4.26 \times 0.015 =$ _____

8. $55 \div 0.11 =$ _____

9. $90 \times \frac{1}{300} \times \frac{20}{3} =$ _____

10. Write $5\frac{3}{4} \div 23$ as a fraction and as a decimal number. _____

11. Write $\frac{7}{100} \div \frac{3}{100}$ as a mixed number. _____

12. Write $\frac{\frac{4}{5}}{20}$ as a simple fraction in lowest terms. _____

13. Write 45% as a fraction in lowest terms. _____

14. Write $2\frac{1}{2}\%$ as a decimal number. _____

15. Write $2\frac{4}{7}$ as an improper fraction. _____

16. 30% of 40 = _____

17. $4.1 + 0.5 + 3 =$ _____

18. $\frac{3}{4} = \frac{?}{8}$ _____

19. Which is larger, 0.4 or 0.21? _____

20. Express the ratio 15 to 20 as a fraction in lowest terms. _____

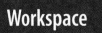

# Changing Decimal Numbers and Whole Numbers to Fractions

A decimal number represents a fraction with a denominator of 10; 100; 1,000; and so on. Each decimal number has three parts: the whole-number part, the decimal point, and the fraction part. Table 1.1 shows the names of the decimal positions.

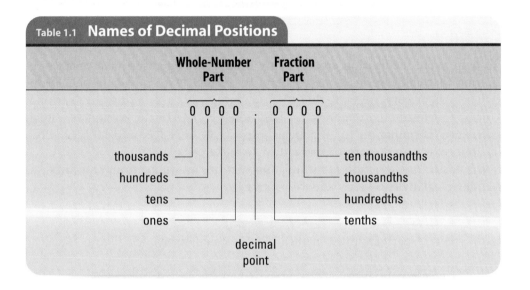

Table 1.1  **Names of Decimal Positions**

Reading a decimal number will help you write it as a fraction.

| Decimal Number | $\longrightarrow$ | Read | $\longrightarrow$ | Fraction |
|---|---|---|---|---|
| 4.1 | $\longrightarrow$ | four and one tenth | $\longrightarrow$ | $4\dfrac{1}{10}$ |
| 0.3 | $\longrightarrow$ | three tenths | $\longrightarrow$ | $\dfrac{3}{10}$ |
| 6.07 | $\longrightarrow$ | six and seven hundredths | $\longrightarrow$ | $6\dfrac{7}{100}$ |
| 0.231 | $\longrightarrow$ | two hundred thirty-one thousandths | $\longrightarrow$ | $\dfrac{231}{1,000}$ |
| 0.0025 | $\longrightarrow$ | twenty-five ten thousandths | $\longrightarrow$ | $\dfrac{25}{10,000}$ |

**NOTE**

A decimal number that is less than 1 is written with a leading zero, for example, 0.3 and 0.0025.

A number can be written in different forms. A decimal number *less than 1*, such as 0.9, is read as *nine tenths* and can also be written as the *proper fraction* $\frac{9}{10}$. In a **proper fraction**, the numerator (the number on the top) of the fraction is smaller than its denominator (the number on the bottom).

A decimal number *greater than 1*, such as 3.5, is read as *three and five tenths* and can also be written as the *mixed number* $3\frac{5}{10}$ or $3\frac{1}{2}$. A **mixed number** combines a whole number and a proper fraction. The *mixed number* $3\frac{1}{2}$, can be changed to an *improper fraction* as follows:

$$3\frac{1}{2} = \frac{3 \times 2 + 1}{2} = \frac{7}{2}$$

The numerator (top number) of an **improper fraction** is larger than or equal to its denominator (bottom number).

Any number can be written as a fraction by writing it over 1. For example, 9 can be written as the improper fraction $\frac{9}{1}$.

## Calculator

**NOTE**

The student CD contains a pull-down calculator.

To help avoid medication errors, many health care agencies have policies requiring that calculations done by hand be verified with a calculator. "Dropdown" calculators are available to candidates who are taking the National Council Licensure Examination for Registered Nurses or the National Council Licensure Examination for Practical Nurses (NCLEX-RN and NCLEX-PN). Therefore, it is important to know how to use a calculator.

A basic, four-function (addition, subtraction, multiplication, and division) handheld calculator with a square-root key

is sufficient to perform most medical dosage calculations. See Figure 1.1.

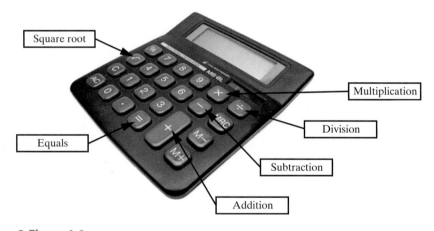

● **Figure 1.1**
**Basic Handheld Calculator**

Some students might prefer a calculator that also has a percent key %, a fraction key $a^{b}c$ , and parentheses keys ( and ) .

To change the improper fraction $\frac{7}{2}$ to a decimal number with a calculator:

First press   7
Then press   ÷
Then press   2
Then press   =
The display shows   3.5

**NOTE**

Some calculators use the Enter key rather than the = key.

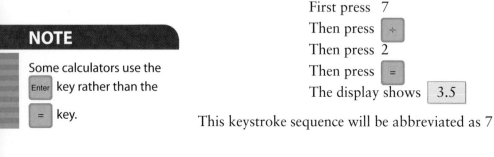

This keystroke sequence will be abbreviated as  7  ÷  2  =   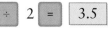 3.5

If the calculator has a fraction key, the mixed-number form of $\frac{7}{2}$ will be obtained by the following keystroke sequence:

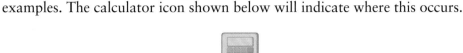

Throughout this chapter, keystroke sequences will be shown for selected examples. The calculator icon shown below will indicate where this occurs.

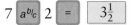

## EXAMPLE 1.1

**Write 2.25 as a mixed number and as an improper fraction.**

The number 2.25 is read *two and twenty-five hundredths* and is written $2\frac{25}{100}$. You can simplify:

$$2\frac{25}{100} = 2\frac{\overset{1}{\cancel{25}}}{\underset{4}{\cancel{100}}} = 2\frac{1}{4} = \frac{2 \times 4 + 1}{4} = \frac{9}{4}$$

So, 2.25 can be written as the mixed number $2\frac{1}{4}$ or as the improper fraction $\frac{9}{4}$.

## Ratios

A **ratio** is a comparison of two numbers.

The ratio of *5 to 10* can also be written as *5:10* or in fractional form as $\frac{5}{10}$. This fraction may be *reduced by cancelling* by a number that evenly divides both the numerator and the denominator. Since 5 evenly divides both 5 and 10, divide as follows:

$$\frac{5}{10} = \frac{5 \div 5}{10 \div 5} = \frac{1}{2}$$

The fraction $\frac{5}{10}$ is *reduced to lowest terms* as $\frac{1}{2}$.

So, the ratio of *5 to 10* can also be written as the ratio of *1 to 2* or *1:2*.

## EXAMPLE 1.2

**Express 6:18 as an equivalent fraction in lowest terms.**

The ratio *6:18*, also written as *6 to 18*, can be written in fractional form as $\frac{6}{18}$. This fraction may be *reduced by cancelling* by a number that evenly divides both the numerator and the denominator. Since 6 divides both 6 and 18, divide as follows:

$$\frac{6}{18} = \frac{6 \div 6}{18 \div 6} = \frac{1}{3}$$

So, the ratio 6 to 18 equals the fraction $\frac{1}{3}$.

**NOTE**

The keystroke sequences presented in this chapter apply to many calculators. But not all calculators work the same way. If you have a problem, consult the user's manual for your calculator. The Student CD is found on the inside back cover.

**NOTE**

In Example 1.1, $\frac{25}{100}$ was simplified by dividing both numerator and denominator by 25. This process is called *cancelling*.

$$\frac{25 \div 25}{100 \div 25} = \frac{1}{4}$$

**Keystroke Sequence for Example 1.1:** To obtain the simplified mixed number, enter the following keystroke sequence.

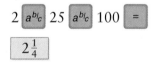

**Keystroke Sequence for Example 1.2:**

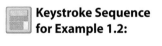
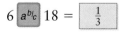

**Keystroke Sequence for Example 1.3:**

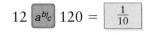

### NOTE

When *reducing* a fraction, you *divide* both numerator and denominator by the same number. This process is called *cancelling*.

When *building* a fraction, you *multiply* both numerator and denominator by the same number.

## EXAMPLE 1.3

Write the ratio 1:10 as an equivalent fraction with 120 in the denominator.

Because 1:10 as a fraction is $\frac{1}{10}$, you need to write this fraction with the larger denominator of 120. Such processes are called **building fractions**.

$$\frac{1}{10} = \frac{?}{120}$$

$\frac{1}{10}$ may be built up by *multiplying top and bottom of the fraction by the same number* (12 in this case) as follows:

$$\frac{1}{10} = \frac{1 \times 12}{10 \times 12} = \frac{12}{120}$$

So, 1:10 is equivalent to $\frac{12}{120}$

## Changing Fractions to Decimal Numbers

To change a fraction to a decimal number, think of the fraction as a division problem. For example:

$$\frac{2}{5} \quad \text{means} \quad 2 \div 5 \quad \text{or} \quad 5\overline{)2}$$

Here are the steps for this division.

**Step 1**   Replace 2 with 2.0 and then place a decimal point directly above the decimal point in 2.0

$$5\overline{)2.0}$$

**Step 2**   Perform the division.

$$\begin{array}{r} 0.4 \\ 5\overline{)2.0} \\ \underline{2\ 0} \\ 0 \end{array}$$

**Keystroke Sequence:**

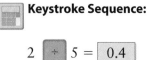

So, $\frac{2}{5} = 0.4$

## EXAMPLE 1.4

Write $\frac{5}{2}$ as a decimal number.

$$\frac{5}{2} \quad \text{means} \quad 5 \div 2 \quad \text{or} \quad 2\overline{)5}$$

**Step 1**   $2\overline{)5.0}^{.}$

$\phantom{Step 1   }2\overline{)5.0}^{2.5}$

**Step 2**   $2\overline{)5.0}$

$\phantom{Step 2   2)}\underline{4}$

$\phantom{Step 2   2)}1\ 0$

$\phantom{Step 2   2)}\underline{1\ 0}$

So, $\dfrac{5}{2} = 2.5$

• 5 ÷ 2 = 2.5

If your calculator has a fraction key, you can also use the keystroke sequence:

• 5 $a^{b/c}$ 2 = $2\frac{1}{2}$

## EXAMPLE 1.5

Write $\dfrac{193}{10}$ as a decimal number.

$$\dfrac{193}{10} \quad \text{means} \quad 193 \div 10 \quad \text{or} \quad 10\overline{)193}$$

**Step 1**   $10\overline{)193.0}^{\,.}$

$\phantom{Step 1   10)}19.3$

**Step 2**   $10\overline{)193.0}$

$\phantom{Step 2   10)}\underline{10}$

$\phantom{Step 2   10)}93$

$\phantom{Step 2   10)}\underline{90}$

$\phantom{Step 2   10)}30$

$\phantom{Step 2   10)}\underline{30}$

$\phantom{Step 2   10)}0$

So, $\dfrac{193}{10} = 19.3$

• 193 ÷ 10 = 19.3

If your calculator has a fraction key, you can also use:

• 193 $a^{b/c}$ 10 = $19\frac{3}{10}$

There is a quicker way to do this problem. To divide a *decimal number by 10*, you *move* the decimal point in the number *one place to the left*. Notice that there is one zero in 10.

$$\dfrac{193}{10} = \dfrac{193.}{10} = 19\underset{\frown}{3}. = 19.3$$

To *divide a number by 100, move* the decimal point in the number *two places to the left* because there are two zeros in 100. So, the quick way to divide by 10; 100; 1,000; and so on is to count the zeros and then move the decimal point to the left the same number of places. The answer should always be a smaller number than the original number. Check your answer to be sure.

**Keystroke Sequences for Example 1.6:**

- 9.25 ÷ 100 =
  
  0.0925

If your calculator has a fraction key, you might try to use the keystroke sequence:

- 9.25 $a^b/_c$ 100 =

But this will probably not work because calculators will not generally permit decimal numbers to be used with the $a^b/_c$ key.

### EXAMPLE 1.6

Write $\frac{9.25}{100}$ as a decimal number.

There are two zeros in 100, so move the decimal point in 9.25 two places to the left, and fill the empty position with a zero.

$$\frac{9.25}{100} = \underset{\curvearrowleft}{.} 9.25 = 0.0925$$

## Rounding Decimal Numbers

Sometimes it is convenient to round an answer—that is, to use an approximate answer rather than an exact one.

### Rounding Off

To round off 1.267 to the *nearest tenth*—that is, to round off the number to one decimal place—do the following:

*Look at the digit after the tenths place (the hundredths place digit). Because this digit (6) is 5 or more, round off 1.267 by adding 1 to the tenths place digit. Finally, drop all the digits after the tenths place. So, 1.267 is approximated by 1.3 when rounded off to the nearest tenth.*

To round off 0.8345 to the *nearest hundredth*—that is, to round off the number to two decimal places—do the following:

*Look at the digit after* the hundredths *place (the thousandths place digit). Because this digit (4) is less than 5, round off 0.8345 by leaving the hundredths digit alone. Finally, drop all the digits after the hundredths place. So, 0.8345 is approximated by 0.83 when rounded off to the nearest hundredth.*

### EXAMPLE 1.7

**Round off 4.8075 to the nearest hundredth, tenth, and whole number.**

4.8075 rounded off to the nearest:   hundredth → 4.81
                                      tenth → 4.8
                                      whole number → 5

Rounding *off* numbers produces results, which can be either larger or smaller than the given numbers. When numbers are rounded *down*, however, the results cannot be larger than the given numbers.

### Rounding Down

**NOTE**

Rounding down is also referred to as *truncating*.

Pediatric dosages are generally *rounded down* rather than *rounded off*. Rounding down is simple to do: part of the number is merely deleted (truncated).

To round down 1.267 to the tenths place—that is, to round down 1.267 to one decimal place—do the following:

*Locate the digit in the tenths place. Delete all the digits after the tenths-place digit.*    1 . 2 6̸ 7̸

*So, 1.267 is approximated by 1.2 when rounded down to the tenths place.*

To round down 0.83452 to the hundredths place—that is, to round down 0.83452 to two decimal places—do the following:

*Locate the digit in the hundredths place. Delete all the digits after the hundredths place digit.*    0 . 8 3 4̸ 5̸ 2̸

*So, 0.83452 is approximated by 0.83 when rounded down to the hundredths place.*

### EXAMPLE 1.8

**Round down 4.8075 to the nearest hundredth, tenth and whole number.**

4.8075 rounded *down* to the nearest:    hundredth → 4.80

tenth → 4.8

whole number → 4

## Adding Decimal Numbers

When adding decimal numbers, write the numbers in a column with the *decimal points lined up under each other*.

### EXAMPLE 1.9

$$3.4 + 0.07 + 6 = \ ?$$

Write the numbers in a column with the decimal points lined up. *Trailing zeros* may be included to give each number the same amount of decimal places. Therefore, write 6 as 6.00 [Think: $6 is equivalent to $6.00].

```
  3.40
  0.07
+ 6.00
  9.47
```

So, the sum of 3.4, 0.07, and 6 is 9.47

## Subtracting Decimal Numbers

When adding or subtracting decimal numbers, write the numbers in a column with the *decimal points lined up under each other*.

**NOTE**

Unless otherwise specified, quantities *less than 1* will generally be rounded to the *nearest hundredth*, whereas quantities *greater than 1* will generally be rounded to the *nearest tenth*. For the sake of uniformity, when rounding numbers in this book, rounding *off* will be used rather than rounding *down*. However, in Chapter 12 *all pediatric dosages will be rounded down*.

**ALERT**

The danger of an overdose must always be guarded against. Therefore, the amount of medication to be administered is often rounded *down* instead of rounded *off*. This rounding down is done routinely in pediatrics and when administering high-alert drugs to adults.

**Keystroke Sequence for Example 1.9:**

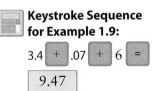

**Keystroke Sequence for Example 1.10:**

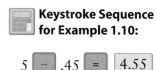

**ALERT**

Be careful: the *subtraction* (minus) key looks like $-$, while the *negative* key looks like $(-)$ or $+/-$.

## EXAMPLE 1.10

$$5 - 0.45 = ?$$

Write the numbers in a column with the decimal points lined up. Include *trailing zeros* to give each number the same amount of decimal places.

$$
\begin{array}{r}
5.00 \\
-\ 0.45 \\
\hline
4.55
\end{array}
$$

So, the difference between 5 and 0.45 is 4.55

# Multiplying Decimal Numbers

To multiply two decimal numbers, first multiply, ignoring the decimal points. Then count the total number of decimal places in the original two numbers. That sum equals the number of decimal places in the answer.

**Keystroke Sequence for Example 1.11:**

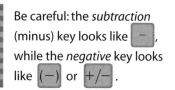

You need not press the leading zero when entering 0.16

## EXAMPLE 1.11

$$304.2 \times 0.16 = ?$$

$$
\begin{array}{r}
304.2 \\
\times\ 0.16 \\
\hline
18252 \\
3042\phantom{0} \\
\hline
48.672
\end{array}
$$

304.2 ← 1 decimal place ⎫ Total of 3
× 0.16 ← 2 decimal places ⎬ decimal places

There are 3 decimal places in the answer.
Place the decimal point here.

So, $304.2 \times 0.16 = 48.672$

**Keystroke Sequence for Example 1.12:**

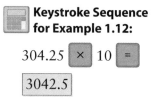

## EXAMPLE 1.12

$$304.25 \times 10 = ?$$

$$
\begin{array}{r}
304.25 \\
\times\phantom{00}10 \\
\hline
3\,042.50
\end{array}
$$

304.25 ← 2 decimal places ⎫ Total of 2
× 10 ← 0 decimal places ⎬ decimal places

There are 2 decimal places in the answer.
Place the decimal point here.

So, $304.25 \times 10 = 3{,}042.50$   or   $3{,}042.5$

There is a quicker way to do this problem. To *multiply any decimal number by 10, move* the decimal point in the number being multiplied *one place to the right*. Notice that there is one zero in 10.

$$304.25 \times 10 = 304.25 \quad \text{or} \quad 3{,}042.5$$

To *multiply a number by 100, move* the decimal point in the number *two places to the right* because there are two zeros in 100. So, the quick way to multiply by 10, 100, 1,000, and so on is to count the zeros and then move the decimal point to the right the same number of places. The answer should always be a larger number than the original. Check your answer to be sure.

### EXAMPLE 1.13

$$23.597 \times 1,000 = ?$$

There are three zeros in 1,000, so move the decimal point in 23.597 three places to the right.

$$23.597 \times 1,000 = 23.597 \quad \text{or} \quad 23,597$$

So, $23.597 \times 1,000 = 23,597$

**Keystroke Sequence for Example 1.13:**

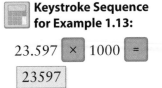

## Dividing Decimal Numbers

When dividing with decimal numbers, be sure that you are careful where you place the decimal point in the answer.

### EXAMPLE 1.14

**Write the fraction $\frac{106.8}{15}$ as a decimal number to the nearest tenth; that is, round off the answer to one decimal place.**

Treat this fraction as a division problem.

$$\frac{106.8}{15} \quad \text{means} \quad 15\overline{)106.8}$$

**Step 1**   $15\overline{)\overset{.}{106.8}}$

**Step 2**   Because you want the answer to the nearest tenth (one decimal place), do the division to two decimal places and then round off the answer. Because the hundredths place digit in the answer is *less than* 5, leave the tenths place digit alone. Finally, drop the digit in the hundredths place.

$$
\begin{array}{r}
7.12 \\
15\overline{)106.80} \\
\underline{105}\phantom{.00} \\
1\,8\phantom{0} \\
\underline{1\,5}\phantom{0} \\
30 \\
\underline{30} \\
0
\end{array}
$$

So, $\frac{106.8}{15}$ is approximated by the decimal number 7.1 to the nearest tenth.

**Keystroke Sequence for Example 1.14:**

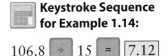

$\approx 7.1$ after rounding off. The symbol "$\approx$" means "is approximately equal to."

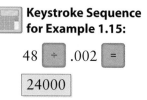

**Keystroke Sequence for Example 1.15:**

48 ÷ .002 =

24000

## EXAMPLE 1.15

Simplify $\frac{48}{0.002}$.

Think of this fraction as a division problem. Since there are three decimal places in 0.002, move the decimal points in both numbers three places to the right.

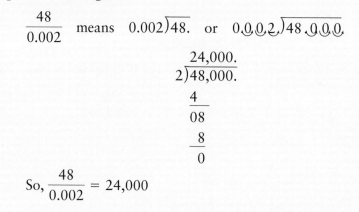

$$\frac{48}{0.002} \quad \text{means} \quad 0.002\overline{)48.} \quad \text{or} \quad 0.002.\overline{)48.000.}$$

$$
\begin{array}{r}
24,000. \\
2\overline{)48,000.} \\
4\phantom{8,000.} \\
\hline
08\phantom{,000.} \\
8\phantom{,000.} \\
\hline
0\phantom{000.}
\end{array}
$$

So, $\dfrac{48}{0.002} = 24{,}000$

# Estimating Answers

When you use a calculator, errors in the keystroke sequence may lead to dangerously high or dangerously low dosages. To help avoid such mistakes:

1. *Carefully enter* the keystroke sequence. A calculator that shows both your entries and the answer in the display is desirable.

2. Think: *Is the answer reasonable?* For example, an oral dosage of 50 tablets is not reasonable!

3. *Use rounding to estimate* the size of the answer. The product of 498 and 49 can be estimated by rounding the numbers off to 500 and 50, respectively. $500 \times 50 = 25{,}000$. Because each factor was made larger, the product of 498 and 49 is a little less than 25,000.

Sometimes it is useful to know whether an answer will be larger or smaller than a given number.

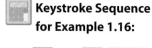

**Keystroke Sequence for Example 1.16:**

.4 ÷ .23 = 1.7

Because 1.7 is larger than 1, the first number entered (0.4) is larger than the second (0.23).

## EXAMPLE 1.16

**Which is larger, 0.4 or 0.23?**

Write the numbers in a column with the decimal points lined up, and include trailing zeros to give each number the same amount of decimal places.

$$0.40$$
$$0.23$$

Since 40 hundredths is larger than 23 hundredths, 0.4 is larger than 0.23

When one number is divided by a second number, if the answer is larger than 1, the first number is the larger. If the answer is less than 1, the second number is larger.

## EXAMPLE 1.17

Is $\frac{0.5}{0.4}$ smaller or larger than 1?

Since the value in the numerator 0.5 is larger than the value in the denominator 0.4, the fraction represents a quantity larger than 1.

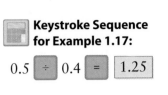

**Keystroke Sequence for Example 1.17:**

$0.5 \div 0.4 = \boxed{1.25}$

## EXAMPLE 1.18

Estimate the value of $\frac{200}{2.2}$.

Because the denominator is approximately equal to 2, the given fraction will be close in value to $\frac{200}{2}$ or 100. In this case, by making the denominator smaller (2 instead of 2.2), you made the value of the entire fraction larger. Therefore, 100 is too large (an overestimate). So, the actual value of $\frac{200}{2.2}$ is a number somewhat less than 100.

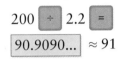

**Keystroke Sequence for Example 1.18:**

$200 \div 2.2 =$
$\boxed{90.9090...} \approx 91$

# Multiplying Fractions

To *multiply fractions*, multiply the numerators to get the new numerator and multiply the denominators to get the new denominator.

## EXAMPLE 1.19

$$\frac{3}{5} \times 6 \times \frac{1}{5} = ?$$

A whole number can be written as a fraction with 1 in the denominator. So, in this example, write 6 as $\frac{6}{1}$ to make all the numbers fractions.

$$\frac{3}{5} \times \frac{6}{1} \times \frac{1}{5} = \frac{3 \times 6 \times 1}{5 \times 1 \times 5} = \frac{18}{25}$$

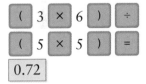

**Keystroke Sequences for Example 1.19:**

- Using parentheses:

$( \; 3 \times 6 \; ) \div$
$( \; 5 \times 5 \; ) =$
$\boxed{0.72}$

- Multiply the numerators, and then divide by each of the denominators:

$3 \times 6 \div 5 \div 5$
$= \boxed{0.72}$

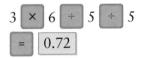

## EXAMPLE 1.20

$$\frac{4}{5} \times \frac{3}{10} \times \frac{20}{7} = ?$$

It is often convenient to cancel before you multiply.

$$\frac{4}{5} \times \frac{3}{\underset{1}{\cancel{10}}} \times \frac{\overset{2}{\cancel{20}}}{7} = \frac{24}{35}$$

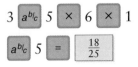

- Using the fraction key:

$3 \; a^{b}/_{c} \; 5 \times 6 \times 1$
$a^{b}/_{c} \; 5 = \boxed{\frac{18}{25}}$

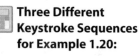
**Three Different Keystroke Sequences for Example 1.20:**

- Multiply the numerators and divide by each of the denominators:

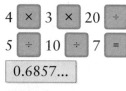

$$0.6857...$$

- Use the fraction key:

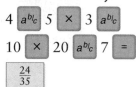

$$\frac{24}{35}$$

- Use parentheses:

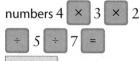

$$0.6857...$$

Do not verify the answer to Example 1.20 on the calculator by using the cancelled numbers 4 $\boxed{\times}$ 3 $\boxed{\times}$ 2 $\boxed{\div}$ 5 $\boxed{\div}$ 7 $\boxed{=}$ $\boxed{0.686...}$ because the calculator will not uncover previous cancellation errors. Therefore, use the original numbers as shown in the keystroke sequences.

**Keystroke Sequence for Example 1.21:**

21 $\boxed{\times}$ 15 $\boxed{\div}$ 7 $\boxed{=}$ $\boxed{45}$

**Keystroke Sequence for Example 1.22:**

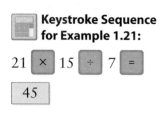

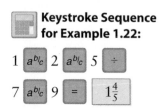

## EXAMPLE 1.21

Simplify $\frac{21 \times 15}{7}$

*Method 1*: Multiply the numbers in the numerator, which yields $\frac{315}{7}$, and then divide 315 by 7, which yields 45

*Method 2*: First cancel by 7, then multiply

$$\frac{\overset{3}{\cancel{21}} \times 15}{\underset{1}{\cancel{7}}} = \frac{3 \times 15}{1} = \frac{45}{1} = 45$$

So, $\frac{21 \times 15}{7} = 45$

# Dividing Fractions

To *divide fractions*, change the division problem to an equivalent multiplication problem by inverting the second fraction.

## EXAMPLE 1.22

$$1\frac{2}{5} \div \frac{7}{9} = ?$$

Write $1\frac{2}{5}$ as the improper fraction $\frac{7}{5}$.

The *division* problem

$$\frac{7}{5} \div \frac{7}{9}$$

Becomes the *multiplication* problem by inverting the second fraction.

$$\frac{7}{5} \times \frac{9}{7}$$

$$\frac{\overset{1}{\cancel{7}}}{5} \times \frac{9}{\underset{1}{\cancel{7}}} = \frac{9}{5} = 1\frac{4}{5}$$

Sometimes you must deal with whole numbers, fractions, and decimal numbers in the same multiplication and division problems.

## EXAMPLE 1.23

**Give the answer to the following problem in simplified fractional form.**

$$\frac{1}{300} \times 60 \times \frac{1}{0.4} = ?$$

Write 60 as a fraction and cancel.

$$\frac{1}{\overset{}{\underset{5}{\cancel{300}}}} \times \frac{\overset{1}{\cancel{60}}}{1} \times \frac{1}{0.4} = \frac{1}{5 \times 0.4} = \frac{1}{2}$$

> **NOTE**
>
> Avoid cancelling decimal numbers. It is a possible source of error.

**Keystroke Sequence for Example 1.23:**

60 ÷ 300 ÷ .4 = 0.5

Sometimes you will need to simplify *fractions that contain decimal numbers*.

## EXAMPLE 1.24

**Give the answer to the following problem in simplified fractional form.**

$$0.35 \times \frac{1}{60} = ?$$

Write 0.35 as the fraction $\frac{0.35}{1}$.

$$\frac{0.35}{1} \times \frac{1}{60} = \frac{0.35}{60}$$

The numerator of this fraction is 0.35, a decimal number. You can write an equivalent form of the fraction by multiplying the numerator and denominator by 100.

$$\frac{0.35}{60} \times \frac{100}{100} = \frac{0\overset{\frown}{.}3\overset{\frown}{5}}{60\overset{\frown}{.}0\overset{\frown}{0}} = \frac{35}{6,000} = \frac{7}{1,200}$$

**Keystroke Sequences for Example 1.24:**

● .35 ÷ 60 = 0.0058...

● If you think of 0.35 as $\frac{35}{100}$, then use the fraction key:

35 $a^{b}/_{c}$ 100 × 1 $a^{b}/_{c}$ 60 = $\frac{7}{1,200}$

## EXAMPLE 1.25

**Give the answer to the following problem in simplified fractional form.**

$$0.88 \times \frac{1}{2.2} = ?$$

$$\frac{0.88}{1} \times \frac{1}{2.2} = \frac{0.88}{2.2}$$

Multiply the numerator and the denominator of this fraction by 100 to eliminate both decimal numbers.

$$\frac{0.88}{2.2} \times \frac{100}{100} = \frac{0\overset{\frown}{.}8\overset{\frown}{8}}{2\overset{\frown}{.}2\overset{\frown}{0}} = \frac{88}{220} = \frac{2}{5}$$

You can simplify $\frac{0.88}{2.2}$ a different way by dividing 0.88 by 2.2

$$2.2\overline{)0.88}^{\,0.4} \quad \text{and} \quad 0.4 = \frac{4}{10} \quad \text{or} \quad \frac{2}{5}$$

**Keystroke Sequence for Example 1.25:**

.88 ÷ 2.2 = 0.4

To change 0.4 to a fraction:

4 $a^{b}/_{c}$ 10 = $\frac{2}{5}$

# Complex Fractions

Fractions that have numerators or denominators that are themselves fractions are called *complex fractions*.

The longest line in the complex fraction separates the numerator (top) from the denominator (bottom) of the complex fraction. As with any fraction, you can write the complex fraction as a division problem [*Top* ÷ *Bottom*].

In the complex fraction $\dfrac{1}{\frac{2}{5}}$, the numerator is 1 and the denominator is $\frac{2}{5}$.

You can simplify this complex fraction as follows:

$$\frac{1}{\frac{2}{5}} \quad \text{means} \quad 1 \div \frac{2}{5} \quad \text{or} \quad 1 \times \frac{5}{2}, \quad \text{which is} \quad \frac{5}{2}$$

In the complex fraction $\dfrac{\frac{1}{2}}{5}$, the numerator is $\frac{1}{2}$ and the denominator is 5.

You can simplify this complex fraction as follows:

$$\frac{\frac{1}{2}}{5} \quad \text{means} \quad \frac{1}{2} \div 5 \quad \text{or} \quad \frac{1}{2} \times \frac{1}{5}, \quad \text{which is} \quad \frac{1}{10}$$

In the complex fraction $\dfrac{\frac{3}{5}}{\frac{2}{5}}$, the numerator is $\frac{3}{5}$ and the denominator is $\frac{2}{5}$.

You can simplify this complex fraction as follows:

$$\frac{\frac{3}{5}}{\frac{2}{5}} \quad \text{means} \quad \frac{3}{5} \div \frac{2}{5} \quad \text{or} \quad \frac{3}{\overset{}{\underset{1}{5\!\!\!/}}} \times \frac{\overset{1}{5\!\!\!/}}{2}, \quad \text{which is} \quad \frac{3}{2}$$

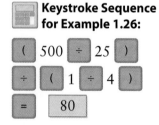

**Keystroke Sequence for Example 1.26:**

( 500 ÷ 25 )
÷ ( 1 ÷ 4 )
= 80

## EXAMPLE 1.26

$$\frac{\dfrac{1}{25} \times 500}{\dfrac{1}{4}} = \,?$$

In this complex fraction, the numerator is $\left(\frac{1}{25} \times 500\right)$ and the denominator is $\frac{1}{4}$. So, you can write the following:

$$\frac{1}{25} \times \frac{500}{1} \div \frac{1}{4} = \,?$$

$$\frac{1}{\underset{1}{25\!\!\!/}} \times \frac{\overset{20}{500\!\!\!/}}{1} \times \frac{4}{1} = 80$$

**EXAMPLE 1.27**

$$\frac{2}{3} \times \frac{1}{\frac{3}{4}} = ?$$

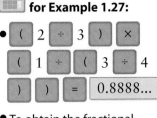

● ( 2 ÷ 3 ) ×
( 1 ÷ ( 3 ÷ 4
) ) =  0.8888...

You can multiply the numerators to get the new numerator and multiply the denominators to get the new denominator, as follows:

$$\frac{2}{3} \times \frac{1}{\frac{3}{4}} = \frac{2 \times 1}{3 \times \frac{3}{4}} = \frac{2}{\frac{9}{4}}$$

● To obtain the fractional form:

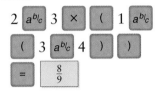
2 $a^{b/c}$ 3 × ( 1 $a^{b/c}$
( 3 $a^{b/c}$ 4 ) )
=  $\frac{8}{9}$

Now, the numerator is 2 and the denominator is $\frac{9}{4}$, so you get

$$\frac{2}{1} \div \frac{9}{4}$$

which becomes 

$$\frac{2}{1} \times \frac{4}{9} = \frac{8}{9}$$

This problem could have been done another way by simplifying $\frac{1}{\frac{3}{4}}$ first.

You can write $\frac{1}{\frac{3}{4}}$ as $1 \div \frac{3}{4}$ as $1 \times \frac{4}{3}$ or $\frac{4}{3}$

Then

$$\frac{2}{3} \times \frac{4}{3} = \frac{8}{9}$$

# Addition and Subtraction of Fractions

Addition and subtraction of fractions in this textbook generally involves fractions with denominators of 2 or 4.

## Same Denominators

When adding or subtracting fractions that have the *same denominators, add or subtract the numerators and keep the common denominator.*

Add $\frac{1}{2}$ and $\frac{1}{2}$

$$\frac{1}{2} + \frac{1}{2} = \frac{1 + 1}{2} = \frac{2}{2}, \text{ which equals } 1$$

From $\frac{11}{4}$ subtract $\frac{5}{4}$

$$\frac{11}{4} - \frac{5}{4} = \frac{11-5}{4} = \frac{6}{4}, \text{ which can be reduced to } \frac{3}{2} \text{ or } 1\frac{1}{2}$$

For *mixed numbers* add (or subtract) the whole number and fraction parts separately.

Add $3\frac{1}{4}$ *and* $2\frac{1}{4}$

$$
\begin{array}{r r}
3 & \dfrac{1}{4} \\[2mm]
+\ 2 & \dfrac{1}{4} \\[1mm]
\hline
5 & \dfrac{1+1}{4} = 5\dfrac{2}{4}, \text{ which equals } 5\dfrac{1}{2}
\end{array}
$$

From $10\frac{3}{4}$, *subtract* $6\frac{1}{4}$

$$
\begin{array}{r r}
10 & \dfrac{3}{4} \\[2mm]
-\ 6 & \dfrac{1}{4} \\[1mm]
\hline
4 & \dfrac{3-1}{4} = 4\dfrac{2}{4}, \text{ which equals } 4\dfrac{1}{2}
\end{array}
$$

## Different Denominators

When adding or subtracting fractions that have *different denominators*, build the fraction(s) so that the denominators are the same (have a common denominator), and proceed as above.

Add $\frac{1}{2}$ and $\frac{1}{4}$

This problem has fractions with different denominators. Recall that $\frac{1}{2} = \frac{2}{4}$. Then the problem becomes

$$\frac{2}{4} + \frac{1}{4} = \frac{2+1}{4} = \frac{3}{4}$$

From $\frac{3}{4}$ subtract $\frac{1}{2}$

Recall that $\frac{1}{2} = \frac{2}{4}$. Then the problem becomes

$$\frac{3}{4} - \frac{2}{4} = \frac{3-2}{4} = \frac{1}{4}$$

For *mixed numbers* add (or subtract) the whole number and fraction parts separately.

Add $9\frac{3}{4}$ and $6\frac{1}{2}$

To make the denominators the same, use $\frac{1}{2} = \frac{2}{4}$

$$
\begin{array}{rcrr}
9 & \frac{3}{4} & = & 9 & \frac{3}{4} \\[2mm]
+\,6 & \frac{1}{2} & = & 6 & \frac{2}{4} \\
\hline
& & & 15 & \frac{3+2}{4} = 15\frac{5}{4}, \text{which equals } 16\frac{1}{4}
\end{array}
$$

From $9\frac{3}{4}$ subtract $6\frac{1}{2}$

To make the denominators the same, use $\frac{1}{2} = \frac{2}{4}$

$$
\begin{array}{rcrr}
9 & \frac{3}{4} & = & 9 & \frac{3}{4} \\[2mm]
-\,6 & \frac{1}{2} & = & 6 & \frac{2}{4} \\
\hline
& & & 3 & \frac{3-2}{4} = 3\frac{1}{4}
\end{array}
$$

From $6\frac{1}{4}$ subtract $4\frac{3}{4}$

*Method 1: Use borrowing (renaming).*

Because $\frac{3}{4}$ is larger than $\frac{1}{4}$, subtraction of the fractions is not possible. Therefore, you may rename $6\frac{1}{4}$ as follows: Borrow 1 from the whole number part (6), and add the 1 to the fractional part ($\frac{1}{4}$). This results in $6\frac{1}{4} = (6-1) + (1 + \frac{1}{4})$ or $5\frac{5}{4}$.

$$
\begin{array}{rcrr}
6 & \frac{1}{4} & = & 5 & \frac{5}{4} \\[2mm]
-\,4 & \frac{3}{4} & = & 4 & \frac{3}{4} \\
\hline
& & & 1 & \frac{5-3}{4} = 1\frac{2}{4} \text{ or } 1\frac{1}{2}
\end{array}
$$

*Method 2: Change the mixed numbers to improper fractions.*

$$
\begin{array}{rcl}
6\frac{1}{4} & = & \frac{25}{4} \\[3mm]
-4\frac{3}{4} & = & \frac{19}{4} \\
\hline
& & \frac{25-19}{4} = \frac{6}{4} \text{ which also equals } 1\frac{1}{2}
\end{array}
$$

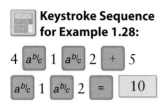

**Keystroke Sequence for Example 1.28:**

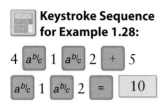

## EXAMPLE 1.28

Add $4\frac{1}{2} + 5\frac{1}{2}$.

$$
\begin{array}{r}
4 \quad \dfrac{1}{2} \\[2mm]
+\ 5 \quad \dfrac{1}{2} \\[1mm]
\hline
9 \quad \dfrac{1+1}{2} = 9\dfrac{2}{2}, \text{ which equals } 9 + 1 \text{ or } 10
\end{array}
$$

# Percentages

> **ALERT**
>
> Calculating with numbers in percent form can be difficult, so percentages should be converted to either fractional or decimal form before performing any calculations.

Percent (%) means *parts per 100* or *divided by 100*. Thus 50% means *50 parts per hundred* or *50 divided by 100*, which can also be written as the fraction $\frac{50}{100}$. The fraction $\frac{50}{100}$ can be changed to the decimal numbers 0.50 and 0.5 or reduced to the fraction $\frac{1}{2}$.

13%     means     $\dfrac{13}{100}$     or     0.13

100%   means     $\dfrac{100}{100}$     or     1

12.3%  means     $\dfrac{12.3}{100}$     or     0.123

$6\dfrac{1}{2}\%$     means     6.5%     or     $\dfrac{6.5}{100}$     or     0.065

## EXAMPLE 1.29

**Write 0.5% as a fraction in lowest terms.**

$$
0.5\% = \frac{0.5}{100} = \frac{5}{1{,}000} = \frac{1}{200}
$$

There is another way to get the answer. Because you understand that $0.5 = \frac{1}{2}$, then

$$
0.5\% = \frac{1}{2}\% = \frac{1}{2} \div 100 = \frac{1}{2} \div \frac{100}{1} = \frac{1}{2} \times \frac{1}{100} = \frac{1}{200}
$$

**Keystroke Sequence for Example 1.30:**

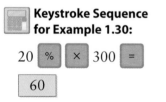

## EXAMPLE 1.30

**What is 20% of 300?**

To find a percent of a number or fraction of a number, translate the "of" as multiplication.

$$20\% \text{ of } 300 \quad \text{means} \quad 20\% \times 300 \text{ or}$$
$$0.20 \times 300 = 60$$

So, 20% of 300 is 60.

## EXAMPLE 1.31

**What is two-thirds of 27?**

To find a percent of a number or fraction of a number, translate the "of" as multiplication.

$$\frac{2}{3} \text{ of } 27 \quad \text{means} \quad \frac{2}{3} \times 27 = 18$$

So, two-thirds of 27 is 18.

**Keystroke Sequence for Example 1.31:**

2 $a^{b}/_{c}$ 3 × 27 =

18

## Percent of Change

It is often useful to determine a *percent of change* (increase or decrease). For example, you might want to know if a 20-pound weight loss for a patient is significant. For an adult patient who was 200 pounds, a 20-pound loss would be a decrease in weight of 10%. However, for a child who was 50 pounds, a 20-pound loss would be a decrease in weight of 40%, which is far more significant than a 10% loss.

To obtain the fraction of change, you may use the formula:

$$\text{Fraction of Change} = \frac{Change}{Old}$$

Then change the fraction to a percent to obtain the percent of change.

## EXAMPLE 1.32

**A daily dosage increases from 4 tablets to 5 tablets. What is the fraction of change and percent of change?**

$$\text{Fraction of Change} = \frac{Change}{Old}$$

Since the original (old) dosage is 4 tablets, and the new dosage is 5 tablets, then the change in dosage is

$$5 \text{ tablets} - 4 \text{ tablets} = 1 \text{ tablet.}$$

$$\text{Fraction of Change} = \frac{Change}{Old} = \frac{1}{4} \text{ or } 25\%.$$

So, the dosage has increased by $\frac{1}{4}$ or 25%.

## EXAMPLE 1.33

**A person was drinking 40 ounces of water per day, but this was reduced to 10 ounces of water per day. What is the percent of change?**

$$\text{Fraction of Change} = \frac{Change}{Old}$$

Since the old amount is 40 ounces, and the new amount is 10 ounces, the change is

$$40 - 10 = 30 \, ounces.$$

$$\text{Fraction of Change} = \frac{Change}{Old} = \frac{30}{40} = \frac{3}{4} \text{ or } 75\%.$$

So, this is a 75% decrease.

# Summary

In this chapter, all the essential mathematical skills that are needed for dosage calculation were reviewed.

When working with fractions:

- Proper fractions have smaller numbers in the numerator than in the denominator.
- Improper fractions have numerators that are larger than or equal to their denominators.
- Improper fractions can be changed to mixed numbers, and vice versa.
- Any number can be changed into a fraction by writing the number over 1.
- Cancel first when you multiply fractions.
- Change a fraction to a decimal number by dividing the numerator by the denominator.
- A ratio may be written as a fraction.
- Simplify complex fractions by dividing the numerator by the denominator.

When working with decimals:

- Line up the decimal points when adding or subtracting.
- Move the decimal point 3 places to the right when multiplying a decimal number by 1,000.
- Move the decimal point 3 places to the left when dividing a decimal number by 1,000.
- Count the total number of places in the numbers you are multiplying to determine the number of decimal places in the answer.
- Avoid cancelling with decimal numbers.

When working with percentages:

- Change to fractions or decimal numbers before doing any calculations.
- "Of" means multiply when calculating a percent of a number.
- Fraction of Change $= \dfrac{Change}{Old}$.

## Workspace

# Practice Sets

The answers to *Try These for Practice* and *Exercises* are found in Appendix A. Ask your instructor for the answers to the *Additional Exercises*.

## Try These for Practice

Test your comprehension after reading the chapter.

1. Write $\frac{5}{16}$ as a decimal number. _____

2. Write $\frac{6.47 \times 2.3}{0.2}$ as a decimal number rounded off to the nearest tenth.

_____

3. Write 40% as a decimal number and as a fraction in lowest terms.

_____

4. $\dfrac{3}{7} \times \dfrac{14}{15} \times \dfrac{5}{6} =$ _____

5. Simplify: $\dfrac{\frac{5}{6}}{\frac{5}{12}}$ _____

## Exercises

Reinforce your understanding in class or at home.

Convert to proper fractions or mixed numbers.

1. $0.85 =$ _____

2. $2\dfrac{1}{2} + 3\dfrac{1}{4} =$ _____

3. $40 \times \dfrac{1}{2} \times \dfrac{9}{16} =$ _____

4. $2\dfrac{3}{5} \div 2 =$ _____

5. $15 \div 3\dfrac{2}{3} =$ _____

6. $9.6 \div \dfrac{3}{7} =$ _____

7. $42 \times \dfrac{1}{9,450} \times \dfrac{3}{0.02} =$ _____

Convert to decimal numbers.

8. $\dfrac{1}{8} =$ _____ (round down to the nearest hundredth)

9. $\dfrac{14}{25} =$ _____

10. $5\dfrac{3}{10} =$ _____

11. $\dfrac{1}{200} =$ _____

12. $\dfrac{1}{75} =$ _____ (round off to the nearest hundredth)

13. $\dfrac{870}{1,000} =$ _____

14. $\dfrac{2.73}{100} =$ _____

15. $\dfrac{14.36}{7} =$ _____ (round down to the nearest tenth)

16. $\dfrac{0.63}{0.9} =$ _____

17. $\dfrac{0.063}{0.09} =$ _____

18. $5\dfrac{1}{2}\% =$ _____

19. $55\% =$ _____

Simplify and write the answer in decimal form.

20. $4.63 \times 6.21 =$ _____ (round off to the nearest hundredth)

21. $0.004 \times 100 =$ _____

22. $2.3456 \times 1,000 =$ _____

23. $0.85 \div 0.03 =$ _____ (round off to the nearest tenth)

24. $8.5 \div 0.12 =$ _____ (round down to the nearest hundredth)

Simplify and write the answer in fractional form and in decimal form rounded off to the nearest tenth.

25. $0.72 \times \dfrac{1}{0.7} = $ _____

26. $\dfrac{\frac{2}{3}}{8} = $ _____

27. $\dfrac{\frac{2}{5}}{100} \times \dfrac{500}{6} = $ _____

28. $\dfrac{26 \times \frac{5}{13}}{\frac{9}{100}} = $ _____

29. $10.3\% = $ _____

30. $99.5\% = $ _____

31. Express the ratio 25:40 as a fraction in lowest terms. _____

32. Express the ratio 60 to 90 as a fraction in lowest terms. _____

33. Find the numerator of the equivalent fraction with the given denominator. $\frac{3}{7} = \frac{?}{21}$ _____

34. Find the numerator of the equivalent fraction with the given denominator. $\frac{6}{11} = \frac{?}{55}$ _____

35. Simplify. $0.3 + 2 + 2.55$ _____

36. Simplify. $2.56 - 1.93$ _____

37. Which is larger, 0.37 or 0.244? _____

38. What is 30% of 500? _____

39. The number of nurses on the night shift has increased from 4 to 5. What is the percent of change? _____

40. A patient was 300 pounds before a diet program. Now she is 240 pounds. What is the percent of change in the patient's weight? _____

## Additional Exercises

Now, test yourself!

Convert the decimal numbers to proper fractions or mixed numbers.

1. $0.62 = $ _____

2. $4\frac{1}{4} - 2\frac{3}{4} = $ _____

Convert the fraction to decimal numbers.

3. $\dfrac{3}{8} = $ _____

4. $\dfrac{7}{25} = $ _____

5. $\dfrac{1}{5} = $ _____

6. $\dfrac{1}{400} = $ _____

7. $\dfrac{1}{150} = $ _____
(round down to the nearest thousandth)

8. $\dfrac{92}{100} = $ _____

9. $\dfrac{3.75}{1,000} = $ _____

10. $\dfrac{193.4}{7} = $ _____
(round off to the nearest tenth)

Convert to decimal numbers.

11. $\dfrac{0.36}{0.4} = $ _____

12. $\dfrac{0.036}{0.04} = $ _____

Multiply the decimal numbers.

13. $278.2 \times 100 =$ _____    14. $10.075 \times 10.3 =$ _____

15. $64.73 \times 1,000 =$ _____

Divide the decimal numbers.

16. $95 \div 0.05 =$ _____    17. $9.5 \div 0.05 =$ _____

Write the answers to Problems 18 through 22 in fractional form.

18. $\dfrac{7}{15} \times 20 \times \dfrac{1}{2} =$ _____    19. $3\dfrac{1}{2} \div 6 =$ _____

20. $13 \div 2\dfrac{1}{3} =$ _____    21. $6.35 \times \dfrac{1}{5} =$ _____

22. $\dfrac{1}{500} \times 1.75 \times \dfrac{1}{0.5} =$ _____

Write the answers to Problems 23 through 26 in fractional form and in decimal form rounded off to the nearest tenth.

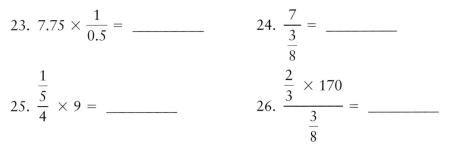

23. $7.75 \times \dfrac{1}{0.5} =$ _____    24. $\dfrac{7}{\frac{3}{8}} =$ _____

25. $\dfrac{\frac{1}{5}}{4} \times 9 =$ _____    26. $\dfrac{\frac{2}{3} \times 170}{\frac{3}{8}} =$ _____

Write the percentages as decimal numbers.

27. $24\dfrac{3}{5}\% =$ _____    28. $63\% =$ _____

Write the percentages as fractions.

29. $2.75\% =$ _____    30. $7.5\% =$ _____

31. Express the ratio 8 to 12 as a fraction in lowest terms. _____

32. Find the numerator of the equivalent fraction with the given denominator. $\frac{5}{8} = \frac{?}{24}$ _____

33. Simplify. $6.2 + 0.04 + 7$ _____

34. Simplify. $15.6 - 0.78$ _____

35. Which is larger, 0.72 or 0.5? _____

36. Is $\dfrac{0.009}{0.01}$ larger than 1? _____

37. What is 4% of 50? _____

38. What is three-eighths of 16? _____

39. The number of capsules a patient received each day has been increased from 1 capsule to 2 capsules. What is the percent of change? _____

40. The number of capsules a patient received each day has been decreased from 2 capsules to 1 capsule. What is the percent of change? _____

**MediaLink**
www.prenhall.com/giangrasso

Animated examples, interactive practice questions with animated solutions, and challenge tests for this chapter can be found on the Pearson Dosage Calculation Tutor that accompanies this text. Additional, unique, interactive resources and activities can be found on the Companion Web site.

Workspace

# Safe and Accurate Drug Administration

## Learning Outcomes

After completing this chapter you will be able to

1. Describe the six "rights" of safe medication administration.
2. Explain the legal implications of medication administration.
3. Describe the routes of medication administration.
4. Identify common abbreviations used in medication administration.
5. Compare the trade name and generic name of drugs.
6. Describe the forms in which medications are supplied.
7. Identify and interpret the components of a Drug Prescription, Physician's Order, and Medication Administration Record.
8. Interpret information found on drug labels and drug package inserts.

This chapter introduces the process of safe and accurate medication administration. Patient safety is a primary goal for all health care providers. Safety in medication administration involves more than merely calculating accurate dosages. Patient rights, knowledge of potential sources of error, critical thinking, and attention to detail are all important in ensuring patient safety. The responsibilities of the people involved in the administration of medication are described.

   The various forms and routes of drugs are presented, as well as abbreviations used in prescribing and documenting the administration of medications. You will learn how to interpret drug orders, drug prescriptions, drug labels, medication administration records, and package inserts.

# The Drug Administration Process

NOTE

For additional information regarding the avoidance of medication errors visit the Companion Web site at www.prenhall.com/giangrasso

Drug administration is a process involving a chain of healthcare professionals. The **prescriber writes** the drug order, the **pharmacist fills** the order, and the **nurse administers** the drug to the patient; each is responsible for the accuracy of the order. To ensure patient safety, they must understand how a patient's drugs act and interact.

Drugs can be life-saving or life-threatening. Every year, thousands of deaths occur because of medication errors. Errors can occur at any point in the medication process.

*Physicians, medical doctors (MD), osteopathic doctors (DO), podiatrists (DPM),* and *dentists (DDS)* can legally prescribe medications. In many states, *physician's assistants, certified nurse midwives,* and *nurse practitioners* can also prescribe a range of medications related to their areas of practice.

Although prescribers may administer drugs to patients, the *registered professional nurse (RN), licensed practical nurse (LPN),* and *licensed vocational nurse (LVN)* are usually responsible for administering drugs ordered by the prescriber.

Personnel who administer medications must be familiar with and follow applicable laws, policies, and procedures relative to the administration of medications, and they have a legal and ethical responsibility to report medication errors. When an error occurs, the patient must be assessed for adverse effects and the prescriber notified. There are many organizations and groups that are striving to reduce medication errors.

# Six Rights of Medication Administration

In order to prepare and administer drugs, it is imperative that you understand and follow the **Six Rights of Medication Administration:**

- Right drug
- Right dose
- Right route
- Right time
- Right patient
- Right documentation

ALERT

The person who administers the drug has the last opportunity to identify an error before a patient might be injured.

These six "rights" should be checked before administering any medications. Failure to achieve any of these rights constitutes a medication error.

Some institutions recognize additional rights, such as the *right to know* and the *right to refuse.* Patients need to be educated about their medications, and if a patient refuses a medication, the reason must be documented and reported.

## The Right Drug

A drug is a chemical substance that acts on the physiological processes in the human body. For example, the drug insulin is given to patients whose bodies do not manufacture sufficient insulin. Some drugs have more than one action.

**NOTE**

A generic drug may be manufactured by different companies under different trade names. For example, the generic drug ibuprofen is manufactured by McNeil PPC under the trade name Motrin, and by Wyeth pharmaceuticals under the trade name Advil. The active ingredients in Motrin and Advil are the same, but the size, shape, color, or fillers may be different. Be aware that patients may become confused and worried about receiving a medication that has a different name or appears to be dissimilar from their usual medication. State and federal governments now permit, encourage, and in some states mandate that the consumer be given the generic form when buying prescription drugs.

Aspirin, for example, is an antipyretic (fever-reducing), analgesic (pain-relieving), and anti-inflammatory drug that also has anticoagulant properties (keeps the blood from clotting). A drug may be taken for one, some, or all its therapeutic properties.

The **generic** name is the official accepted name of a drug, as listed in the United States Pharmacopeia (USP). The designation of USP after a drug name indicates that the drug meets government standards. A drug has only one generic name, but can have many trade names. By law, generic names must be identified on all drug labels.

Many companies may manufacture the same drug using different **trade** (patented, brand, or proprietary) names. The drug's trade name is followed by the trademark symbol™ or the registration symbol®. For example, **Avodart®** is the trade name and **dutasteride** is the generic name for the drug shown in ● **Figure 2.1**.

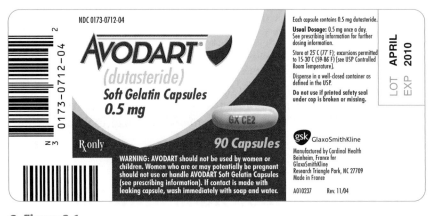

● **Figure 2.1**
**Drug label for Avodart.**
*(Reproduced with permission of GlaxoSmithKline.)*

**Dosage strength** indicates the amount of drug in a specific unit of measurement. The dosage strength of Avodart is 0.5 mg per capsule.

Each drug has a unique identification number. This number is called the **National Drug Code (NDC) number.** The NDC number for Avodart is 0173-0712-04. It is printed in two places on the label and is also encoded in the bar code. The *Food and Drug Administration (FDA)* regulates the manufacturing, sale, and effectiveness of all medications sold in the United States. Legislatures and other governmental agencies also regulate the administration of medications. The FDA estimates that the bar coding of prescription drugs reduces medication errors by as much as 50 percent.

To help avoid errors, drugs should be prescribed using only the generic name or by using both the generic and trade names. Many drugs have names that sound alike, or have names or packaging that look alike. A healthcare organization must develop its own list of "look-alike/sound-alike drugs" in order to meet the *National Patient Safety Goals* of the *Joint Commission*. The Joint Commission was formerly known as the *Joint Commission on Accreditation of Healthcare Organizations (JCAHO)*. Table 2.1 includes a sample list of drugs whose names may be confused.

| Table 2.1    **Look-Alike/Sound-Alike Drugs** | |
| --- | --- |
| **Drug Name** | **Look-Alike/Sound-Alike Drug Name*** |
| Acetazolamide* | acetohexamide |
| ceftazidime (Tazidime) | ceftizoxime sodium (Cefizox) |
| ceftin (cefuroxime axetil) | Cefzil (cefprozil) |
| cephalexin hydrochloride (Keftab) | cephalexin monohydrate (Keflex) |
| dactinomycin | daptomycin |
| DiaBeta* | Zebeta |
| ephedrine* | epinephrine |
| Evista* | Avinza |
| fluconazole (Diflucan) | fluorouracil (Adrucil) |
| folic acid* | folinic acid (leucovorin calcium) |
| glipizide (Glucotrol) | glyburide (Micronase) |
| heparin* | Hespan |
| Humalog* | Humulin |
| hydralazine hydrochloride (Apresoline) | hydroxyzine embonate (Atarax) |
| indarubicin* | daunorubicin |
| Inderal (propanolol hydrochloride) | Inderide (propanolol hydrochlorothiazide) |
| nizatidine (Axid) | nifedipine (Procardia) |
| Novolin 70/30* | Novolog Mix 70/30 |
| Protapam Chloride (pralidoxime chloride) | protamine sulfate |
| Retrovir* | ritonvair |
| vinblastine* | vincristine |

*These drug names are included on the JCAHO's list of look-alike or sound-alike drug names.

**ALERT**

*Giving the wrong drug is a common medication error.* In order to avoid errors, carefully read drug labels at the following times, even if the dose is prepackaged, labeled, and ready to be administered:

- When reaching for the container.
- Immediately before preparing the dose.
- When replacing or discarding the container.

These are referred to as the *three checks.*
*Always question the patient concerning any allergies to medications!* Make sure the drug is not expired, and never give a drug from a container that is unlabeled or has an unreadable label.

## The Right Dose

A person prescribing or administering medications has the *legal responsibility* of knowing the correct dose. Calculations may be necessary, and appropriate equipment must be used to measure the dose. Since no two people are exactly alike, and no drug affects every human body in exactly the same way, drug doses must be individualized. Responses to drug actions may differ according to the gender, race, genetics, nutritional and health status, age and weight of the patient (especially children and the elderly), as well as the route and time of administration.

The **standard adult dosage** for each drug is determined by its manufacturer. A standard adult dosage is recommended based on the requirements of an average-weight adult, and may be stated either as a *set dose* (20 mg) or as a *range* (150–300 mg). In the latter case, the minimum and maximum recommended dosages given are referred to as the **safe dosage range.** Recommended dosage may be found in many sources, including the package insert, the Hospital Formulary, and the manufacturer's Web site.

**Body surface area (BSA)** is an estimate of the total skin area of a person measured in meters squared ($m^2$). Body surface area is determined by formulas based on height and weight or by the use of a BSA nomogram (see Chapter 6). Many drug doses administered to children or used for cancer therapy are calculated based on BSA.

**ALERT**

The calibrated dropper *supplied with a medication* should be used ONLY for that medication. For example, the dropper that is supplied with digoxin (Lanoxin) can not be used to measure furosemide (Lasix).

**ALERT**

Be very attentive when reading the drug label. You might make a serious error if you mistake the total amount in a *multi-dose* container for a *unit dose*.

Carefully read the drug label to determine the *dosage strength*. Perform and *check calculations* and pay special attention to decimal points. When giving an IV drug to a pediatric patient or giving a high-alert drug (one that has a high risk of causing injury), always *double check the dosage and pump settings*, and confirm these with a colleague. Be sure to check for the recommended *safe dosage range* based on the patient's age, BSA, or weight. After you have calculated the dose, be certain to administer using standard measuring devices such as calibrated medicine droppers, syringes, or cups.

Medications may be prepared by the pharmacist or drug manufacturer in unit-dose packaging or multiple-dose packaging. **Unit-dose** medications may be in the forms of single tablets, capsules, or a liquid dosage sealed in an individual package. Unit-dose medications may be packaged in vials, bottles, prefilled syringes, or ampules, each of which contains only one dosage of a medication. When more than one dose is contained in a package, this is referred to as **multi-dose** packaging. See ● **Figures 2.2** and **2.3**.

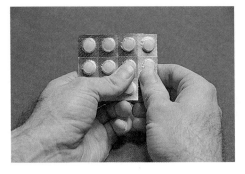 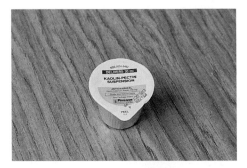

● **Figure 2.2**
**Unit-dose packages.**

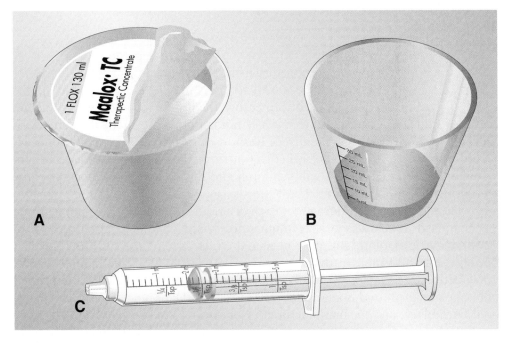

● **Figure 2.3**
**Liquid medication in a**
**a. single dose package**
**b. medication cup**
**c. oral syringe**

## The Right Route

Medications must be administered *in the form* and *via the route specified by the prescriber*. Medications are manufactured in the **form** of tablets, capsules, liquids, suppositories, creams, patches, or injectable medications (which are supplied in solution or in a powdered form to be reconstituted). The form (preparation) of a drug affects its speed of onset, intensity of action, and route of administration. The **route** indicates the site of the body and method of drug delivery.

**Oral Medications.** Oral medications are administered **by mouth** (PO) and are supplied in both solid and liquid form. The most common solid forms are *tablets* (tab), *capsules* (cap), and *caplets* (● **Figure 2.4**).

**Scored** tablets have a groove down the center so that the tablet can be easily broken in half. To avoid an incorrect dose, unscored tablets should never be broken.

**Enteric-coated** tablets are meant to dissolve in the intestine rather than in the stomach. Therefore, they should neither be chewed nor crushed. A **capsule** is a gelatin case containing a powder, liquid, or granules (pulverized fragments of solid medication). When a patient cannot swallow, certain capsules may be opened and their contents mixed in a liquid or sprinkled on a food, such as apple sauce. Theo-dur Sprinkles is an example of such a medication.

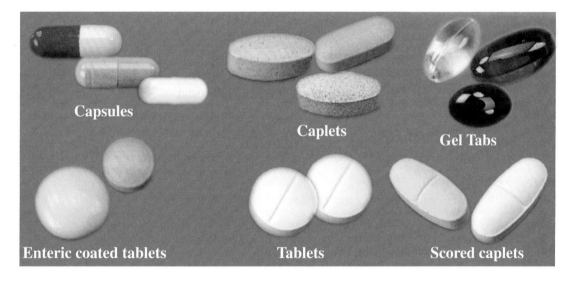

● **Figure 2.4**
**Forms of oral medications.**

**Sustained-release** (SR), **extended-release** (XL), **or delayed-release** (DR) tablets or capsules slowly release a controlled amount of medication into the body over a period of time. Therefore, these drugs *should not be opened, chewed, or crushed.*

Tablets for **buccal** administration are absorbed by the mucosa of the mouth (see ● **Figure 2.5**). Tablets for **sublingual** (SL) administration are absorbed under the tongue (see ● **Figure 2.6**). Tablets for buccal or sublingual administration should never be swallowed.

Oral drugs also come in liquid forms: *elixirs*, *syrups*, and *suspensions*. An **elixir** is an alcohol solution, a **syrup** is a medication dissolved in a sugar-and-water solution, and a **suspension** consists of an insoluble drug in a liquid base.

**ALERT**

*DO NOT* substitute a different route for the prescribed route because a serious overdose or underdose may occur.

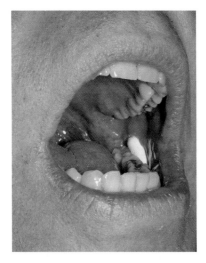

● **Figure 2.5**
**Buccal route: Tablet between cheek and teeth.**

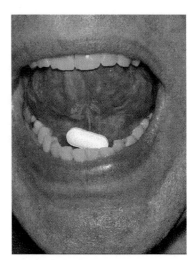

● **Figure 2.6**
**Sublingual route: Tablet under tongue.**

Liquid medications may also be administered **enterally** into the gastrointestinal tract via a specially placed tube, such as a *nasogastric (NG), gastrostomy (GT), or percutaneous endoscopic gastrostomy (PEG) tube* (see Chapter 10).

**Parenteral Medications.** Parenteral medications are those that are injected (via needle) into the body by various routes. They are absorbed faster and more completely than drugs given by other routes. Drug forms for parenteral use are sterile and must be administered using aseptic (sterile) technique. See Chapters 7 and 9.

The most common parenteral sites are the following:

- **Epidural:** into the epidural space (in the lumbar region of the spine)
- **Intramuscular (IM):** into the muscle
- **Subcutaneous (subcut):** into the subcutaneous tissue
- **Intravenous (IV):** into the vein
- **Intradermal (ID):** beneath the skin
- **Intracardiac (IC):** into the cardiac muscle
- **Intrathecal:** into the spinal column

**Cutaneous Medications.** Cutaneous medications are those that are administered through the skin or mucous membrane. Cutaneous routes include the following:

- **Topical:** administered *on the skin surface* and may provide a *local* or *systemic* effect. Those drugs applied for a **local** effect are absorbed very slowly, and amounts reaching the general circulation are minimal. Those administered for a **systemic** effect provide a slow release and absorption in the general circulation.
- **Transdermal:** contained *in a patch or disk and applied to the skin.* These are administered for their *systemic* effect. Patches allow constant, controlled amounts of drug to be released over 24 hours or more. Examples include nitroglycerin for angina or chest pain, nicotine to control the urge to smoke, and fentanyl for chronic pain. See ● **Figure 2.7.**

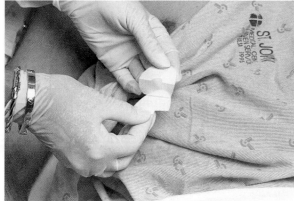
(a)

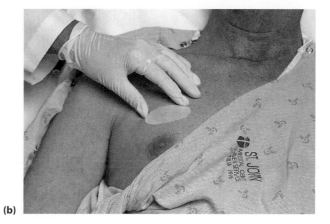
(b)

● **Figure 2.7**
Transdermal patch: (a) protective coating removed; (b) patch immediately applied to clean, dry, hairless skin and labeled with date, time, and initials.

- **Inhalation:** breathed into the respiratory tract through the nose or mouth. *Nebulizers, dry powder inhalers (DPI), and metered dose inhalers (MDI) are* types of devices used to administer drugs via inhalation. A **nebulizer** vaporizes a liquid medication into a fine mist that can then be inhaled using a face mask or handheld device. A **DPI** is a small device used for solid drugs. The device is activated by the process of inhalation, and a fine powder is inhaled. An **MDI** uses a propellant to deliver a measured dose of medication with each inhalation. See ● **Figure 2.8**.

- **Solutions and ointments:** applied to the mucosa of the eyes (optic), nose (nasal), ears (otic), or mouth

- **Suppositories:** are shaped for insertion into a body cavity (vagina, rectum, or urethra) and dissolve at body temperature

Some drugs are supplied in multiple forms and therefore can be administered by a variety of routes. For example, Tigan (trimethobenzamide HCl) is supplied as a capsule, suppository, or solution for injection.

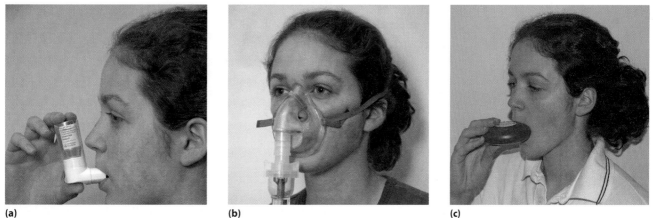
(a)     (b)     (c)

● **Figure 2.8**
Inhalation devices: (a) metered dose inhaler; (b) nebulizer with face mask; (c) dry powder inhaler.

## ALERT

Timing of medication administration can be critical for maintaining a stable concentration of the drug in the blood and avoiding interactions with other drugs. Usually a dose should be given within 30 minutes of the time specified by the prescriber— up to 30 minutes before or 30 minutes after.

Know the agency policy and always administer the dose immediately after it is prepared.

## ALERT

The patient's bed number or room number is *not* to be used for patient identification. Know and use the identifiers recognized and required by your agency.

## The Right Time

The prescriber will indicate when and how often a medication should be administered. Oral medications can be given either before or after meals, depending on the action of the drug. Medications can be ordered *once a day* (daily), *twice a day* (b.i.d.), *three times a day* (t.i.d.), and *four times a day* (q.i.d). Most healthcare facilities designate specific times for these administrations. To maintain a more stable level of the drug in the patient, the period between administrations of the drug should be prescribed at regular intervals, such as q4h (every four hours), q6h, q8h, or q12h.

Be aware that b.i.d. is not necessarily the same as q12h. B.I.D. may mean administer at 10 A.M. and 6 P.M., whereas q12h may mean administer at 10 A.M. and 10 P.M. (depending on the particular facility's policy). Drugs can also be ordered prn to be administered as needed.

## The Right Patient

Before administering any medication, it is essential to determine the identity of the recipient. Administering a medication to a patient other than the one for whom it was ordered is one example of a medication error. The Joint Commission continues to include proper patient identification in its National Patient Safety Goals, and it requires the use of at least two forms of patient identification. Suggested identifiers include: the patient identification bracelet information, verbalization of the patient's name by the patient or parent, the patient's home telephone number, or the patient's hospital number.

After identifying the patient, match the drug order, patient's name, and age to the **Medication Administration Record (MAR)**. To help reduce errors many agencies now use computers at the bedside, and/or use handheld devices (scanners) to read the bar code on a patient's identification bracelet and on the medication packages. See ● **Figure 2.9**.

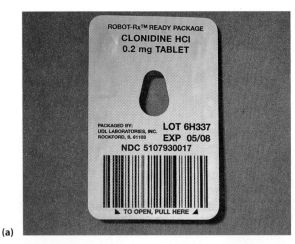
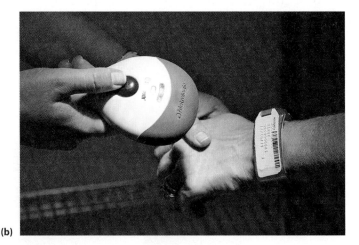

(a)　　　　　　　　　　　　　　　　　　　(b)

● **Figure 2.9**
**Bar codes: (a) unit-dose drug; (b) scanner reading a patient's identification band.**

## The Right Documentation

Always document the name and dosage of the drug, as well as the route and time of administration on the MAR. Sign your initials *immediately after, but never before*, the dose is given. It is important to include any relevant information. For example, document patient allergies to medications, heart rate (when giving digoxin), and blood pressure (when giving antihypertensive drugs). All documentation must be legible. Remember the axiom, "If it's not documented, it's not done."

*Anticipate side effects!* A **side effect** is an undesired physiologic response to a drug. For example, codeine relieves pain, but its side effects include constipation, nausea, drowsiness, and itching. Be sure to record any observed side effects and discuss them with the prescriber.

Safe drug administration requires a knowledge of common abbreviations. For instance, when the prescriber writes **"Demerol 75 mg IM q4h prn pain,"** the person administering the drug reads this as **"Demerol, 75 milligrams, intramuscular, every four hours, as needed for pain."** Be cautious with abbreviations because they can be a source of medication error. Only approved abbreviations should be used (Table 2.2).

| Table 2.2 **Common Abbreviations Used for Medication Administration** | | | |
|---|---|---|---|
| **Abbreviation** | **Meaning** | **Abbreviation** | **Meaning** |
| **Route:** | | Q.I.D. or q.i.d. | four times per day |
| GT | gastrostomy tube | Stat | immediately |
| ID | intradermal | T.I.D. or t.i.d. | three times per day |
| IM | intramuscular | | |
| IV | intravenous | **General:** | |
| IVP | intravenous push | c | with |
| IVPB | intravenous piggyback | cap | capsule |
| NGT | nasogastric tube | d.a.w. | dispense as written |
| PEG | percutaneous endoscopic gastrostomy | DR | delayed release |
| | | ER | extended release |
| PO | by mouth | g | gram |
| PR | by rectum | gr | grain |
| SL | sublingual | gtt | drop |
| Supp | suppository | kg | kilogram |
| | | L | liter |
| **Frequency:** | | mcg | microgram |
| ac | before meals | mg | milligram |
| ad lib | as desired | mL | milliliter |
| B.I.D. or b.i.d. | two times a day | NKA | no known allergies |
| h, hr | hour | NPO | nothing by mouth |
| pc | after meals | s | without |
| prn | whenever needed or necessary | Sig | directions to patient |
| | | Susp | suspension |
| q | every | SR | sustained release |
| q2h | every two hours | t or tsp | teaspoon |
| q4h | every four hours | T or tbs | tablespoon |
| q6h | every six hours | tab | tablet |
| q8h | every eight hours | XL or XR | extended release |
| q12h | every twelve hours | | |

The Joint Commission requires healthcare organizations to follow its official "*Do Not Use List*" that applies to all medication orders and all medication documentation. See Table 2.3.

| Table 2.3  JCAHO Official "Do Not Use List"[1] | | |
| --- | --- | --- |
| **Do Not Use** | **Potential Problem** | **Use Instead** |
| U (for unit) | Mistaken for "0" (zero), the number "4" (four) or "cc" | Write "unit" |
| IU (International Unit) | Mistaken for IV (intravenous) or the number 10 (ten) | Write "International Unit" |
| Q.D., QD, q.d., qd (daily) | Mistaken for each other | Write "daily" |
| Q.O.D., QOD, q.o.d, qod (every other day) | Period after the Q mistaken for "I" and the "O" mistaken for "I" | Write "every other day" |
| Trailing zero (X.0 mg)[2] | Decimal point is missed | Write X mg |
| Lack of leading zero (.X mg) | | Write 0.X mg |
| MS | Can mean morphine sulfate or magnesium sulfate | Write "morphine sulfate" Write "magnesium sulfate" |
| $MSO_4$ and $MgSO_4$ | Confused for one another | |

[1]Applies to all orders and all medication-related documentation that is handwritten (including free-text computer entry) or on preprinted forms.

[2] **Exception:** A "trailing zero" may be used only where required to demonstrate the level of precision of the value being reported, such as for laboratory results, imaging studies that report size of lesions, or catheter/tube sizes. It may not be used in medication orders or other medication-related documentation.

Additional Abbreviations, Acronyms, and Symbols
(For *possible* future inclusion in the Official "Do Not Use" List)

| **Do Not Use** | **Potential Problem** | **Use Instead** |
| --- | --- | --- |
| > (greater than) | Misinterpreted as the number | Write "greater than" |
| < (less than) | "7" (seven) or the letter "L" Confused for one another | Write "less than" |
| Abbreviations for drug names | Misinterpreted due to similar abbreviations for multiple drugs | Write drug names in full |
| Apothecary units | Unfamiliar to many practitioners Confused with metric units | Use metric units |
| @ | Mistaken for the number "2" (two) | Write "at" |
| cc | Mistaken for U (units) when poorly written | Write "mL" or "milliliters" |
| μg | Mistaken for mg (milligrams) resulting in one thousand-fold overdose | Write "mcg" or "micrograms" |

# Drug Prescriptions

Before anyone can administer any medication, there must be a legal order or prescription for the medication.

A **drug prescription** is a directive to the pharmacist for a drug to be given to a patient who is being seen in a medical office or clinic, or is being discharged from a healthcare facility. A prescription can be written, faxed, phoned, or emailed from a secure encrypted computer system to a pharmacist. There are many varieties of prescription forms. All prescriptions should contain the following:

- Prescriber's full name, address, telephone number, and (when the prescription is given for a controlled substance), the Drug Enforcement Administration (DEA) number
- Date the prescription is written
- Patient's full name, address, and age or date of birth
- Drug name (generic name should be included), dosage, route, frequency, and amount to be dispensed
- When only the trade name is written, the prescriber must indicate whether it is acceptable to substitute a generic form
- Directions to the patient that must appear on the drug container
- Number of refills permitted

Every state has a drug substitution law that either mandates or may permit a less-expensive generic drug substitution by the pharmacist. If the prescriber has an objection to a generic drug substitute, the prescriber will write "do not substitute," "dispense as written," "no generic substitution," or "medically necessary" (● Figure 2.10). Some states require bar codes on prescription forms.

**Adam Smith, M.D.**
**100 Main Street**
**Utopia, New York 10000**

Phone (212) 345-6789                    License # 123456

Name: _Joan Soto_                    Date: _November 24, 2010_

Address: _4205 Main Street_          Age/DOB: _04/20/48_
_____ _Utopia, NY 10000_

**R𝗑**      _Glucotrol 5 mg tablets_
     Sig: _1 tablet PO, daily, 30 minutes before breakfast_

Dispense: _90_
Refills: _1_

**THIS PRESCRIPTION WILL BE FILLED GENERICALLY UNLESS THE PRESCRIBER WRITES "d a w" IN THE BOX BELOW.**

| | _d a w_ | |
|---|---|---|
| | _Adam Smith MD_ | |

● Figure 2.10
**Drug prescription for Glucotrol.**

This prescription is interpreted as follows:

- Prescriber:                                         Adam Smith, M.D.

- Prescriber address:                          100 Main Street., Utopia, NY 10000

- Prescriber phone number:              (212) 345-6789

- Date prescription written:             November 24, 2010

- Patient's full name:                         Joan Soto

- Patient address:                              4205 Main Street, Utopia NY 10000

- Patient date of birth:                      April 20, 1948

- Drug name:                                     Glucotrol (trade name)

- Dosage:                                          5 mg

- Route:                                            by mouth (PO)

- Frequency:                                      once a day

- Amount to be dispensed:              90 tablets

- Acceptable to substitute              no, the prescriber has written "d a w"
  a generic form?

- Directions to the patient:             take 1 tablet by mouth daily 30 minutes before
                                                       breakfast

- Refill instructions:                         one refill permitted

## EXAMPLE 2.1

Read the prescription in ● Figure 2.11 and complete the following information.

- Date prescription written: _____

- Patient full name: _____

- Patient address: _____

- Patient date of birth: _____

- Generic drug name: _____

- Dosage: _____

- Route: _____

- Frequency: _____

- Amount to be dispensed: _____

- Acceptable to substitute a generic form? _____

- Directions to the patient: _____

- Refill instructions: _____

---

### Primary Care Associates
**1234 Spring Street, Manhattan, Kansas 10001**
**(913) 999-5678**

Name: _Mary Moral_                    Date: _10/22/10_

Address: _124 Winding Lane_           Date of Birth: _4/29/52_

_Manhattan, Kansas 10001_

**R̶x**   _doxycycline (Vibra-Tabs) 100 mg_

_Disp # 14_

_Sig: Take 1 capsule PO b.i.d. for 7 days_

Refills: _0_

_Alicia Rodriguez,_ ARNP

**Alicia Rodriguez, Adult Registered Nurse Practitioner**

**Substitution is mandatory**
**unless the words "no substitution" appear in the box above.**

---

● **Figure 2.11**
**Drug prescription for doxycycline.**

This is what you should have found:

- Date prescription written:       10/22/2010
- Patient full name:               Mary Moral
- Patient address:                 124 Winding Lane, Manhattan, Kansas 10001
- Patient date of birth:           4/29/52
- Generic drug name:               doxycycline
- Dosage:                          100 mg
- Route:                           by mouth
- Frequency:                       two times a day
- Amount to be dispensed:          14 capsules
- Acceptable to substitute a generic form?       yes
- Directions to the patient:       take one capsule twice a day for 7 days
- Refill instructions:             cannot be refilled

# Medication Orders

**Medication orders** are directives to the pharmacist for the drugs used in a hospital or other healthcare facility. The terms _medication orders, drug orders,_ and _physician's orders_ are used interchangeably, and the forms used will vary

**ALERT**

If persons administering medications have difficulty understanding or interpreting the orders, it is their responsibility to clarify the orders with the prescribers.

from agency to agency. No medication should be given without a medication order. Medication orders can be *written* or *verbal*. Each medication order should follow a specific sequence: drug name, dose, route, and frequency.

**Written** medication orders are documented in a special book for doctor's orders, on a physician's order sheet in the patient's chart, or in a computer.

A **verbal** order must contain the same components as a written order or else it is invalid. In order to provide for the safety of the patient, generally verbal orders may be taken only in an emergency. The verbal order must eventually be written and signed by the physician.

## Types of Medication Orders

The most common type of medication order is the **routine order**, which indicates that the ordered drug is administered until a discontinuation order is written or until a specified date is reached.

A **standing order** is prescribed in anticipation of sudden changes in a patient's condition. Standing orders are used frequently in critical care units, where a patient's condition may change rapidly, and immediate action would be required. Standing orders may also be used in long-term care facilities where a physician may not be readily available; for example, "*Tylenol (acetaminophen) 650 mg PO q4h for temperature of 101°F or higher.*"

A **prn order** is written by the prescriber for a drug to be given when a patient needs it; for example, "*Codeine 30 mg PO q4h prn mild–moderate pain.*"

A **stat order** is an order that is to be administered immediately. Stat orders are usually written for emergencies or when a patient's condition suddenly changes; for example, "*Lasix 80 mg IV stat.*"

## Components of a Medication Order

The essential components of a medication order are the following:

- **Patient's full name and date of birth:** Often this information is stamped or imprinted on the medication order form. Additional information may include the patient's admission number, religion, type of insurance, and physician's name.

- **Date and time the order was written:** This includes the month, day, year, and time of day. Many institutions use military time, which is based on a "24-hour clock" that does not use A.M. or P.M. (●**Figure 2.12**). Military

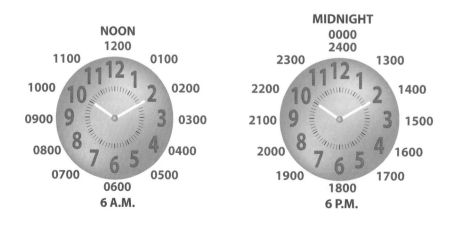

● **Figure 2.12**
**Clocks Showing 10:10** A.M.
**(1010h) and 10:10** P.M. **(2210h).**

times are written as four-digit numbers. Thus, 2:00 A.M. in military time is 0200h (pronounced "Oh two hundred hours"), 12 noon is 1200h (pronounced twelve hundred hours), 2:00 P.M. is 1400h (pronounced *fourteen hundred hours*), and midnight is 2400h.

There is confusion between the meanings of 12 A.M. and 12 P.M. Twelve noon, for example, is literally neither A.M. (ante meridiem: before midday), nor is it P.M. (post meridiem: after midday). Noon *is* midday! Therefore, to avoid confusion when administering medications, for noon and midnight use *12 noon* and *12 midnight*, or use military time (*1200h* and *2400h*).

- **Name of the medication:** The generic name is recommended. If a prescriber desires to prescribe a trade name drug, "no generic substitution" must be specified.
- **Dosage of the medication:** The amount of the drug.
- **Route of administration.**
- **Time and frequency of administration.**
- **Signature of the prescriber:** The medication order is not legal without the signature of the prescriber.
- **Signature of the person transcribing the order:** This may be the responsibility of a nurse or others identified by agency policy.

The physician's order in ● **Figure 2.13** can be interpreted as follows:

**Name of patient:** John Camden
**Birth date:** Feb. 11, 1955
**Date of admission:** Nov. 20, 2010
**Admission number:** 602412
**Religion:** Roman Catholic (RC)
**Insurance:** Blue Cross Blue Shield (BCBS)
**Date and time the order was written:** 11/20/2010 at 0800h or 8:00 A.M.

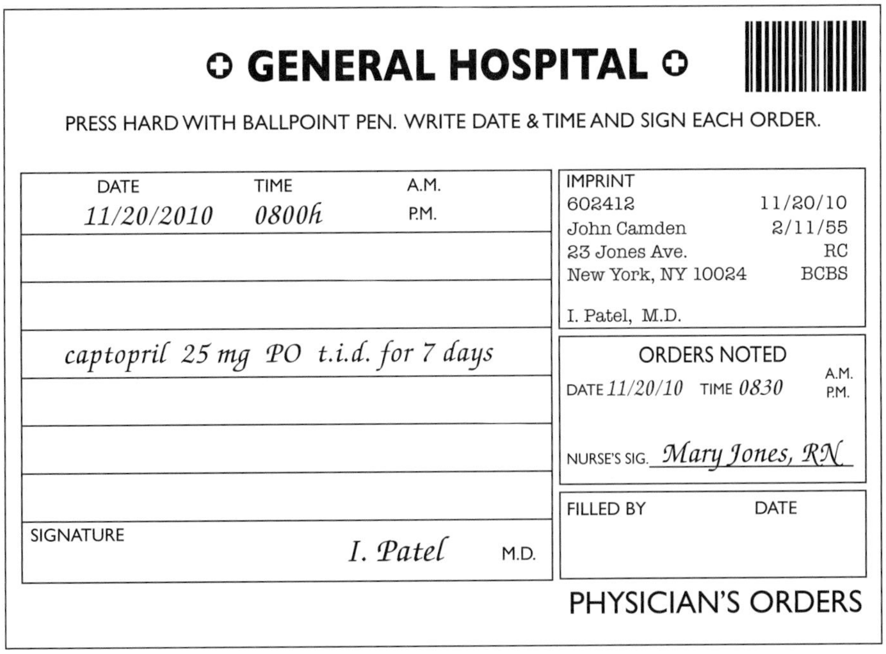

● **Figure 2.13**
Physician's order for captopril.

**NOTE**
Drug orders follow a specific sequence: drug name, dosage, route, and frequency.

Name of the medication: captopril

Dosage: 25 mg

Route of administration: PO (by mouth)

Frequency of administration: t.i.d., three times a day for 7 days

Signature of person writing the order: I. Patel, MD

Person who transcribed the order: Mary Jones, RN

## EXAMPLE 2.2

Interpret the physician's order sheet shown in ● Figure 2.14 and record the following information:

Date order written: _____

Time order written: _____

Name of drug: _____

Dosage: _____

Route of administration: _____

Frequency of administration: _____

Name of prescriber: _____

Name of patient: _____

Birth date: _____

Religion: _____

Type of insurance: _____

Person who transcribed the order: _____

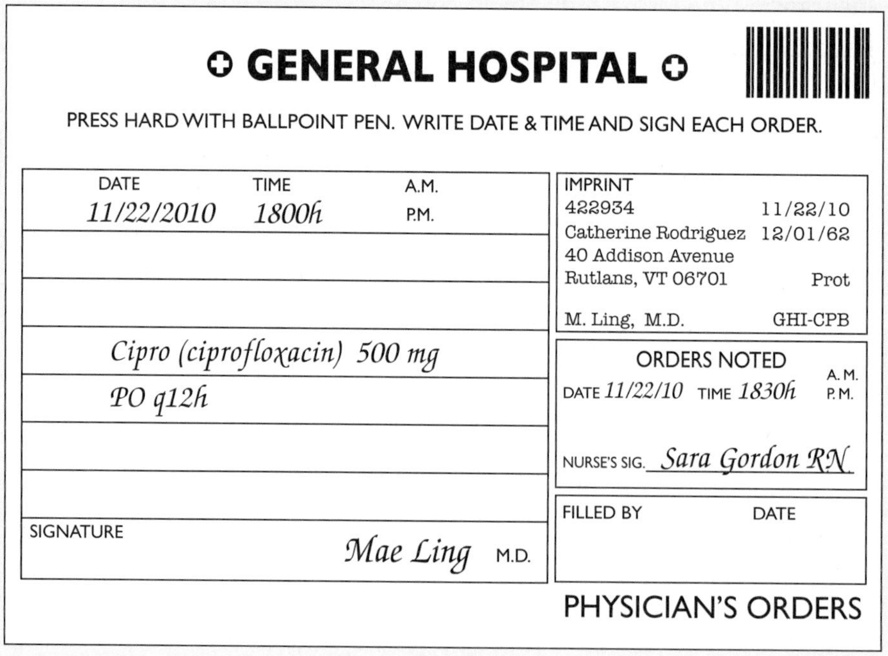

**⊕ GENERAL HOSPITAL ⊕**

PRESS HARD WITH BALLPOINT PEN. WRITE DATE & TIME AND SIGN EACH ORDER.

| DATE | TIME | A.M. |
|------|------|------|
| 11/22/2010 | 1800h | P.M. |

| IMPRINT | |
|---------|---|
| 422934 | 11/22/10 |
| Catherine Rodriguez | 12/01/62 |
| 40 Addison Avenue | |
| Rutlans, VT 06701 | Prot |
| M. Ling, M.D. | GHI-CPB |

Cipro (ciprofloxacin) 500 mg

PO q12h

| ORDERS NOTED | A.M. |
|--------------|------|
| DATE 11/22/10 TIME 1830h | P.M. |

NURSE'S SIG. _Sara Gordon RN_

SIGNATURE

_Mae Ling_ M.D.

| FILLED BY | DATE |
|-----------|------|

**PHYSICIAN'S ORDERS**

● **Figure 2.14**
**Physician's order for Cipro.**

This is what you should have found:

- Date order written:            11/22/2010
- Time order written:            1800h or 6:00 P.M.
- Name of drug:                  Cipro (ciprofloxacin)
- Dosage:                        500 mg
- Route:                         by mouth
- Frequency of administration:   every 12 hours
- Name of prescriber:            Mae Ling, M.D.
- Name of patient:               Catherine Rodriguez
- Birth date:                    December 1, 1962
- Religion:                      Protestant
- Type of insurance:             GHI-CBP
- Person who transcribed the order:  Sara Gordon, RN

## Medication Administration Records

A **Medication Administration Record (MAR)** is a form used by healthcare facilities to document all drugs administered to a patient. It is a legal document, part of the patient's medical record, and the format varies from agency to agency. Every agency develops policies related to using the *MAR* including: how to add new medications, discontinue medications, document one-time or stat medications, the process to follow if a medication is not administered or a patient refuses a medication, and how to correct an error on the *MAR*.

*Routine*, *PRN*, and *STAT* medications all may be written in separate locations on the *MAR*. *PRN* and *STAT* medications may also have a separate form. If a medication is to be given regularly, a complete schedule is written for all administration times. Each time a dose is administered, the healthcare worker initials the time of administration. The full name, title, and initials of the person who gave the medication must be recorded on the MAR.

After a prescriber's order has been verified, a nurse or other healthcare provider transcribes the order to the MAR. This record is used to check the medication order; prepare the correct medication dose; and record the date, time, and route of administration.

The essential components of the MAR include the following:

- **Patient information:** a stamp or printed label with patient identification (name, date of birth, medical record number).
- **Dates:** when the order was written, when to start the medication, and when to discontinue it.
- **Medication information:** full name of the drug, dose, route, and frequency of administration.
- **Time of administration:** frequency as stated in the prescriber's order; for example, t.i.d. Times for *PRN* and *one-time doses* are recorded *precisely* at the time they are administered.
- **Initials:** the initials and the signature of the person who administered the medication are recorded.
- **Special instructions:** instructions relating to the medication; for example, "Hold if systolic BP is less than 100."

**ALERT**

Before administering any medication, always compare the label on the medication with the information on the MAR. If there is a discrepancy, you must check the prescriber's original order.

## EXAMPLE 2.3

Study the MAR in ● Figure 2.15, then complete the following chart and answer the questions.

| | | | | | | | |
|---|---|---|---|---|---|---|---|

**UNIVERSITY HOSPITAL**

789652
Wendy Kim
44 Chester Avenue
New York, NY 10003

9/11/2010
12/20/60
RC
Medicaid

**DAILY MEDICATION ADMINISTRATION RECORD**

Dr. Juan Rodriguez, M.D.

PATIENT NAME _____ *Wendy Kim* _____

ROOM # _____ *422* _____

IF ANOTHER RECORDS IS IN USE ☐

ALLERGIC TO (RECORD IN RED): _____ *tomato, codeine* _____

DATES GIVEN ⁝ ▼          DATE DISCHARGED:

| RED CHECK INITIAL | ORDER DATE | INITIAL | EXP DATE | MEDICATION, DOSAGE, FREQUENCY AND ROUTE | HOURS | 12 | 13 | 14 | 15 | | | | | | |
|---|---|---|---|---|---|---|---|---|---|---|---|---|---|---|---|
| | 9/12 | JY | 9/19 | Pepcid (famotidine) 20 mg | 0600 | / | MC | MC | | | | | | | |
| | | | | IVPB q12h for 7 days begin at 1800h | 1800 | MJ | SG | SG | | | | | | | |
| | | | | | | | | | | | | | | | |
| | 9/12 | JY | 9/18 | digoxin 0.125 mg PO daily | 0900 | JY | JY | JY | | | | | | | |
| | | | | | | | | | | | | | | | |
| | 9/12 | JY | 9/18 | Lotensin (benazepril hydrochloride) | 0900 | JY | JY | JY | | | | | | | |
| | | | | 20 mg PO q12h | 2100 | MJ | SG | SG | | | | | | | |
| | | | | | | | | | | | | | | | |
| | 9/12 | JY | 9/18 | Ticlid (ticlopidine hydrocholoride) | 0900 | JY | JY | JY | | | | | | | |
| | | | | 250 mg PO daily | | | | | | | | | | | |
| | | | | | | | | | | | | | | | |
| | 9/12 | JY | 9/18 | Xanax (alprazolam) 0.5 mg PO HS | 2100 | MJ | SG | SG | | | | | | | |
| | | | | | | | | | | | | | | | |

| INT. | NURSES' FULL SIGNATURE AND TITLE | INT. | CODES FOR INJECTION SITES | |
|---|---|---|---|---|
| JY | Jim Young, RN | | A- left anterior thigh | H- right anterior thigh |
| MC | Marie Colon, RN | | B- left deltoid | I- right deltoid |
| MJ | Mary Jones, LPN | | C- left gluteus medius | J- right gluteus medius |
| SG | Sara Gordon, RN | | D- left lateral thigh | K- right lateral thigh |
| | | | E- left ventral gluteus | L- right ventral gluteus |
| | | | F- left lower quadrant | M- right lower quadrant |
| | | | G- left upper quadrant | N- right upper quadrant |

● **Figure 2.15**
**MAR for Wendy Kim.**

| Name of Drug | Dose | Route of Administration | Time of Administration |
|---|---|---|---|
|  |  |  |  |
|  |  |  |  |
|  |  |  |  |
|  |  |  |  |
|  |  |  |  |
|  |  |  |  |

1. Identify the drugs and their doses administered at 9:00 A.M.

_____

2. Identify the drugs and their doses administered at 9:00 P.M.

_____

3. Who administered the ticlopidine hydrochloride on 9/14?

_____

4. What is the route of administration for famotidine?

_____

5. What is the time of administration for Pepcid?

_____

This is what you should have found:

| Name of Drug | Dose | Route of Administration | Time of Administration |
|---|---|---|---|
| Pepcid (famotidine) | 20 mg | IVPB | 0600h (6 A.M.) & 1800h (6 P.M.) |
| digoxin | 0.125 mg | PO | 0900h (9 A.M.) |
| Lotensin(benazepril hydrochloride) | 20 mg | PO | 0900h (9 A.M.) and 2100h (9 P.M.) |
| Ticlid (ticlopidine hydrochloride) | 250 mg | PO | 0900h (9 A.M.) |
| Xanax (alprazolam) | 0.5 mg | PO | 2100h (9 P.M.) |

1. digoxin 0.125 mg; Lotensin 20 mg; Ticlid 250 mg
2. Lotensin 20 mg, Xanax 0.5mg
3. Jim Young, RN
4. IVPB
5. 0600h (6 A.M.) and 1800h (6 P.M.)

## EXAMPLE 2.4

Study the MAR in ● Figures 2.16a and 2.16b, then fill in the following chart and answer the questions.

| Name of Routine Drug | Dose | Route of Administration | Time of Administration |
|---|---|---|---|
| | | | |
| | | | |
| | | | |
| | | | |
| | | | |
| | | | |
| | | | |

1. Which drugs were administered at 10:00 A.M. on 11/23?

   _____

2. Which drug was given stat and what was the route; date and time?

   _____

3. Who administered the captopril at 2:00 P.M. on 11/21?

   _____

4. What is the route of administration for Epogen?

   _____

5. How many doses of Capoten did the patient receive by 7:00 P.M. on 11/24?

   _____

Here is what you should have found:

| Name of Routine Drug | Dose | Route of Administration | Time of Administration |
|---|---|---|---|
| Coumadin (warfarin sodium) | 10 mg | PO | 10:00 A.M. |
| Capoten (captopril) | 25 mg | PO | 10:00 A.M., 2:00 P.M., 6:00 P.M. |
| Lasix (furosemide) | 20 mg | PO | 10:00 A.M. |
| Maxipime (cefepime hydrochloride) | 1g | IVPB | 10:00 A.M. and 10:00 P.M. |
| Epogen (erythropoietin) | 3,000 units | subcutaneously | three times a week at 10:00 A.M. |
| digoxin | 0.125 mg | PO | 10:00 A.M. |

1. Coumadin 10 mg; Capoten 25 mg; Lasix 20 mg; Maxipime 1g, Epogen 3,000 units, digoxin 0.125 mg, Dilaudid 2 mg.

2. Dilaudid IV on 11/23 at 10:00 A.M.

3. Marie Colon, RN

4. subcutaneous

5. 14

---

**UNIVERSITY HOSPITAL**

**DAILY MEDICATION ADMINISTRATION RECORD**

659204
Mohammad Kamal
4103 Ely Avenue
Bronx, NY 10466

11/20/2010
10/2/52
Musl
GHI-CBP

Dr. Indu Patel, M.D.

PATIENT NAME ___Mohammad Kamal___

ROOM # ___302___

IF ANOTHER RECORDS IS IN USE ☐

ALLERGIC TO (RECORD IN RED): ___sulfa, fish___

DATES GIVEN ⬇ MONTH/DAY    YEAR: _2010_

| RED CHECK INITIAL | ORDER DATE | INITIAL | EXP DATE | MEDICATION, DOSAGE, FREQUENCY AND ROUTE | TIME | 11/20 | 11/21 | 11/22 | 11/23 | 11/24 | 11/25 | 11/26 |
|---|---|---|---|---|---|---|---|---|---|---|---|---|
| | 11/20 | MC | 11/26 | Coumadin (warfarin sodium) 10 mg | 10AM | — | MC | MC | MC | MJ | MJ | JY |
| | | | | PO daily | | | | | | | | |
| | 11/20 | MC | 11/26 | Capoten (captopril) 25 mg | 10AM | — | MC | MC | MC | MJ | MJ | JY |
| | | | | PO t.i.d. | BP | — | 160/110 | 150/70 | 160/110 | 138/86 | 130/80 | 130/80 |
| | | | | | 2PM | MC | MC | MC | MC | MJ | MJ | JY |
| | | | | | BP | 150/90 | 140/80 | 140/90 | 140/80 | 130/84 | 130/82 | 128/76 |
| | | | | | 6PM | MC | MC | MC | MC | MJ | MJ | JY |
| | | | | | BP | 160/100 | 150/90 | 160/100 | 140/80 | 130/80 | 128/80 | 128/80 |
| | 11/20 | MC | 11/26 | Lasix (furosemide) 20 mg PO daily | 10AM | — | MC | MC | MC | MJ | MJ | JY |
| | 11/20 | SG | 11/27 | Maxipime (cefepime hydrochloride) | 10AM | — | MC | MC | MC | MJ | MJ | JY |
| | | | | 1g IVPB q12hr for 7 days | 10PM | — | SG | SG | SG | SG | SG | SG |
| | 11/21 | MC | 11/27 | Epogen (erythropoietin) 3,000 units | 10AM | — | MC | | MC | | MJ | |
| | | | | subcutaneous, three times per week, | | | | | | | | |
| | | | | start on 11/21 | | | | | | | | |
| | 11/21 | MC | 11/27 | digoxin, 0.125 mg PO daily | 10AM | — | MC | MC | MC | MJ | MJ | JY |
| | | | | | HR | — | 72 | 70 | 96 | 76 | 80 | 80 |
| | | | | | | | | | | | | |

| INT. | NURSES' FULL SIGNATURE AND TITLE | INT. | NURSES' FULL SIGNATURE AND TITLE |
|---|---|---|---|
| MC | Marie Colon, RN | | |
| SG | Sara Gordon, RN | | |
| MJ | Mary Jones, LPN | | |
| JY | Jim Young, RN | | |

● **Figure 2.16a**
**MAR for Mohammad Kamal.**

### UNIVERSITY HOSPITAL

### DAILY MEDICATION ADMINISTRATION RECORD

659204
Mohammad Kamal
4103 Ely Avenue
Bronx, NY 10466

11/20/2010
10/2/52
Musl
GHI-CBP

Dr. Indu Patel, M.D.

PATIENT NAME _Mohammad Kamal_

ROOM # _302_

ALLERGIC TO (RECORD IN RED): _sulfa, fish_

IF ANOTHER RECORDS IS IN USE ☐

DATES GIVEN    MONTH/DAY    YEAR: _2010_

**PRN MEDICATION**

| ORDER DATE | EXPIRATION DATE/TIME | MEDICATION, DOSAGE, FREQUENCY AND ROUTE | | DOSES GIVEN | | | | | | |
|---|---|---|---|---|---|---|---|---|---|---|
| 11/20 | 11/27 | Tylenol (acetaminophen) 650 mg PO q 3-4 h prn pain | DATE | 11/20 | 11/20 | 11/20 | | | | |
| | | | TIME | 6 PM | 10 AM | 6 PM | | | | |
| | | | INIT | MJ | MC | 6 PM | | | | |
| 11/20 | 11/27 | Robitussin DM 10 ml | DATE | 11/20 | 11/21 | | | | | |
| | | | TIME | 10 AM | 10 PM | | | | | |
| | | | INIT | MJ | SG | | | | | |
| | | PO q12h prn | DATE | | | | | | | |
| | | | TIME | | | | | | | |
| | | | INIT | | | | | | | |
| 11/20 | 11/27 | Tylenol (acetaminophen) 325 mg PO q 3-4 h prn | DATE | | | | | | | |
| | | | TIME | | | | | | | |
| | | | INIT | | | | | | | |
| | | Temp above 101° F | DATE | | | | | | | |
| | | | TIME | | | | | | | |
| | | | INIT | | | | | | | |

**STAT-ONE DOSE-PRE-OPERATIVE MEDICATIONS**

◯ Check here if additional sheet in use.

| ORDER DATE | MEDICATION-DOSAGE ROUTE | DATE | TIME | INIT | ORDER DATE | MEDICATION-DOSAGE ROUTE | DATE | TIME | INIT |
|---|---|---|---|---|---|---|---|---|---|
| 11/23 | Dilaudid (hydromorphone) 2 mg IV now | 11/23 | 10AM | MC | | | | | |
| | | | | | | | | | |

| INT. | NURSES' FULL SIGNATURE AND TITLE | INT. | NURSES' FULL SIGNATURE AND TITLE |
|---|---|---|---|
| MJ | Mary Jones, RN | | |
| MC | Marie Colon, RN | | |
| SG | Sara Gordon, RN | | |

● **Figure 2.16b** MAR for Mohammad Kamal.

## Technology in the Medication Administration Process

Many healthcare agencies have computerized the medication process. Those who prescribe or administer medications must use security codes and passwords to access the computer system. Prescribers input orders and all other essential patient information directly into a computer terminal. This system may be referred to as **Computerized Physician Order Entry (CPOE)**. The order is received in the pharmacy, where a patient's drug profile (list of drugs) is maintained. The nurse verifies the order in the computer and inputs his/her digital ID after the medication is administered. A computer printout replaces the handwritten MAR.

One advantage of a computerized system is that handwritten orders do not need to be deciphered or transcribed. The computer program can also identify possible interactions among the patient's medications and automatically alert the pharmacist and persons administering the drugs.

Some institutions use *Automated Medication Dispensing Machines (ADC)* to dispense medications. See ● **Figure 2.17**. The healthcare provider must still

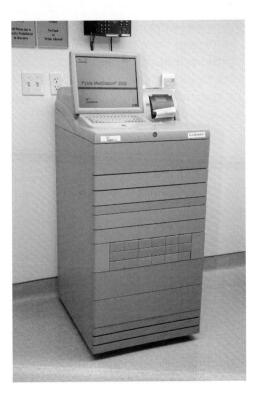

● **Figure 2.17**
**Automated Medication Dispensing**
**Machine (ADC).**

be vigilant when using such technology, and must be sure to follow the "Six Rights of Medication Administration."

● **Figure 2.18** is a portion of a *computerized MAR* for a 24-hour period stated in military time. This MAR divides the day into three shifts. Note that no medications have yet been recorded for the 3:01 P.M.–11:00 P.M. shift (1501h–2300h).

| SCHEDULED | 12/06/10–12/07/10 2301–0700 | 12/07/10 0701–1500 | 12/07/10 1501–2300 |
|---|---|---|---|
| ℞ Cefepime (Maxipime) | | 0840 2 g TVPB MAB | 2015 |
| ℞ Emoxaparin Na (Lovenox) | | 1026 40 mg subcutaneous MAB | |
| ℞ Furosemide (Lasix) | 0611 20 mg IVP DJS | | |
| ℞ Hetastarch (he SPAN) | | 0920 250 mL IVPB MAB | |
| ℞ KCl (Potassium chloride) | | 1026 20 mEq ER tab PO MAB | |
| ℞ Metoprolol XL (Toprol XL) | | 1000 CANCEL MAB | 2200 |
| ℞ Metronidazole (Flagyl) | 0611 500 mg IVPB DJS | 1324 500 mg IVPB MAB | 2200 |
| ℞ NTG (Nitroglycerin) | 0110 15 mg oint topical DJS 0611 15 mg oint topical DJS | 1231 15 mg oint topical MAB | 1800 |
| ℞ Pantoprazole (Protonix) 40 mg IVPB | | 1026 40 mg IVPB MAB | |
| PRN | 12/06/10–12/07/10 2301–0700 | 12/07/10 0701–1500 | 12/07/10 1501–2300 |
| ℞ Saline flush | 0110 2 mL IV flush DJS | 0829 2 mL IV flush MAB | 1600 |
| ℞ Morphine | 0115 4 mg IVP DJS 0439 4 mg IVP DJS | 1306 2 mg IVP MAB | |
| IV | 12/06/10–12/07/10 2301–0700 | 12/07/10 0701–1500 | 12/07/10 1501–2300 |
| ℞ NS (NaCl, 0.9%, 1 L) | | 0810 | 2130 |

| PRN ORDERS | |
|---|---|
| Hydrocodone 5 mg and Acetaminophen 500 mg | x 1–2 tab PO q4h prn process if pain |
| Saline flush | 2 mL IV flush q8 at 0000/0800/1600 and prn |
| Insulin, human regular sliding scale {Novolin R SS} | See scale prn if BS 200–249 mg/dL give 4 Units of Reg insulin subcut |

● **Figure 2.18**
**A portion of a computerized MAR.**

Scheduled (routine), IV, and PRN orders are shown. For each order administered, the MAR indicates the time, order, and the nurse's digital identification. Currently there is a variety of computerized medication systems in use. The healthcare provider has a responsibility to be both knowledgeable of the facility's policies and proficient in using its system.

### EXAMPLE 2.5

Use the MAR in Figure 2.18 to answer the following questions:

1. Which drug was ordered in milliequivalents?

_____

2. What drugs were administered at 6:11 A.M. on 12/06/2010?

_____

3. Identify the dosage, route, and time that Flagyl was administered before noon on 12/07/2010.

_____

4. Identify the name, dosage, route, and time of administration of the PRN drugs administered after noon on 12/07/2010.

_____

5. How many times did the patient receive NTG (Nitroglycerin) on 12/07/2010?

_____

This is what you should have found:

1. KCl (Potassium chloride)
2. Furosemide (Lasix), Metronidazole (Flagyl), and NTG (Nitroglycerin)
3. 500 mg, IVPB at 0611h (6:11 A.M.)
4. Morphine 2 mg IVP was given at 1306h (1:06 P.M.)
5. Three times

# Drug Labels

You will need to understand the information found on drug labels in order to calculate drug dosages. The important features of a drug label are identified in
● Figure 2.19.

1. **Name of drug:** Mycobutin is the trade name. In this case, the name begins with an uppercase letter, is in large type, and is boldly visible on the label. The generic name is rifabutin, written in lowercase letters.
2. **Form of drug:** The drug is in the form of a capsule.
3. **National Drug Code (NDC) number:** 0013-5301-17.
4. **Bar code:** Has the NDC number encoded in it.
5. **Dosage strength:** 150 mg of the drug are contained in one capsule.

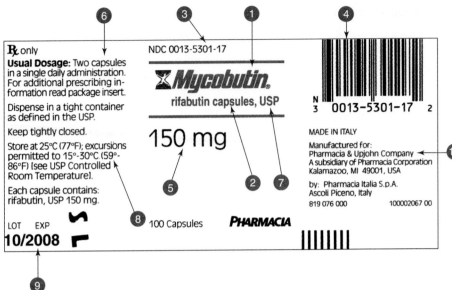

**ALERT**

Always read the expiration date! After the expiration date, the drug may lose its potency or act differently in a patient's body. Discard expired drugs. Never give expired drugs to patients!

● **Figure 2.19**
**Drug label for Mycobutin.**
*(Reg. Trademark of Pfizer Inc. Reproduced with permission.)*

6. **Dosage recommendations:** 2 capsules in a single daily administration. Note that the manufacturer informs you to read the package insert.

7. **USP:** This drug meets the standards of the United States Pharmacopeia.

8. **Storage directions:** Some drugs have to be stored under controlled conditions if they are to retain their effectiveness. This drug should be stored at 25°C (77°F).

9. **Expiration date:** The expiration date specifies when the drug should be discarded. After 10/2008 (October 31, 2008), the drug cannot be dispensed and should be discarded. For the sake of simplicity, not every drug label in this textbook will have an expiration date.

10. **Manufacturer:** Pharmacia & Upjohn.

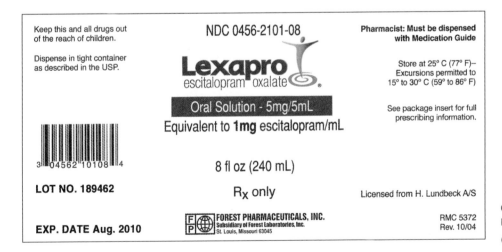

● **Figure 2.20**
**Drug label for Lexapro.**
*(Courtesy of Forest Pharmaceuticals, Inc.)*

The label in ● **Figure 2.20** indicates the following information:

1. **Trade name:** Lexapro

2. **Generic name:** escitalopram oxalate

3. **Form:** oral solution

4. **Dosage strength:** 5 mg/5 mL, equivalent to 1 mg of escitalopram per mL

5. **Dosage recommendations:** See package insert for full prescribing information

6. **NDC number:** 0456-2101-08

7. **Expiration date:** August 2010

8. **Total volume in container:** 8 fl oz (240 mL)

9. **Manufacturer:** Forest Pharmaceuticals, Inc.

10. **Lot number** or **Control number:** The lot number of this drug is 189462. This number identifies where and when a drug was manufactured. When there is a problem with particular batches of a drug and these batches must be recalled, lot numbers are useful for identifying which items are to be taken off the market.

### EXAMPLE 2.6

Read the label in ● Figure 2.21 and find the following:

1. Trade name: _____

2. Generic name: _____

3. Form: _____

4. Dosage strength: _____

5. NDC number: _____

6. Dosage and use: _____

7. Instructions for dispensing: _____

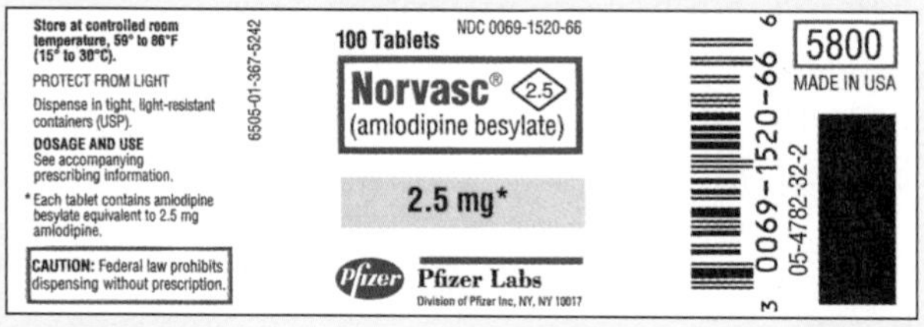

● **Figure 2.21**
**Drug label for Norvasc.**
*(Reg - Trademark of Pfizer Inc. Reproduced with permission.)*

The label for the antihypertensive drug Norvasc in Figure 2.21 indicates the following:

1. **Trade name:** Norvasc

2. **Generic name:** amlodipine besylate

3. **Form:** Tablets

4. **Dosage strength:** 2.5 mg per tablet

5. **NDC number:** 0069152066

6. **Dosage and use:** See accompanying information

7. **Instructions for dispensing:** Dispense in tight, light-resistant container

## EXAMPLE 2.7

Examine the label shown in ● Figure 2.22 and record the following information:

1. Trade name: _____
2. Generic name: _____
3. Form: _____
4. Dosage strength: _____
5. Amount of drug in container: _____
6. Storage temperature: _____
7. Special instructions: _____

This is what you should have found:

1. **Trade name:** Norvir
2. **Generic name:** ritonavir
3. **Form:** Oral solution
4. **Dosage strength:** 80 mg per mL
5. **Amount of drug in container:** 240 mL
6. **Storage temperature:** Do not refrigerate
7. **Special instructions:** Shake well before use. ALERT: Find out about medicines that should NOT be taken with Norvir.

**NDC** 0074-1940-63
**240 mL**

# NORVIR®

## (RITONAVIR ORAL SOLUTION)

## 80 mg per mL

Shake well before each use.
**DO NOT REFRIGERATE**
Use by product expiration date.

Ⓐ    ℞ only    02-8410-2/R4

**ALERT**
Find out about medicines
that should NOT be taken
with NORVIR.

Note to Pharmacist: Do not cover ALERT
box with pharmacy label.

**EXP. MARCH 2010**
**LOT**

● **Figure 2.22**
**Drug label for Norvir.**

*(Reproduced with permission of Abbott Laboratories.)*

## EXAMPLE 2.8

Examine the label shown in ● Figure 2.23 and record the following information:

1. Trade name: _____
2. Generic name: _____
3. Form: _____
4. Dosage strength: _____
5. Usual adult dosage: _____

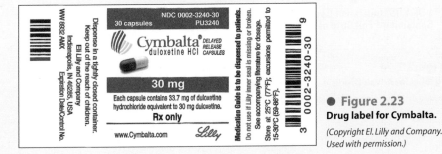

● **Figure 2.23**
**Drug label for Cymbalta.**

*(Copyright El. Lilly and Company. Used with permission.)*

This is what you should have found:

1. **Trade name:** Cymbalta
2. **Generic name:** duloxetine HCl
3. **Form:** Delayed-Release capsules
4. **Dosage strength:** 30 mg per capsule
5. **Usual adult dosage:** See package insert

## Combination Drugs

Combination drugs contain two or more generic drugs in one form. Both names and strengths of each drug are on the label. Two such medication labels follow.

Examine the label shown in ● **Figure 2.24.** The label for this anti-asthma combination drug indicates that each blister contains 250 micrograms of fluticasone and 50 micrograms of salmeterol.

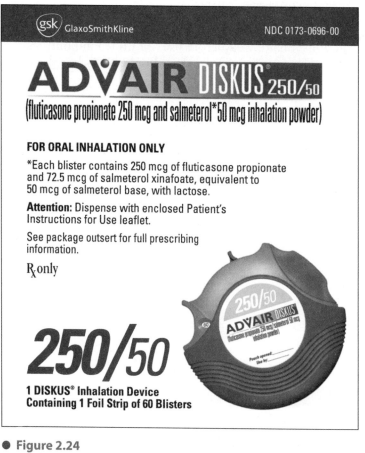

● **Figure 2.24**
**Drug label for Advair Diskus.**
*(Reproduced with the permission of GlaxoSmithKline.)*

## EXAMPLE 2.9

Examine the label shown in ● Figure 2.25 and answer the following questions:

1. What is the trade name and dosage strength of the drug?

_____

2. What is the dosage strength of acetaminophen?

_____

3. What is the route of administration?

_____

4. What is the amount of drug in the container?

_____

5. What is the usual dosage?

_____

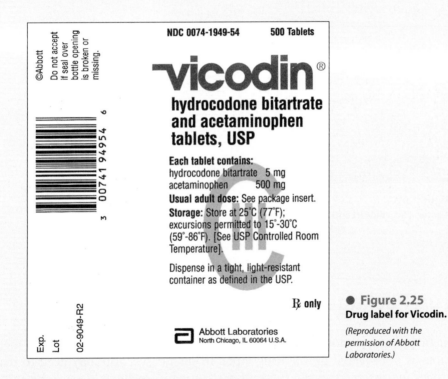

● Figure 2.25
**Drug label for Vicodin.**

*(Reproduced with the permission of Abbott Laboratories.)*

This is what you should have found:

1. Vicodin is the trade name, and the dosage strength is 5 mg/500 mg per tablet
2. 500 mg of acetaminophen per tablet
3. By mouth
4. 500 tablets
5. See package insert

# Controlled Substances

Certain drugs which can lead to abuse or dependence are classified by law as **controlled substances**. These drugs are divided into five categories, called schedules. Schedule I drugs are those with the highest potential for abuse (for example, heroin, marijuana). Schedule V drugs are those with the lowest potential for abuse (for example, cough medications containing codeine). *Controlled substance*s must be stored, handled, disposed of, and administered according to regulations established by the *U.S. Drug Enforcement Agency (DEA)*. Hospitals and pharmacies must register with the *DEA* and use their assigned numbers to purchase scheduled drugs. Those who prescribe medications must have a *DEA* number in order to prescribe *controlled substances*.

The *controlled substance* OxyContin (oxycodone hydrochloride) is a Schedule II drug, as indicated by the Cɪɪ on the label. (See the arrow in ● **Figure 2.26**.)

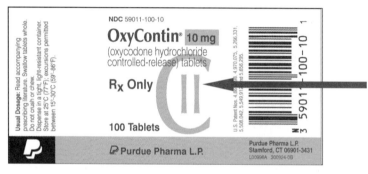

● **Figure 2.26**
**OxyContin, a Schedule II controlled substance.**

*(Reprinted with permission of Purdue Pharma.)*

# Drug Package Inserts

Sometimes information needed to safely prepare, administer, and store medications is not located on the drug label. In such cases, you may need to read the **package insert**. The pharmaceutical company includes a package insert with each container of a prescription drug. The information on a drug package insert is intended for the prescriber, pharmacist, and the person who administers the drug. It contains descriptions of a drug's chemistry and how it acts in the body. ● **Figure 2.27** shows an excerpt from a drug package insert for Avodart.

Always consult the package insert when you need information about

- mixing and storing a drug
- preparing a drug dose
- recommended safe dose and range
- indications, contraindications, and warnings
- side effects and adverse reactions

## AVODART®
(dutasteride)
**Soft Gelatin Capsules**

### DESCRIPTION

AVODART (dutasteride) is a synthetic 4-azasteroid compound that is a selective inhibitor of both the type 1 and type 2 isoforms of steroid 5α-reductase (5AR), an intracellular enzyme that converts testosterone to 5α-dihydrotestosterone (DHT).

Dutasteride is chemically designated as (5α,17β)-N-{2,5 bis(trifluoromethyl)phenyl}-3-oxo-4-azaandrost-1-ene-17-carboxamide. The empirical formula of dutasteride is $C_{27}H_{30}F_6N_2O_2$, representing a molecular weight of 528.5 with the following structural formula:

$$NOHHHHNOHCF_3HCF_3**$$

Dutasteride is a white to pale yellow powder with a melting point of 242° to 250°C. It is soluble in ethanol (44 mg/mL), methanol (64 mg/mL), and polyethylene glycol 400 (3 mg/mL), but it is insoluble in water.

AVODART Soft Gelatin Capsules for oral administration contain 0.5 mg of the active ingredient dutasteride in yellow capsules with red print. Each capsule contains 0.5 mg of dutasteride dissolved in a mixture of mono-di-glycerides of caprylic/capric acid and butylated hydroxytoluene. The inactive excipients in the capsule shell are gelatin (from certified BSE-free bovine sources), glycerin, and ferric oxide (yellow). The soft gelatin capsules are printed with edible red ink.

### INDICATIONS AND USAGE

AVODART is indicated for the treatment of symptomatic benign prostatic hyperplasia (BPH) in men with an enlarged prostate to:

- Improve symptoms
- Reduce the risk of acute urinary retention
- Reduce the risk of the need for BPH-related surgery

### CONTRAINDICATIONS

AVODART is contraindicated for use in women and children.

AVODART is contraindicated for patients with known hypersensitivity to dutasteride, other 5a-reductase inhibitors, or any component of the preparation.

### PRECAUTIONS

**General:** Lower urinary tract symptoms of BPH can be indicative of other urological diseases, including prostate cancer. Patients should be assessed to rule out other urological diseases prior to treatment with AVODART. Patients with a large residual urinary volume and/or severely diminished urinary flow may not be good candidates for 5α-reductase inhibitor therapy and should be carefully monitored for obstructive uropathy.

**Blood Donation:** Men being treated with dutasteride should not donate blood until at least 6 months have passed following their last dose. The purpose of this deferred period is to prevent administration of dutasteride to a pregnant female transfusion recipient.

**Use in Hepatic Impairment:** The effect of hepatic impairment on dutasteride pharmacokinetics has not been studied. Because dutasteride is extensively metabolized and has a half-life of approximately 5 weeks at steady state, caution should be used in the administration of dutasteride to patients with liver disease.

**Use with Potent CYP3A4 Inhibitors:** Although dutasteride is extensively metabolized, no metabolically based drug interaction studies have been conducted. The effect of potent CYP3A4 inhibitors has not been studied. Because of the potential for drug-drug interactions, care should be taken when administering dutasteride to patients taking potent, chronic CYP3A4 enzyme inhibitors (e.g., ritonavir).

**Effects on Prostate-Specific Antigen and Prostate Cancer Detection:** Digital rectal examinations, as well as other evaluations for prostate cancer, should be performed on patients with BPH prior to initiating therapy with AVODART and periodically thereafter.

Dutasteride reduces total serum PSA concentration by approximately 40% following 3 months of treatment and approximately 50% following 6, 12, and 24 months of treatment. This decrease is predictable over the entire range of PSA values, although it may vary in individual patients. Therefore, for interpretation of serial PSAs in a man taking AVODART, a new baseline PSA concentration should be established after 3 to 6 months of treatment, and this new value should be used to assess potentially cancer-related changes in PSA. To interpret an isolated PSA value in a man treated with AVODART for 6 months or more, the PSA value should be doubled for comparison with normal values in untreated men.

The free-to-total PSA ratio (percent free PSA) remains constant at Month 12, even under the influence of AVODART. If clinicians elect to use percent free PSA as an aid in the detection of prostate cancer in men receiving AVODART, no adjustment to its value appears necessary.

### DOSAGE AND ADMINISTRATION

The recommended dose of AVODART is 1 capsule (0.5 mg) taken orally once a day. The capsules should be swallowed whole. AVODART may be administered with or without food. No dosage adjustment is necessary for subjects with renal impairment or for the elderly (see CLINICAL PHARMACOLOGY: Pharmacokinetics: Special Populations: Geriatric and Renal Impairment). Due to the absence of data in patients with hepatic impairment, no dosage recommendation can be made (see PRECAUTIONS: General).

### HOW SUPPLIED

AVODART Soft Gelatin Capsules 0.5 mg are oblong, opaque, dull yellow, gelatin capsules imprinted with "GX CE2" in red ink on one side packaged in bottles of 30 (NDC 0173-0712-15) and 90 (NDC 0173-0712-04) with child-resistant closures.

**Storage and Handling:** Store at 25°C(77°F); excursions permitted to 15-30°C(59-86°F) [see USP Controlled Room Temperature].

Dutasteride is absorbed through the skin. AVODART Soft Gelatin capsules should not be handled by women who are pregnant or who may become pregnant because of the potential for absorption of dutasteride and the subsequent potential risk to a developing male fetus (see CLINICAL PHARMACOLOGY: Pharmacokinetics, WARNINGS: Exposure of Women—Risk to Male Fetus, and PRECAUTIONS: Information for Patients and Pregnancy).

Manufactured by Cardinal Health
Beinheim, France for
GlaxoSmithKline
Research Triangle Park, NC 27709
©2005, GlaxoSmithKline. All rights reserved.
May 2005 RL-2188

● **Figure 2.27**
**Excerpts of Avodart package insert.**

*(Reproduced with permission of GlaxoSmithKline.)*

## EXAMPLE 2.10

Read the package insert in Figure 2.27 and fill in the requested information.

1. What is the generic name of the drug?

_____

2. For what condition is Avodart used?

_____

3. How long after Avodart has been discontinued can a patient donate blood?

_____

4. What is the recommended dose of the drug?

_____

5. What is the drug form?

_____

This is what you should have found:

1. dutasteride.
2. Benign prostatic hyperplasia (BPH).
3. Men being treated with dutasteride should not donate blood until at least 6 months have passed following their last dose.
4. The recommended dose of Avodart is 1 capsule (0.5 mg) orally once a day.
5. The drug is supplied in the form of soft gelatin capsules.

## Summary

In this chapter, the Medication Administration Process was discussed, including those who may administer drugs; the "six rights" and "three checks" of medication administration; and how to interpret prescriptions, medication orders, medication administration records, drug labels, and drug package inserts.

■ The six rights of medication administration serve as a guide for *safe* administration of medications to patients.

■ Failure to achieve any of the six rights constitutes a medication error.

■ A person administering medications has a legal and ethical responsibility to report medication errors.

■ Medication errors can occur at any point in the medication process.

■ A drug should be prescribed using its generic name.

■ Understanding drug orders requires the interpretation of common abbreviations.

■ Never use any abbreviations on the JCAHO "Official Do Not Use" list.

■ Read drug labels carefully; many drugs have look-alike/sound-alike names.

■ Carefully read the label to determine dosage strength and check calculations, paying special attention to decimal points.

■ Medications must be administered in the form and via the route specified by the prescriber.

■ The form of a drug affects its speed of onset, intensity of action, and route of administration.

■ The *oral (PO)* route is the one most commonly used.

■ *Buccal* and *sublingual* medications must be kept in the mouth until they are completely dissolved.

■ *Topical* medications may have local and systemic effects. *Transdermal patches* are applied for their systemic effect.

■ *Inhalation* medications may be administered with various devices, such as *nebulizers, dry powder* and *metered dose inhalers.*

■ *Parenteral* medications are injected into the body. In order to prevent infection, sterile technique must be used for their administration.

■ Before administering any medication, it is essential to identify the patient.

- Medications should be documented immediately after, but never before, they are administered.
- No medication should be given without a legal order.
- If persons administering medications have difficulty understanding or interpreting the order, they must clarify the order with the prescriber.
- Medication administration is rapidly becoming computerized.
- Drug package inserts contain detailed information about the drug, including mixing, storing a drug, preparing a drug dose, indications, contraindications, warnings, side effects, adverse reactions, and the recommended safe dose range.

# Practice Sets

The answers to *Try These for Practice* and *Exercises* are found in Appendix A. Ask your instructor for the answers to the *Additional Exercises*.

## Try These for Practice

Test your comprehension after reading the chapter.

Study the drug labels in ● **Figures 2.28** to **2.32** and answer the following five questions.

1. What is the route of administration for montelukast sodium?

   _____

2. How many tablets are contained in the container for Zocor?

   _____

3. What is the quantity of drug in each 5 mL of EryPed?

   _____

4. What is the trade name for valproic acid?

   _____

5. What is contained in 1 mL of the drug Kaletra?

   _____

## Exercises

Reinforce your understanding in class or at home.

Use the information from drug labels in Figures 2.28 to 2.32 to complete Exercises 1 to 5.

1. Write the generic name for Kaletra.

   _____

2. Write the trade name for the drug whose NDC number is 0006-0117-31.

   _____

3. What is the total amount of solution in the bottle of Kaletra?

   _____

Workspace

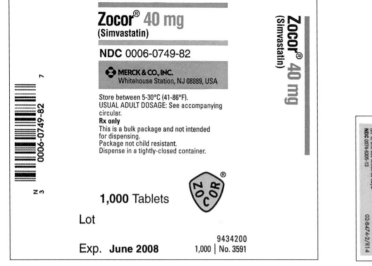

**● Figure 2.28**
**Drug label for Zocor.**

*(The labels for the products Zocor 40mg are reproduced with permission of Merck & Co., Inc., copyright owner.)*

**● Figure 2.29**
**Drug label for EryPed.**

*(Reproduced with permission of Abbott Laboratories.)*

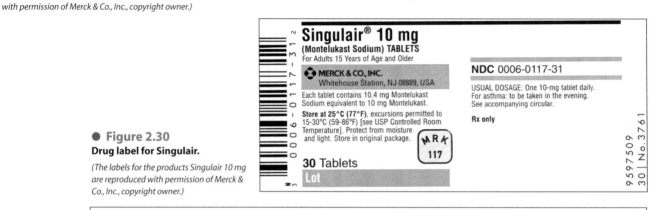

**● Figure 2.30**
**Drug label for Singulair.**

*(The labels for the products Singulair 10 mg are reproduced with permission of Merck & Co., Inc., copyright owner.)*

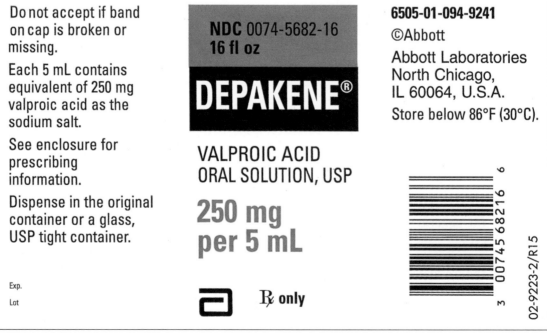

**● Figure 2.31**
**Drug label for Depakene.**

*(Reproduced with the permission of Abbott Laboratories.)*

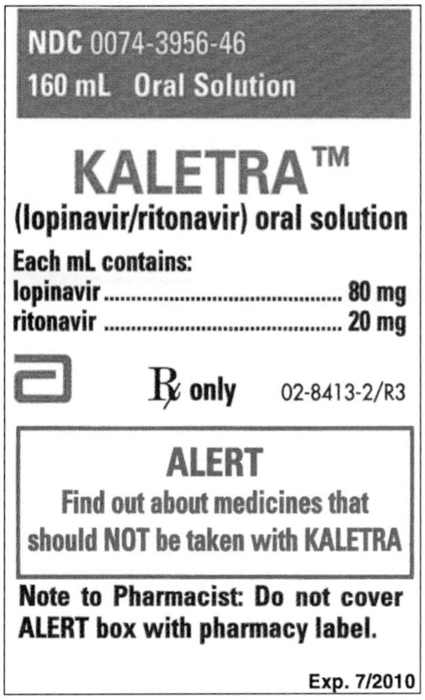

● Figure 2.32
**Drug label for Kaletra.**
*(Reproduced with permission of Abbott Laboratories.)*

4. What is the dosage strength of EryPed?

   _____

5. What is the dosage strength of the drug whose NDC number is 0006-0749-82?

   _____

6. Study the MAR in ● **Figures 2.33a** and **2.33b** and answer the questions.

   (a) Which drugs were administered at 10 P.M. on 12/10/2010?

   _____

   (b) Designate the time of the day the patient received ibandronate sodium.

   _____

   (c) How many doses of Dilantin were administered to the patient by nurse Young?

   _____

   (d) What drugs must be taken before breakfast?

   _____

   (e) What is the last date on which the patient will receive Bactrim?

   _____

7. Study the physician's order sheet in ● **Figure 2.34** and then answer the following questions.

   (a) Which drugs are ordered to be given once daily?

   _____

   (b) Which drug should be given four times a day?

   _____

   (c) What is the dose and route of administration of metoclopramide?

   _____

# UNIVERSITY HOSPITAL

324689
Jane Ambery
2336 17th Avenue
Brooklyn, NY 10001

12/7/2010
5/01/47
Protestant
HIP

## DAILY MEDICATION ADMINISTRATION RECORD

Dr. Mae Ling

PATIENT NAME _____ Jane Ambery _____

ROOM # _____ 112 _____

IF ANOTHER RECORDS IS IN USE ☐

ALLERGIC TO (RECORD IN RED): _____ sulfa, fish _____

DATES GIVEN ⋮ MONTH/DAY   YEAR: _____ 2010 _____

| RED CHECK INITIAL | ORDER DATE | INITIAL | EXP DATE | MEDICATION, DOSAGE, FREQUENCY AND ROUTE | TIME | 12/7 | 12/8 | 12/9 | 12/10 | 12/11 | 12/12 | 12/13 |
|---|---|---|---|---|---|---|---|---|---|---|---|---|
| | 12/7 | MC | 12/13 | Dilantin (phenytoin) 100 mg | 10AM | MC | MC | MC | MC | | | |
| | | | | PO t.i.d. | 2PM | MC | MC | MC | MC | | | |
| | | | | | 6PM | JY | JY | JY | JY | | | |
| | 12/7 | SG | 12/16 | Bactrim DS 2tabs PO q12h | 8AM | SG | SG | SG | SG | | | |
| | | | | for 10 days | 8PM | JY | JY | JY | JY | | | |
| | 12/7 | SG | 12/13 | Bonivar (ibandronate sodium) | 6AM | SG | SG | SG | SG | | | |
| | | | | 2.5 mg PO daily. Take 60 minutes | | | | | | | | |
| | | | | before first food or drink of day | | | | | | | | |
| | | | | (except plain water) | | | | | | | | |
| | 12/7 | SG | 12/13 | Humulin N insulin 15 units subcut | 7:30AM | SG | SG | SG | SG | | | |
| | | | | every morning | | | | | | | | |
| | | | | 30 minutes before breakfast | | | | | | | | |
| | 12/7 | SG | 12/13 | Humulin R insulin 8 units subcut | 7:30AM | SG | SG | SG | SG | | | |
| | | | | every morning | | | | | | | | |
| | | | | 30 minutes before breakfast | | | | | | | | |

| INT. | NURSES' FULL SIGNATURE AND TITLE | INT. | NURSES' FULL SIGNATURE AND TITLE |
|---|---|---|---|
| SG | Sara Gordon, RN | | |
| MC | Marie Colon, RN | | |
| JY | Jim Young, RN | | |
| | | | |
| | | | |

● **Figure 2.33a**
Medication Administration Record for Jane Ambery.

---

# UNIVERSITY HOSPITAL

324689
Jane Ambery
2336 17th Avenue
Brooklyn, NY

12/7/2010
5/01/47
Protestant
HIP

## DAILY MEDICATION ADMINISTRATION RECORD

Dr. Mae Ling, M.D.

PATIENT NAME _____ Jane Ambery _____

ROOM # _____ 112 _____

IF ANOTHER RECORDS IS IN USE ☐

ALLERGIC TO (RECORD IN RED): _____ sulfa, fish _____

DATES GIVEN ⋮ MONTH/DAY   YEAR: _____ 2010 _____

### PRN MEDICATION

| ORDER DATE | EXPIRATION DATE/TIME | MEDICATION, DOSAGE, FREQUENCY AND ROUTE | | DOSES GIVEN | | | | | | | |
|---|---|---|---|---|---|---|---|---|---|---|---|
| 12/10 | 12/17 | | DATE | 12/10 | | | | | | | |
| | | Anusol supp 1 PR q4–6h prn | TIME | 10 PM | | | | | | | |
| | | | INIT | JY | | | | | | | |
| | | | DATE | | | | | | | | |
| | | | TIME | | | | | | | | |
| | | | INIT | | | | | | | | |

STAT-ONE DOSE-PRE-OPERATIVE MEDICATIONS        ◯  Check here if additional sheet in use.

| ORDER DATE | MEDICATION–DOSAGE ROUTE | DATE | TIME | INIT | ORDER DATE | MEDICATION–DOSAGE ROUTE | DATE | TIME | INIT |
|---|---|---|---|---|---|---|---|---|---|
| | | | | | | | | | |
| | | | | | | | | | |

| INT. | NURSES' FULL SIGNATURE AND TITLE | INT. | NURSES' FULL SIGNATURE AND TITLE |
|---|---|---|---|
| JY | Jim Young, RN | | |

● **Figure 2.33b**
Medication Administration Record for Jane Ambery.

**PHYSICIAN'S ORDERS**

| ORDER DATE | DATE DISC | | |
|---|---|---|---|
| 4/20/10 | 4/30/10 | Omnicef (cefdinir) 300 mg PO q12h for 10 days | |
| 4/20/10 | 4/27/10 | digoxin 0.125 mg PO daily | |
| 4/20/10 | 4/27/10 | Glucophage (metformin HCl) 850 mg PO b.i.d. with breakfast and dinner | |
| 4/20/10 | 4/27/10 | Reglan (metoclopramide) 10 mg PO 30 minutes before meals and at bedtime | |
| 4/20/10 | 4/23/10 | Duragesic transdermal film ER 25 mg per hour. Remove in 72 hours. | |
| 4/20/10 | 4/27/10 | Lasix 40 mg PO daily | |
| **PLEASE INDICATE BEEPER #** → | | | 222 |

2/28/52
Episcopal
Aetna

4/20/2010

Jane Myers
23 College Ave
Salt Lake City
Utah 46022

Dr. Juan Rodriguez
#212332

Workspace

● **Figure 2.34**
**Physician's order sheet for patient Jane Myers.**

 (d) What is the route of administration for Duragesic?

_____

 (e) Which drug is given every 12 hours?

_____

8. Use the package insert shown in ● **Figure 2.35** to answer the following questions.

 (a) What is an appropriate dose for relief of skeletal muscle spasm?

_____

 (b) What tests are advisable during long-term therapy?

_____

 (c) What is the dosage strength of the Diazepam Oral Solution?

_____

 (d) What is the NDC number of the Intensol Oral Solution (Concentrate)?

_____

9. Fill in the following table with the equivalent times.

| Standard Time | Military Time |
|---|---|
| 9 A.M. | _____ |
| _____ | 1500h |
| | 1200h |
| 6 P.M. | _____ |
| | 2015h |
| 2:30 A.M. | _____ |
| | 1645h |
| 6 A.M. | _____ |
| _____ | 0000h |

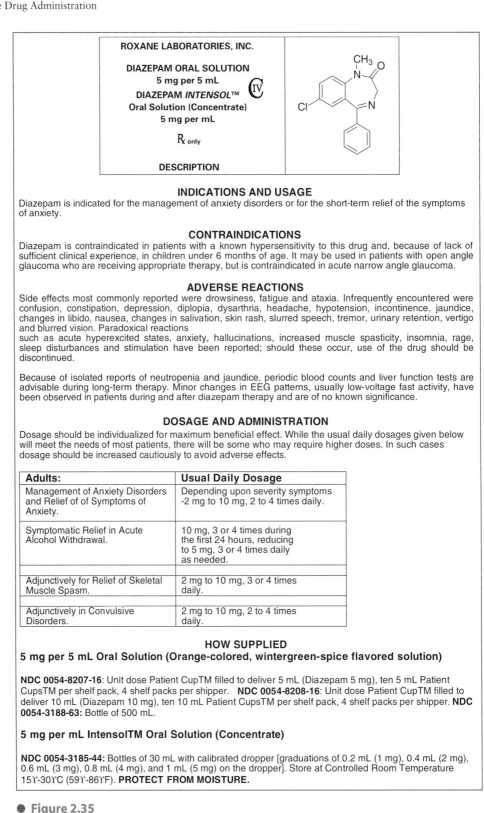

### ROXANE LABORATORIES, INC.

**DIAZEPAM ORAL SOLUTION**
5 mg per 5 mL
**DIAZEPAM *INTENSOL*™**
Oral Solution (Concentrate)
5 mg per mL

R$_x$ only

**DESCRIPTION**

### INDICATIONS AND USAGE

Diazepam is indicated for the management of anxiety disorders or for the short-term relief of the symptoms of anxiety.

### CONTRAINDICATIONS

Diazepam is contraindicated in patients with a known hypersensitivity to this drug and, because of lack of sufficient clinical experience, in children under 6 months of age. It may be used in patients with open angle glaucoma who are receiving appropriate therapy, but is contraindicated in acute narrow angle glaucoma.

### ADVERSE REACTIONS

Side effects most commonly reported were drowsiness, fatigue and ataxia. Infrequently encountered were confusion, constipation, depression, diplopia, dysarthria, headache, hypotension, incontinence, jaundice, changes in libido, nausea, changes in salivation, skin rash, slurred speech, tremor, urinary retention, vertigo and blurred vision. Paradoxical reactions
such as acute hyperexcited states, anxiety, hallucinations, increased muscle spasticity, insomnia, rage, sleep disturbances and stimulation have been reported; should these occur, use of the drug should be discontinued.

Because of isolated reports of neutropenia and jaundice, periodic blood counts and liver function tests are advisable during long-term therapy. Minor changes in EEG patterns, usually low-voltage fast activity, have been observed in patients during and after diazepam therapy and are of no known significance.

### DOSAGE AND ADMINISTRATION

Dosage should be individualized for maximum beneficial effect. While the usual daily dosages given below will meet the needs of most patients, there will be some who may require higher doses. In such cases dosage should be increased cautiously to avoid adverse effects.

| Adults: | Usual Daily Dosage |
|---|---|
| Management of Anxiety Disorders and Relief of of Symptoms of Anxiety. | Depending upon severity symptoms -2 mg to 10 mg, 2 to 4 times daily. |
| Symptomatic Relief in Acute Alcohol Withdrawal. | 10 mg, 3 or 4 times during the first 24 hours, reducing to 5 mg, 3 or 4 times daily as needed. |
| Adjunctively for Relief of Skeletal Muscle Spasm. | 2 mg to 10 mg, 3 or 4 times daily. |
| Adjunctively in Convulsive Disorders. | 2 mg to 10 mg, 2 to 4 times daily. |

### HOW SUPPLIED
**5 mg per 5 mL Oral Solution (Orange-colored, wintergreen-spice flavored solution)**

**NDC 0054-8207-16**: Unit dose Patient Cup™ filled to deliver 5 mL (Diazepam 5 mg), ten 5 mL Patient Cups™ per shelf pack, 4 shelf packs per shipper.   **NDC 0054-8208-16**: Unit dose Patient Cup™ filled to deliver 10 mL (Diazepam 10 mg), ten 10 mL Patient Cups™ per shelf pack, 4 shelf packs per shipper. **NDC 0054-3188-63**: Bottle of 500 mL.

**5 mg per mL Intensol™ Oral Solution (Concentrate)**

**NDC 0054-3185-44:** Bottles of 30 mL with calibrated dropper [graduations of 0.2 mL (1 mg), 0.4 mL (2 mg), 0.6 mL (3 mg), 0.8 mL (4 mg), and 1 mL (5 mg) on the dropper]. Store at Controlled Room Temperature 15Υ-30Υ°C (59Υ-86Υ°F). **PROTECT FROM MOISTURE.**

● **Figure 2.35**
**Excerpts from package insert for Diazepam.**

*(Courtesy of Roxane Laboratories Inc.)*

10. Interpret the following drug orders:

    (a) *digoxin 0.25 mg PO daily, hold if heart rate less then 60*

    (b) *Toradol (ketorolac) 15 mg IVP q6h × 4 doses*

    (c) *Milk of Magnesia 30 mL PO daily prn constipation*

    (d) *ibuprofen 800 mg PO t.i.d.*

    (e) *Novolin R insulin 5 units subcut stat*

11. Determine which part is missing for each of the following drug orders:

    (a) 01/02/2010              2310h
        *Amoxicillin 500 mg q.i.d.*

    (b) *enalapril 10 mg via NGT daily*
            I. Patel MD

    (c) 3/22/2010
        *metroprolol 25 mg via PEG hold for HR less than 60 and SBP
        less than 100*

    (d) *1900h*
        *Solu-Medrol 60 mg IVPB*
            J.Rodriguez MD

    (e) 12/28/2010              10:00am
        *aspirin po daily*
            A.Rodriguez RN ANP

## Additional Exercises

Now, test yourself!
Study the drug labels shown in ● **Figure 2.36** to answer questions 1–5.

1. Write the generic name for Atarax.

   _____

2. Write the trade name for ziprasidone HCl.

   _____

3. Which drug can be administered by injection?

   _____

4. What is the route of administration for furosemide?

   _____

5. Write a trade name for the drug whose NDC number is 0049-5590-93.

   _____

Workspace

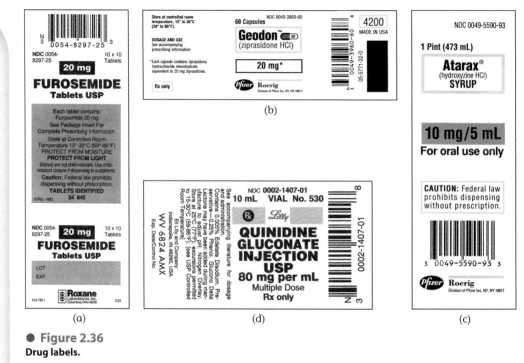

● **Figure 2.36**
**Drug labels.**

*2-36a (Courtesy of Roxane Laboratories Inc.) 2-36b (Reg. Trademark of Pfizer Inc. Reproduced with permission.) 2-36c (Reg. Trademark of Pfizer Inc. Reproduced with permission.) 2-36d (Copyright Eli Lilly and Company. Used with permission.)*

6. Study the MAR in ● **Figure 2.37**. Fill in the following chart and answer the questions.

| Name of Drug | Dose | Route of Administration | Time of Administration | Date Started | Expiration Date |
|---|---|---|---|---|---|
| Celebrex | | | | | |
| Flomax | | | | | |
| Ditropan | | | | | |
| Zoloft | | | | | |
| Seroquel | | | | | |
| Valium | | | | | |
| fluconazole | | | | | |

(a) Which drug(s) was administered at 8 P.M. on 12/7/2010?

_____

(b) How many doses of Valium did the patient receive in seven days?

_____

(c) What is the name of the drug administered IV?

_____

(d) How many medications were administered at 5 P.M.? Name the medication(s).

_____

## MEDICATION RECORD

| DIAGNOSIS | urinary tract infection |
| | cronic depression |
| | osteoarthritis |

Jim Ellington
2335 15ª Ave
Queens, NY
10221

12/20/20
Protestant
BCBS

ALLERGIES
(LIST IN RED)

Mae Ling, MD
#324689

12/07/2010

KNOWN ALLERGIES  Yes ☐  No ☒    WEIGHT _____ 104 lb _____

| ORDER DATE | EXP. DATE | MEDICATION, DOSAGE, FREQUENCY & ROUTE | HOURS | December DATES GIVEN |||||||||||||| DO NOT WRITE IN THIS COLUMN |
| | | | | 7 | 8 | 9 | 10 | 11 | 12 | 13 | 14 | 15 | 16 | 17 | 18 | 19 | 20 | |
| --- | --- | --- | --- | --- | --- | --- | --- | --- | --- | --- | --- | --- | --- | --- | --- | --- | --- | --- |
| 12/7 | 12/18 | Celebrex 100 mg PO | 8AM | RG | RG | RG | RG | RG | MD | MD | | | | | | | | |
| | | b.i.d. q12h | 8PM | TK | TK | TK | TK | TK | JO | JO | | | | | | | | |
| | | | | | | | | | | | | | | | | | | |
| 12/7 | 12/13 | Flomax 0.4 mg | 5PM | RD | RD | RD | RD | RD | JO | JO | | | | | | | | |
| | | PO 30 min AC dinner | | | | | | | | | | | | | | | | |
| | | | | | | | | | | | | | | | | | | |
| 12/7 | 12/13 | Ditropan 5 mg | 8AM | RG | RG | RG | RG | RG | MD | MD | | | | | | | | |
| | | PO daily | | | | | | | | | | | | | | | | |
| | | | | | | | | | | | | | | | | | | |
| 12/8 | 12/14 | Zoloft 100 mg PO | 8AM | X | RG | RG | RG | RG | MD | MD | | | | | | | | |
| | | q AM | | | | | | | | | | | | | | | | |
| | | | | | | | | | | | | | | | | | | |
| 12/7 | 12/13 | Seroquel 100 mg | 9PM | RD | RD | RD | RD | RD | JO | JO | | | | | | | | |
| | | PO hs | | | | | | | | | | | | | | | | |
| | | | | | | | | | | | | | | | | | | |
| 12/9 | 12/16 | Valium 10 mg PO | | | | | | | | | | | | | | | | |
| | | prn q hs | 9PM | X | X | RD | X | RD | JO | JO | | | | | | | | |
| | | | | | | | | | | | | | | | | | | |
| 12/8 | 12/15 | 100 ml D5/NS with | 8AM | X | X | RG | RG | RG | MD | MD | | | | | | | | |
| | | fluconazole 400 mg | 8PM | X | RD | RD | RD | RD | JO | JO | | | | | | | | |
| | | IV q12h | | | | | | | | | | | | | | | | |
| | | | | | | | | | | | | | | | | | | |

| INIT. | NURSES' FULL SIGNATURE & TITLE | INIT. | NURSES' FULL SIGNATURE & TITLE | INIT. | NURSES' FULL SIGNATURE & TITLE |
| --- | --- | --- | --- | --- | --- |
| RG | Robert Graham, RN | JO | Joan Olsen | | |
| MD | Martha Daly, RN | | | | |
| TK | Taylore Keife, RN | | | | |
| RD | Rachel Dugas, RN | | | | |

● **Figure 2.37**
**Medication record.**

(e) Designate the time of day the patient received Ditropan.

_____

(f) Identify the nurse who administered the medication on 12/7/07 at 8 A.M.

_____

(g) Identify the medication(s) administered at 9 P.M. on 12/08/07.

_____

(h) What is the name of the patient's physician?

_____

**Workspace**

| | | PHYSICIAN'S ORDERS | CHART COPY |
|---|---|---|---|

FORM 01 109

| ORDER DATE | DATE DISC | | |
|---|---|---|---|
| 4/20/10 | 4/27/10 | Cefaclor 250 mg q8h PO for 7 days | |
| 4/20/10 | 4/27/10 | nitroglycerin transdermal 10 cm² daily | |
| | | remove from 10 PM – 7 AM daily | |
| 4/20/10 | 4/27/10 | Diabenase 0.1g daily PO AC breakfast | |
| 4/22/10 | 4/29/10 | furosemide 80 mg PO b.i.d | |
| 4/23/10 | 4/30/10 | Monopril 20 mg PO daily | |

PATIENT CERTIFCATION

2/28/52  Episcopal  Aetna

4/20/2010

Jane Myers
23 College Ave
Salt Lake City
Utah 46022

Dr. D. Looby
#212332

**PLEASE INDICATE BEEPER #** → | 222 |

● **Figure 2.38**
**Physician's order sheet.**

7. Study the physician's order sheet in ● **Figure 2.38**; then answer the following questions.

   (a) What is the route of administration for nitroglycerin?

   _____

   (b) How many doses of Cefaclor would the patient receive in 1 week?

   _____

   (c) Which drugs are to be given daily?

   _____

   (d) Which drug was ordered on April 22, 2010?

   _____

   (e) Which drug is to be given every 8 hours?

   _____

   (f) Identify the drug(s) that are to be administered before breakfast?

   _____

8. Use the package insert shown in ● **Figure 2.39** to answer the following questions.

   (a) What is the generic name of the drug?

   _____

   (b) What is the form of the drug?

   _____

   (c) On what type of diet should the patient, who is receiving Lipitor, be placed?

   _____

   (d) What is the maximum daily dose of Lipitor recommended for heterozygous familial hypercholesterolemia in pediatric patients (10–17 years of age)?

   _____

# Lipitor®
## (Atorvastatin Calcium)
## Tablets

**DESCRIPTION**

LIPITOR® (atorvastatin calcium) is a synthetic lipid-lowering agent. Atorvastatin is an inhibitor of 3-hydroxy-3-methylglutaryl-coenzyme A (HMG-CoA) reductase. This enzyme catalyzes the conversion of HMG-CoA to mevalonate, an early and rate-limiting step in cholesterol biosynthesis.

**DOSAGE AND ADMINISTRATION**

The patient should be placed on a standard cholesterol-lowering diet before receiving LIPITOR and should continue on this diet during treatment with LIPITOR.

**Hypercholesterolemia (Heterozygous Familial and Nonfamilial) and Mixed Dyslipidemia (*Fredrickson* Types IIa and IIb)**

The recommended starting dose of LIPITOR is 10 or 20 mg once daily. Patients who require a large reduction in LDL-C (more than 45%) may be started at 40 mg once daily. The dosage range of LIPITOR is 10 to 80 mg once daily. LIPITOR can be administered as a single dose at any time of the day, with or without food. The starting dose and maintenance doses of LIPITOR should be individualized according to patient characteristics such as goal of therapy and response (see *NCEP Guidelines,* summarized in Table 5). After initiation and/or upon titration of LIPITOR, lipid levels should be analyzed within 2 to 4 weeks and dosage adjusted accordingly.

Since the goal of treatment is to lower LDL-C, the NCEP recommends that LDL-C levels be used to initiate and assess treatment response. Only if LDL-C levels are not available, should total-C be used to monitor therapy.

**Heterozygous Familial Hypercholesterolemia in Pediatric Patients (10-17 years of age)**

The recommended starting dose of LIPITOR is 10 mg/day; the maximum recommended dose is 20 mg/day (doses greater than 20 mg have not been studied in this patient population). Doses should be individualized according to the recommended goal of therapy (see NCEP Pediatric Panel Guidelines[1], CLINICAL PHARMACOLOGY, and...

[1] National Cholesterol Education Program (NCEP): Highlights of the Report of the Expert Panel on Blood Cholesterol Levels in Children Adolescents, *Pediatrics.* 89(3):495-501. 1992.

● **Figure 2.39**

**Excerpts from package insert for Lipitor.**

*(Reg. Trademark of Pfizer Inc. Reproduced with permission.)*

9. Interpret the following drug orders:

    (a) 7/20/2010           0400h

              *Lasix (furosemide) 60 mg IVP stat*

                    A.Smith MD

    (b) 4/03/2010           1200h

            *digoxin 0.125 mg PO daily*

                 Mae Ling MD

    (c) 12/22/2010        0800h

            *heparin 5000 units subcut q12h*

               A.Rodriguez RN, ANP

(d) 07/72/2010

*Compazine (prochlorperazine) 7 mg IM q4h prn*

I.*Patel* DO

(e) 11/14/2010

*nitroglycerin 0.3 mg SL prn anginal pain, repeat q5min., up to 15 min.*

J.*Rodriguez* MD

10. Determine which part is missing for each of the following drug orders:

(a) *heparin 5000 units stat*

(b) 01/01/2010

*Novolin 70/30 15 units daily*

A.*Smith* MD

(c) 03/14/2010                0200h

*meperidine 50 mg for pain stat*

*Mae Ling* MD

(d) 1500h

*acetaminophen 125 mg q4h prn*

(e) 09/09/2010        0900h

*cefaclor 125 mg po*

J.*Rodriguez* MD

**MediaLink**

www.prenhall.com/giangrasso

Animated examples, interactive practice questions with animated solutions, and challenge tests for this chapter can be found on the Pearson Dosage Calculation Tutor that accompanies this text. Additional, unique, interactive resources and activities can be found on the Companion Web site.

# Ratio and Proportion

## Learning Outcomes

$24 = 8\,x$

After completing this chapter, you will be able to

1. Solve problems using ratio and proportion.
2. Identify some common units of measurement and their abbreviations.
3. Convert a quantity expressed with a single unit of measurement to an equivalent quantity with a different single unit of measurement.
4. Convert a quantity expressed as a rate to another rate.

In this chapter, you will learn to use ratio and proportion. This simple approach to drug calculations largely frees you from the need to memorize formulas. This method involves setting up appropriate proportions and using basic mathematics to solve the proportions. Once this technique is mastered, you will be able to calculate drug dosages quickly and safely.

# Ratios

A **ratio** compares two quantities. Ratios can be expressed in a variety of ways, including fractional form. For this reason, fractions are sometimes referred to as *ratio*nal numbers.

Suppose a recipe indicates that 1 cup of sugar and 2 cups of flour are needed to make a certain type of cake. The relative amounts of sugar and flour in the cake are crucial to its quality. To compare the amount of sugar to the amount of flour in this recipe, any of the following equivalent *sugar-flour ratios* could be used:

1 cup of sugar *for every* 2 cups of flour
1 cup of sugar *per* 2 cups of flour
1 cup of sugar *to* 2 cups of flour
1 cup to 2 cups
1 to 2
1:2
$\frac{1}{2}$

On the other hand, to compare the amount of flour to the amount of sugar in this recipe, the following equivalent *flour-sugar ratios* could be used:

2 cups of flour *for every* 1 cup of sugar
2 cups of flour *per* 1 cup of sugar
2 cups of flour *to* 1 cup of sugar
2 cups to 1 cup
2 to 1
2:1
$\frac{2}{1}$

As you can see, the order of the numbers in the flour-sugar ratio is the reverse of the order in the sugar-flour ratio.

Now, if twice the amount of this cake were needed, the baker would need to double the amount of each of the ingredients in the recipe.

Therefore, instead of

*1 cup of sugar and 2 cups of flour,*
*2 cups of sugar and 4 cups of flour*

would be required, and the *sugar-flour ratio* would now be 2 to 4. Although the quantities of sugar and flour have each been increased, the ratio of sugar to flour has not changed; the ratio 1:2 is equivalent to the ratio 2:4. It is easy to see this equivalency when both the ratios are written in fractional form because $\frac{1}{2} = \frac{2}{4}$.

Recall that in Chapter 1 both *building and reducing* fractions were discussed, and $\frac{1}{2}$ could be "*built*" into $\frac{2}{4}$ by multiplying both numerator and denominator by 2, as follows:

$$\frac{1}{2} = \frac{1 \times 2}{2 \times 2} = \frac{2}{4}$$

Similarly, $\frac{2}{4}$ could be "*reduced*" to $\frac{1}{2}$ by dividing both numerator and denominator by 2 as follows:

$$\frac{2}{4} = \frac{2 \div 2}{4 \div 2} = \frac{1}{2}$$

So, $\frac{1}{2}$ and $\frac{2}{4}$ are equivalent ratios.

Next, suppose that three times the amount of the cake were needed. The baker would need to multiply the amount of each ingredient in the recipe by three.

Therefore, instead of using

*1 cup of sugar and 2 cups of flour,*

*3 cups of sugar and 6 cups of flour*

would be required.

Continuing this process, a table could be constructed showing the amount of sugar and the corresponding amount of flour needed in order to make various amounts of this cake. See Table 3.1.

**Table 3.1 Some Corresponding Amounts of Sugar and Flour for a 1 to 2 Sugar-Flour Ratio**

| Cups of Sugar | Cups of Flour |
|---|---|
| 1 | 2 |
| 2 | 4 |
| 3 | 6 |
| 4 | 8 |
| 5 | 10 |
| 6 | 12 |

**Units of measurement** are the "*labels*," such as inches, ounces, minutes, and hours, that are sometimes written after a number. Units of measurement are also referred to as *dimensions*, or simply *units*. For example, in the quantity 3 cups the unit of measurement is *cups*.

## EXAMPLE 3.1

Suppose a recipe indicates that 1 cup of sugar and 2 cups of flour are needed to make a certain type of cake. If the baker wants to make some of this cake and decides to use 10 cups of flour, how much sugar would be needed?

| Cups of Sugar | Cups of Flour |
|---|---|
| 1 | 2 |
| 2 | 4 |
| 3 | 6 |
| 4 | 8 |
| ⑤ ← | ⑩ |
| 6 | 12 |

The baker could look at Table 3.1 and see that for 10 cups of flour, 5 cups of sugar are needed.

Another way to solve the problem is to realize that the amount of flour (10 cups) is 5 times the amount of flour (2 cups) in the recipe. Whenever the amount of flour in the recipe is multiplied by 5, the amount of sugar in the recipe must also be multiplied by 5.

So, the terms in the ratio of

*1 cup of sugar to 2 cups of flour*

are each multiplied by 5 to yield

*5 cups of sugar to 10 cups of flour*

and 5 cups of sugar would be needed.

## EXAMPLE 3.2

Mary prepares her morning coffee by combining 5 parts black coffee with 2 parts milk.

(a) What is the black coffee-milk ratio expressed in colon [:] form and in fractional form?

(b) Mary wants to make some of her morning coffee and take it along in a thermos bottle. If she used 8 ounces of milk, how much black coffee must be added to the bottle?

(a) The drink has 5 parts black coffee to 2 parts milk. This is a ratio of *5 parts to 2 parts* or a ratio of *5 to 2*. This ratio can also be written in colon form as *5:2* or in fractional form as $\frac{5}{2}$.

(b) A table could be constructed showing the amount of black coffee and the corresponding amount of milk needed in order to make various amounts of this drink. See Table 3.2.

**Table 3.2  Some Corresponding Amounts of Black Coffee and Milk in a 5 to 2 Ratio**

| Ounces of Black Coffee | Ounces of Milk |
|:---:|:---:|
| 5 | 2 |
| 10 | 4 |
| 15 | 6 |
| 20 | 8 |
| 25 | 10 |
| 30 | 12 |

Mary could look at Table 3.2 and see that for 8 ounces of milk, 20 ounces of black coffee are needed.

| Ounces of Black Coffee | Ounces of Milk |
|:---:|:---:|
| 5 | 2 |
| 10 | 4 |
| 15 | 6 |
| (20) ← | → (8) |
| 25 | 10 |
| 30 | 12 |

# Rates

**Rates** are like ratios except that they compare two quantities with *different units of measurement.*

For example, a car might be traveling on a highway at a constant rate of speed of *50 miles per hour.* This rate has two different units of measurement, *miles* and *hours.* To compare the number of *miles* traveled to the number of *hours* driven, any of the following equivalent *rates of speed* could be used:

> 50 miles for every 1 hour driven
>
> 50 miles per each hour driven
>
> 50 miles per hour
>
> 50 miles:1 hour
>
> 50 miles/1 hour
>
> 50 miles/hour

Notice that if the car drove twice the number of hours (2 hours), then the car would travel twice the distance (100 miles). However, the rate of speed would be the same.

Now, consider a worker's rate of pay. Suppose the pay rate is $60 for every 2 hours worked. To compare the amount of *dollars* paid to the number of *hours* worked, any of the following equivalent *rates of pay* could be used:

> $60 for every 2 hours worked
>
> $60 per 2 hours
>
> $60:2 hours
>
> $60/2 hours
>
> $30 for every 1 hour worked
>
> $30 per hour
>
> $30:1 hour
>
> $30/hour

Notice that if a person worked 2 hours for $60, or if the person worked 1 hour for $30, the rate of pay would be the same.

## EXAMPLE 3.3

**Each can of cola contains 12 ounces.**

**(a) How many ounces are contained in 6 cans?**

**(b) How many cans would contain 18 ounces?**

| Cans of Cola | Ounces of Cola |
|---|---|
| 1 | 12 |
| 2 | 24 |
| 3 | 36 |
| 4 | 48 |
| 5 | 60 |
| 6 | 72 |

(a) A table could be constructed showing the number of 12-oz cans and the corresponding number of ounces. The last line of the table indicates that 6 cans contain 72 ounces.

Another way to do the problem is to realize that the rate is 12 ounces per 1 can. In this case the number of cans is multiplied by 6, so the number of ounces must also be multiplied by 6.

So, the terms in the rate of

*12 ounces per 1 can*

are each multiplied by 6 to yield

*72 ounces per 6 cans*

(b) If the number of cans in the rate is multiplied by $\frac{1}{2}$, the number of ounces must also be multiplied by $\frac{1}{2}$.

So, the terms in the rate of

*12 ounces per 1 can*

are each multiplied by $\frac{1}{2}$ to yield

*6 ounces per $\frac{1}{2}$ can*

Put these two rates into a table as follows:

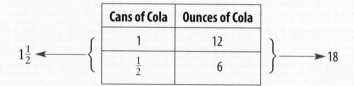

| Cans of Cola | Ounces of Cola |
|---|---|
| 1 | 12 |
| $\frac{1}{2}$ | 6 |

By adding the two rows of the above table, it can be concluded that 18 ounces of cola are contained in $1\frac{1}{2}$ cans.

## EXAMPLE 3.4

(a) **An object is moving at a rate of 72 inches in 2 hours. Express this rate in terms of inches/hour.**

(b) **An object is moving at a rate of 240 inches per hour. Express this rate in terms of inches/min.**

(c) **An object is moving at a rate of 2 feet per minute. Express this rate in terms of feet/hour.**

You can do this problem in many different ways.

(a) The rate *72 inches in 2 hours*, in fractional form, is $\frac{72\ in}{2\ h}$.

It is already in the form of inches/hour, so merely reduce the fraction as follows:

$$\frac{72\ in}{2\ h} = \frac{72}{2}\ \frac{in}{h} = 36\ in/h$$

(b) To change *240 inches/hour* to *inches/minute*, substitute 60 minutes for 1 hour as follows:

$$\frac{240\ in}{1\ h} = \frac{240\ in}{60\ min} = \frac{240}{60}\ \frac{in}{min} = 4\ in/min$$

(c)  To change *2 feet/minute* to *feet/hour*, multiply both numerator and denominator by 60 because 60 min = 1h.

$$\frac{2 \; ft \times 60}{1 \; min \times 60} = \frac{120 \; ft}{60 \; min} = \frac{120 \; ft}{1 \; h} = 120 \text{ ft/h}$$

# Proportions

A **proportion** is a statement or equation indicating that two ratios or two rates are equal. For example,

$$\frac{2}{4} = \frac{5}{10} \text{ is a proportion.}$$

True proportions have an interesting property. If the true proportion is written in fractional form, when you cross multiply, the products obtained are equal.

Cross multiply:

$$\frac{2}{4} \diagdown \frac{5}{10}$$

$$(5)(4) = (2)(10)$$
$$20 = 20$$

The products each equal 20.

The proportion $\frac{2}{4} = \frac{5}{10}$ may also be written using the colon form as follows:

$$2 : 4 = 5 : 10$$

In this form, the equivalent to cross multiplication is to multiply the means and the extremes (inside numbers and outside numbers) as follows:

$$2 \times 10 = 20$$
$$2 : 4 = 5 : 10$$
$$4 \times 5 = 20$$

Again, these products are both equal to 20.

> **NOTE**
>
> This book will use the fractional form of proportions rather than the colon form.

### EXAMPLE 3.5

**Verify that $\frac{30}{1,000} = \frac{6}{200}$ is a true portion.**

To verify that this proportion is true, cross multiply. If the products obtained are equal, then the proportion is true.

Cross multiply

$$\frac{30}{1,000} \diagdown \frac{6}{200}$$

$$(6)(1000) = (30)(200)$$
$$6,000 = 6,000$$

Because the products are equal, it is a true proportion.

### EXAMPLE 3.6

**Is $\frac{30}{120} = \frac{6}{18}$ a true portion?**

To determine if this proportion is true, cross multiply. If the products obtained are equal, then the proportion is true.

Cross multiply

$$\frac{30}{120} = \frac{6}{18}$$

$$(6)(120) = (30)(18)$$

$$720 \neq 540$$

Because the products are not equal, $\frac{30}{120} = \frac{6}{18}$ is not a true proportion.

# The Mathematics Needed to Solve Proportions

Your first step toward understanding how to solve proportions is a review of a few basic arithmetic and algebraic concepts.

## Using Parentheses to Indicate Multiplication

In algebra, letters are used to stand for numbers. The letter $x$ is the symbol most commonly used to represent an unknown number, but the times sign $\times$ is also a symbol for multiplication. To avoid confusion between the two meanings of the same symbol, *the times sign $\times$ will generally be avoided* throughout the remainder of the textbook. Instead of using $\times$ to represent multiplication, a pair of parentheses will be used.

So, $3 \times 4 = 12$ will often be written as $(3)(4) = 12$.

## Multiplying by 1

The rules of algebra are generalizations of the rules of arithmetic. In arithmetic, when 1 is multiplied by 7, the result is 7. When 1 is multiplied by 52, the result is 52. In general, *when 1 is multiplied by any number, the result is that same number*. In algebraic terms, 1 multiplied by $x$ equals $x$. This can be summarized as:

$$(1)(x) = x$$

## Dividing by 1

In arithmetic, when 9 is divided by 1 the result is 9, and when 23 is divided by 1 the result is 23. In general, *when any number is divided by 1 the result is that same number*. In algebraic terms, $x$ divided by 1 equals $x$. This can be summarized as:

$$\frac{x}{1} = x$$

## Shorthand for Multiplication

When a known number is multiplied by an unknown number, 7 times $x$, for example, this product could be represented as $(7)(x)$. The product of the two numbers $(7)$ and $(x)$ is usually written in the shorthand $7x$. This can be summarized as:

$$(7)(x) = 7x$$

**EXAMPLE 3.7**

**Simplify the expression: $(45)(x)$**

When a known number $(45)$ is multiplied by an unknown number $(x)$, the product may be written in the simplified shorthand form of $45x$.

## Commutative Property

In arithmetic, when you multiply numbers, the order of the factors does not matter. You may **commute** the factors (*switch their positions*) without changing the product. For example,

$$3 \times 4 = 12 \quad \text{and} \quad 4 \times 3 = 12,$$

therefore,

$$3 \times 4 = 4 \times 3$$

You may want to use this commutative property when you have to multiply an unknown number by a known number. To multiply an unknown number by 12, you could write $(x)(12)$. But reversing the order of the factors gives $(12)(x)$, and the shorthand for this is $12x$.

Similarly,

$$(x)(37) = (37)(x) = 37x$$

**EXAMPLE 3.8**

**Simplify the expression: $(x)(13)$**

Since the order does not matter when you multiply two numbers, you may write

$$(x)(13) \text{ as } (13)(x)$$

The shorthand for $(13)(x)$ is $13x$.

## Cancelling

In arithmetic a fraction can be reduced by cancelling. For example, the fraction $\frac{21}{28}$ could be reduced as follows. Write the numerator and denominator in factored form.

$$\frac{21}{28} = \frac{(7)(3)}{(7)(4)}$$

Now cancel the (7)'s.

$$\frac{21}{28} = \frac{(\cancel{7})(3)}{(\cancel{7})(4)} = \frac{3}{4}$$

So, $\frac{21}{28} = \frac{3}{4}$

This cancelling technique will be used in solving simple equations.

## Solving Simple Equations

In the process of solving proportions, you will frequently encounter simple equations like:

$$3x = 6$$

This equation states that 3 times a number equals 6. To solve this equation means to find a value of $x$ that will make the equation true. Because 3 times 2 equals 6, the solution is 2.

Not every simple equation can easily be solved mentally. So, the technique for solving such equations is to manipulate them so that $x$ is alone on one side of the equal sign. This can be accomplished by dividing both sides of the equation by the **coefficient of $x$** (the number multiplying the $x$).

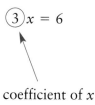

$$\textcircled{3}x = 6$$

coefficient of $x$

In the term $3x$, the coefficient of $x$ is 3, so you should divide both sides of the equation by 3.

$$\frac{3x}{3} = \frac{6}{3}$$

Now cancel the 3s

$$\frac{\cancel{3}x}{\cancel{3}} = \frac{6}{3}$$

This gives

$$x = \frac{6}{3}$$

Simplify $\frac{6}{3}$

$$x = 2$$

### EXAMPLE 3.9

**Solve the equation $5x = 35$**

To solve this equation means to find the value of $x$ that will make the equation true. The technique is to manipulate the equation so that $x$ is alone on one side of the equation. This can be accomplished by dividing both sides of the equation by the coefficient of $x$, which is 5 in this case.

$$\text{⑤}x = 35$$

coefficient of $x$

Divide by 5

$$\frac{5x}{5} = \frac{35}{5}$$

Now cancel

$$\frac{\cancel{5}x}{\cancel{5}} = \frac{35}{5}$$

This gives

$$x = 7$$

# Solving Proportions

Throughout the textbook you will encounter **proportions** in which one of the four numbers in the proportion is unknown. For example,

$$\frac{2}{?} = \frac{5}{10}.$$

In this proportion, the denominator of the first fraction is not known. Unknown numbers are often represented by letters of the alphabet, $x$ in particular. So this equation might also be written as

$$\frac{2}{x} = \frac{5}{10}$$

Finding this unknown number $x$ that makes the proportion true is called "*solving the proportion.*" In general, solving a proportion involves two steps:

1. *Cross multiply* to obtain a simple equation
2. To solve the simple equation, *divide both sides of the equation by the coefficient of $x$*

Since the proportion is written in fractional form, when you cross multiply, the products obtained are equal.

$$\frac{2}{x} = \frac{5}{10}$$

$$(5)(x) = (2)(10)$$

Simplifying, you get the simple equation

$$5x = 20$$

Divide by 5, the coefficient of $x$

$$\frac{5x}{5} = \frac{20}{5}$$

Cancel

$$\frac{\cancel{5}x}{\cancel{5}} = \frac{20}{5}$$

This gives

$$x = 4$$

So, 4 is the solution of the equation.

You may *check your answer* by substituting 4 for $x$ in the original proportion as follows:

$$\frac{2}{④} = \frac{5}{10}$$

Now cross multiply

$$\frac{2}{4} = \frac{5}{10}$$

$$(5)(4) = (2)(10)$$

$$20 = 20$$

Since the products are equal, the solution 4 is correct.

**NOTE**

You should always check your answers to proportion problems by substituting the answer into the proportion, cross multiplying, and seeing if the products are equal.

**EXAMPLE 3.10**

**Solve the proportion $\frac{5}{12} = \frac{x}{6}$**

The first step in solving the proportion is to cross multiply

$$\frac{5}{12} = \frac{x}{6}$$

$$(12)(x) = (5)(6)$$

Simplify

$$12x = 30$$

Divide both sides by 12, the coefficient of $x$

$$\frac{12x}{12} = \frac{30}{12}$$

Cancel

$$\frac{\cancel{12}x}{\cancel{12}} = \frac{30}{12}$$

This gives

$$x = \frac{30}{12}$$

Simplify

$$x = 2.5$$

## EXAMPLE 3.11

**Solve:** $\frac{x}{26} = \frac{10.1}{13}$

Cross multiply

$$\frac{x}{26} = \frac{10.1}{13}$$

$$(10.1)(26) = 13x$$

At this point, there are two different approaches that may be used to finish the problem.

*Method 1*: Multiply 10.1 by 26 to obtain 262.6

$$262.6 = 13x$$

Divide both sides by 13, which is the coefficient of $x$

$$\frac{262.6}{13} = \frac{13x}{13}$$

Cancel

$$\frac{262.6}{13} = \frac{\cancel{13}x}{\cancel{13}}$$

Simplify

$$20.2 = x$$

*Method 2*: Do not multiply 10.1 by 26 to obtain 262.6, but leave the left side of the equation in factored form as follows:

$$(10.1)(26) = 13x$$

Divide both sides by 13 which is the coefficient of $x$

$$\frac{(10.1)(26)}{13} = \frac{13x}{13}$$

Cancel

$$\frac{(10.1)(\cancel{26}^{2})}{\cancel{13}_{1}} = \frac{\cancel{13}x}{\cancel{13}}$$

$$(10.1)(2) = x$$

Multiply

$$20.2 = x$$

The advantage of *Method 2* in this case is that it avoids the creation of the large number 262.6 and its subsequent division by 13.

# Changing Quantities with Single Units of Measurement

Many problems in dosage calculation require changing a quantity with a single unit of measurement into an equivalent quantity with a different single unit of measurement. To accomplish these changes, you will need to know the relationship between the units involved.

| Table 3.3  **Equivalents for Common Units** |
| --- |
| 12 inches (in) = 1 foot (ft) |
| 2 pints (pt) = 1 quart (qt) |
| 16 ounces (oz) = 1 pound (lb) |
| 60 seconds (sec) = 1 minute (min) |
| 60 minutes (min) = 1 hour (h or hr) |
| 24 hours (h or hr) = 1 day (d) |
| 7 days (d) = 1 week (wk) |
| 12 months (mon) = 1 year (yr) |

Table 3.3 contains equivalents for several common units of measurement including the equivalence 7 *days* = 1 *week*.

This equivalence can be used to determine the solution to the problem of finding the number of weeks in 21 days. In this problem there are two quantities: *weeks* and *days*. You know that 1 week is equivalent to 7 days, and you need to find the unknown number of weeks which would contain 21 days.

Think of the problem this way:

$$7 \text{ days} = 1 \text{ week}$$

$$21 \text{ days} = ? \text{ weeks}$$

To determine if a proportion exists between *days* and *weeks*, ask yourself the question "if the number of *weeks* is doubled, is the number of *days* doubled?" If the answer were no, then days and weeks would not be proportional and a proportion would not be used to solve the problem.

But the answer is yes because for a given period of time, whenever the number of weeks is doubled, the number of days would be doubled. So the number of days and the number of weeks are proportional, and a proportion could be used to solve the problem.

The proportion could be set up in either of the following two ways:

$$\frac{weeks}{days} = \frac{weeks'}{days'}$$

or

$$\frac{days}{weeks} = \frac{days'}{weeks'}$$

The same answer will be obtained regardless of which of the two forms is used.

In mathematics the **prime notation** (') is commonly used to link together two quantities. The primed quantities are linked together, and the unprimed quantities are linked. In this case *days* and *weeks* are associated together, while *days'* (read, *days prime*) is associated with *weeks'*.

Because you know that 1 week equals 7 days, you can substitute those numbers, *1 and 7, for weeks and days*, respectively. Because you need to find the number of weeks ($x$) containing 21 days, you can substitute those quantities, *$x$ and 21, for weeks' and days'*, respectively.

Substituting into the second form $\dfrac{days}{weeks} = \dfrac{days'}{weeks'}$

you obtain

$$\frac{7 \ days}{1 \ week} = \frac{21 \ days}{x \ weeks}$$

Eliminate the units of measurement

$$\frac{7}{1} = \frac{21}{x}$$

cross multiply

$$\frac{7}{1} = \frac{21}{x}$$

$$(21)(1) = (7)(x)$$

Simplify

$$21 = 7x$$

Divide both sides by 7, the coefficient of $x$

$$\frac{21}{7} = \frac{7x}{7}$$

Cancel

$$\frac{21}{7} = \frac{\cancel{7}x}{\cancel{7}}$$

Simplify

$$3 = x$$

You have just used the ratio and proportion method to convert a given amount of time measured in one unit of measurement (21 days) to an equivalent amount of time measured in another unit of measurement (3 weeks).

## Solving One-Step Problems with Single Units of Measurement

Suppose that you want to express 18 months as an equivalent amount of time measured in years. That is,

$$18 \ months = ? \ years$$

Both *18 months* and *? years* are quantities that have single units of measurement. This problem can be solved by using a proportion. The steps to follow in solving a proportion problem are:

1. *Identify the two units of measurement in the problem.*
   In this problem there are two quantities: *months* and *years*.

2. *Write a known equivalence between the units of measurement.*
   You need to know that 12 months is equivalent to 1 year.

3. *Let x stand for the amount you are trying to find and write an equivalence involving x*
   You have to find the unknown number of years $(x)$ that would contain 18 months.
   So, think of the problem this way:

   $$12 \text{ months} = 1 \text{ year}$$
   $$18 \text{ months} = x \text{ years}$$

4. *Write a proportion using the two units of measurement.*
   Because the number of months and the number of years are proportional, a proportion could be used to solve the problem. The proportion could be set up in either of the following two ways:

   $$\frac{yr}{mon} = \frac{yr'}{mon'}$$

   or

   $$\frac{mon}{yr} = \frac{mon'}{yr'}$$

   You will get the same answer regardless of which of the two forms you use.

5. *Substitute into the proportion.*
   Because you know that 1 year equals 12 months, you can substitute those numbers, *1 and 12, for years and months,* respectively. And because you need to find the number of years $(x)$ containing 18 months, you can substitute those quantities *(x and 18) for years' and months',* respectively.

   Substituting into the second form $\dfrac{mon}{yr} = \dfrac{mon'}{yr'}$

   you obtain

   $$\frac{12 \ mon}{1 \ yr} = \frac{18 \ mon}{x \ yr}$$

6. *Eliminate the units of measurement*

   $$\frac{12}{1} = \frac{18}{x}$$

7. *Cross multiply*

   $$\frac{12}{1} \diagdown \frac{18}{x}$$

   $$(18)(1) = (12)(x)$$

   Simplify

   $$18 = 12x$$

8. *Divide both sides of the equation by 12, the coefficient of x.*

$$\frac{18}{12} = \frac{12x}{12}$$

9. *Cancel*

$$\frac{18}{12} = \frac{\cancel{12}x}{\cancel{12}}$$

*Simplify*

$$1\tfrac{1}{2} = x$$

So, 18 months is equivalent to $1\tfrac{1}{2}$ years.

10. *Check your answer*

In the proportion, replace $x$ by $1\tfrac{1}{2}$, cross multiply, and see if the cross products are equal.

$$\frac{12}{1} = \frac{18}{1\tfrac{1}{2}}$$

Cross multiply

$$(18)(1) = (12)(1\tfrac{1}{2})$$

Simplify

$$18 = 18$$

Because the products are equal, the answer is verified.

In summary the steps in solving a proportion are:

1. Identify the two units of measurement in the problem
2. Write a known equivalence between the units of measure
3. Let $x$ stand for the amount you are trying to find and write an equivalence involving $x$
4. Write a proportion using the two units of measurement
5. Substitute into the proportion
6. Eliminate the units
7. Cross multiply
8. Divide both sides of the equation by the coefficient of $x$ (unless it is 1)
9. Cancel and simplify
10. Check your answer by substituting and cross multiplying

## EXAMPLE 3.12

**Change $2\tfrac{1}{4}$ hours to an equivalent amount of time in *minutes*.**

In this problem there are two quantities: *minutes* and *hours*. You need to know that 60 minutes is equivalent to 1 hour, and you have to find the unknown number of minutes that would contain $2\tfrac{1}{4}$ hours.

So, think of the problem this way:

$$60 \text{ minutes} = 1 \text{ hour}$$
$$? \text{ minutes} = 2\tfrac{1}{4} \text{ hours}$$

Because the number of minutes and the number of hours are proportional, a proportion could be used to solve the problem. The proportion could be set up as

$$\frac{min}{hr} = \frac{min'}{hr'}$$

Because 60 minutes equals 1 hour, you can substitute the numbers *60 and 1 for minutes and hours*, respectively. And because you need to find the number of minutes $(x)$ equal to $2\frac{1}{4}$ hours, you can substitute those quantities $(x$ and $2\frac{1}{4})$ *for minutes' and hours', respectively.*

Substituting, you get

$$\frac{60\ min}{1\ hr} = \frac{x\ min}{2\frac{1}{4}\ hr}$$

Eliminate the units of measurement

$$\frac{60}{1} = \frac{x}{2\frac{1}{4}}$$

cross multiply

$$\frac{60}{1} \diagdown \frac{x}{2\frac{1}{4}}$$

$$(x)(1) = (60)(2\tfrac{1}{4})$$

Simplify

$$x = 135$$

So, $2\frac{1}{4}$ hours is equivalent to 135 minutes.

## EXAMPLE 3.13

**Change 5.5 feet to an equivalent length in inches.**

In this problem there are two quantities: *inches* and *feet*. You need to know that 12 inches is equivalent to 1 foot, and you have to find the unknown number of inches that would be equivalent to 5.5 feet.

So, think of the problem this way:

$$12 \text{ inches} = 1 \text{ feet}$$
$$x \text{ inches} = 5.5 \text{ feet}$$

Because the number of inches and the number of feet are proportional, a proportion could be used to solve the problem. The proportion could be set up as

$$\frac{in}{ft} = \frac{in'}{ft'}$$

Because 12 inches equals 1 foot, you can substitute those numbers, 12 and *1*, *for feet* and *inches*, respectively. And because you need to find the number of inches (*x*) containing 5.5 feet, you can substitute those quantities, *x* and 5.5, for *inches'* and *feet'*, respectively.

Substituting you get

$$\frac{12 \; in}{1 \; ft} = \frac{x \; in}{5.5 \; ft}$$

Eliminate the units of measurement

$$\frac{12}{1} = \frac{x}{5.5}$$

cross multiply

$$\frac{12}{1} \times \frac{x}{5.5}$$

$$(x)(1) = (12)(5.5)$$

Simplify

$$x = 66$$

So, 5.5 feet is equivalent to 66 inches.

## EXAMPLE 3.14

**An infant weighs 6 pounds 5 ounces. What is the weight of the infant in ounces?**

Because *6 pounds 5 ounces* means *6 pounds + 5 ounces*, you need to first convert 6 pounds to ounces.

There are two quantities: *ounces* and *pounds*. You need to know that 16 ounces is equivalent to 1 pound, and you have to find the unknown number of ounces that would be equivalent to 6 pounds.

So, think of the problem this way:

$$16 \text{ ounces} = 1 \text{ pound}$$

$$x \text{ ounces} = 6 \text{ pounds}$$

Because the number of ounces and the number of pounds are proportional, a proportion could be set up as

$$\frac{oz}{lb} = \frac{oz'}{lb'}$$

Because 16 ounces equals 1 pound, you can substitute those numbers, 16 and *1*, for *ounces* and *pound*, respectively. And because you need to find the number of ounces (*x*) containing 6 pounds, you can substitute those quantities, *x* and 6, for *ounces'* and *pound'*, respectively.

Substituting, you get

$$\frac{16 \; oz}{1 \; lb} = \frac{x \; oz}{6 \; lb}$$

Eliminate the units of measurement and cross multiply

$$\frac{16}{1} = \frac{x}{6}$$

$$(x)(1) = (16)(6)$$

Simplify

$$x = 96$$

Because 6 pounds equals 96 ounces, the infant weighs 96 ounces + 5 ounces, or 101 ounces.

As part of Example 3.14, the number of ounces that is equivalent to 6 pounds was found. The proportion used was in the form:

(1)
$$\frac{oz}{lb} = \frac{oz'}{lb'}$$

Other proportions which students may choose to use to solve the problem are:

(2)
$$\frac{lb}{oz} = \frac{lb'}{oz'}$$

(3)
$$\frac{oz}{oz'} = \frac{lb}{lb'}$$

(4)
$$\frac{lb}{lb'} = \frac{oz}{oz'}$$

Any of these forms will give the correct answer. However, for simplicity, this textbook uses only types 1 and 2.

Ratio and proportion can be applied to a wide variety of problems, as illustrated in the next example.

## EXAMPLE 3.15

**If the currency exchange rate in a country is 9 pesos for 1 dollar, how many pesos will be exchanged for 45 dollars?**

In this problem there are two quantities: *pesos* and *dollars*. You know that 9 pesos is equivalent to 1 dollar, and you have to find the unknown number of pesos that would be equivalent to 45 dollars.

So think of the problem this way:

9 pesos = 1 dollar

? pesos = 45 dollars

Because the number of pesos and the number of dollars are proportional, a proportion could be set up as

$$\frac{pesos}{dollars} = \frac{pesos'}{dollars'}$$

Because you know that 1 dollar equals 9 pesos, you can substitute those numbers, *1* and *9*, for *dollars and pesos*, respectively. And because you need to find the number of pesos (*x*) containing 45 dollars, you can substitute those quantities, *x* and 45, for *pesos'* and *dollars'*, respectively.

Substituting, you obtain

$$\frac{9 \ pesos}{\$1} = \frac{x \ pesos}{\$45}$$

Eliminate the units of measurement and cross multiply

$$\frac{9}{1} = \frac{x}{45}$$

$$(x)(1) = (9)(45)$$

Simplify

$$x = 405$$

So, $45 will be exchanged for 405 pesos.

## EXAMPLE 3.16

**A hospital administrator would like to have a *4 to 1* patient-nurse ratio in the emergency room at all times. At that rate, how many nurses would be needed when there are 20 emergency room patients?**

In this problem there are two quantities: *nurses* and *patients*. You need to know that 1 nurse is required for 4 patients, and you have to find the unknown number of nurses that would be needed for 20 patients.

So, think of the problem this way:

$$1 \ nurse = 4 \ patients$$
$$x \ nurses = 20 \ patients$$

Because the number of nurses and the number of patients are proportional, a proportion could be set up as

$$\frac{patients}{nurses} = \frac{patients'}{nurses'}$$

Because you know that 1 nurse "equals" 4 patients, you can substitute those numbers, *1* and *4*, *for nurses and patients*, respectively. And because you need to find the number of nurses (*x*) needed for 20 patients, you can substitute those quantities, *x* and 20, for *nurses'* and *patients'*, respectively.

Substituting, you get

$$\frac{4 \ patients}{1 \ nurse} = \frac{20 \ patients}{x \ nurses}$$

Eliminate the units of measurement and cross multiply

$$\frac{4}{1} = \frac{20}{x}$$

$$(20)(1) = (4)(x)$$

Simplify

$$20 = 4x$$

Divide both sides by 4 and cancel

$$\frac{\overset{5}{\cancel{20}}}{\underset{1}{\cancel{4}}} = \frac{\cancel{4}x}{\cancel{4}}$$

$$5 = x$$

So, 5 nurses would be needed when there are 20 emergency room patients.

# Solving Multi-Step Problems with Single Units of Measurement

Sometimes you will encounter more complicated problems whose solution will require the use of more than one proportion.

### EXAMPLE 3.17

**Change 4 hours to an equivalent amount of time in seconds.**

In this problem there are two quantities: *seconds* and *hours*. Most people have not memorized the direct equivalence between seconds and hours. But they do know equivalences between *hours* and *minutes* and between *minutes* and *seconds*, namely,

$$1 \text{ hour} = 60 \text{ minutes}$$

and

$$1 \text{ minute} = 60 \text{ seconds}$$

This problem will be done in two steps; first change the *4 hours* to *minutes*, and then change the resulting *minutes* to *seconds*.

Think of *Step 1* this way:

$$1 \text{ hour} = 60 \text{ minutes}$$
$$4 \text{ hours} = x \text{ minutes}$$

The first proportion could be

$$\frac{min}{h} = \frac{min'}{h'}$$

Substitute *60* and *1 for min* and *h*, and *x* and *4 for min'* and *h'*.

$$\frac{60 \ min}{1 \ h} = \frac{x \ min}{4 \ h}$$

Eliminate the units of measurement and cross multiply

$$\frac{60}{1} = \frac{x}{4}$$

$$(x)(1) = (60)(4)$$
$$x = 240$$

So, 4 hours is equivalent to 240 minutes.
   In *Step 2*, change *240 minutes to seconds*.

Think of *Step 2* this way:

$$1 \text{ minute} = 60 \text{ seconds}$$
$$240 \text{ minutes} = x \text{ seconds}$$

The second proportion could be

$$\frac{\text{min}}{\text{sec}} = \frac{\text{min}'}{\text{sec}'}$$

Substitute 1 and 60 for *min* and *sec*, and *240* and *x* for *min'* and *sec'*.

$$\frac{1 \ min}{60 \ sec} = \frac{240 \ min}{x \ sec}$$

Eliminate the units of measurement and cross multiply.

$$\frac{1}{60} = \frac{240}{x}$$

$$(240)(60) = (1)(x)$$
$$14{,}400 = x$$

So, 4 hours is equivalent to 14,400 seconds.

## EXAMPLE 3.18

**Convert 50,400 minutes to an equivalent amount of time in days.**

In this problem, there are two quantities: *minutes* and *days*. Most people have not memorized the direct equivalence between minutes and days. But they do know that

$$60 \text{ minutes is equivalent to 1 hour}$$

and

$$24 \text{ hours is equivalent to 1 day}$$

This problem will be done in two steps; first change the *50,400 minutes to hours*, and then change the resulting *hours to days*.
   Think of *Step 1* this way:

$$60 \text{ minutes} = 1 \text{ hour}$$
$$50{,}400 \text{ minutes} = x \text{ hours}$$

The first proportion could be

$$\frac{min}{h} = \frac{min'}{h'}$$

You can substitute those numbers *1* and *60 for h* and *min*, and *x* and *50,400 for h'* and *min'*.

$$\frac{60\ min}{1\ h} = \frac{50,400\ min}{x\ h}$$

Eliminate the units of measurement and cross multiply

$$\frac{60}{1} = \frac{50,400}{x}$$

$$(50,400)(1) = (60)(x)$$
$$50,400 = 60x$$

Divide by 60 and cancel.

$$\frac{50,400}{60} = \frac{\cancel{60}x}{\cancel{60}}$$
$$840 = x$$

So 50,400 minutes is equivalent to 840 hours.
In *Step 2* you change the *840 hours* to *days*

Think of *Step 2* this way:

$$24\ hours = 1\ day$$
$$840\ hours = x\ days$$

The second proportion could be

$$\frac{d}{h} = \frac{d'}{h'}$$

Substitute those numbers *1* and *24 for d* and *h*, and you can substitute *x* and *840 for d'* and *h'*.

$$\frac{1\ d}{24\ h} = \frac{x\ d}{840\ h}$$

Eliminate the units of measurement and cross multiply

$$\frac{1}{24} = \frac{x}{840}$$

$$(x)(24) = (1)(840)$$
$$24x = 840$$

Divide by 24 and cancel.

$$\frac{\cancel{24}x}{\cancel{24}} = \frac{840}{24}$$
$$x = 35$$

So, 50,400 minutes is equivalent to 35 days.

## EXAMPLE 3.19

**Kim is having a party for 24 people and is serving hot dogs. Each person will eat 2 hot dogs. How much will the hot dogs for the party cost if a package of 8 hot dogs costs $2.50?**

In this problem, there are three important quantities: *people*, *hot dogs*, and *dollars*. Here are the relationships given in the problem:

> *24 people* will require *?* *dollars*
> *1 person* eats *2 hot dogs*
> *8 hot dogs* cost *$2.50*

This problem will be done in two steps; first determine the number of hot dogs 24 people will eat, and then determine the cost of those hot dogs.

Think of *Step 1* this way:

$$1 \text{ person} = 2 \text{ hot dogs}$$
$$24 \text{ persons} = x \text{ hot dogs}$$

The first proportion could be

$$\frac{person}{hot\ dogs} = \frac{person'}{hot\ dogs'}$$

Substituting, you get

$$\frac{1\ person}{2\ hot\ dogs} = \frac{24\ persons}{x\ hot\ dogs}$$

Eliminate the units of measurement and cross multiply

$$\frac{1}{2} \underset{=}{\overset{24}{\diagup}} \ \frac{}{x}$$

$$48 = x$$

So, 48 hot dogs are needed.

In *Step 2*, you "change" 48 hot dogs to dollars.

Think of *Step 2* this way:

$$48 \text{ hot dogs} = x \text{ dollars}$$
$$8 \text{ hot dogs} = 2.50 \text{ dollars}$$

The second proportion could be set up as

$$\frac{hot\ dogs}{dollars} = \frac{hot\ dogs'}{dollars'}$$

Substituting you get

$$\frac{48\ hot\ dogs}{x\ dollars} = \frac{8\ hot\ dogs}{2.50\ dollars}$$

Eliminate the units of measurement and cross multiply

$$\frac{48}{x} \underset{=}{\overset{8}{\diagup}} \ \frac{}{2.50}$$

$$(8)(x) = (48)(2.50)$$
$$8x = 120$$

Divide by 8 and cancel

$$\frac{\cancel{8}x}{\cancel{8}} = \frac{120}{8}$$

$$x = 15$$

So, the hot dogs for the party will cost $15.

# Changing One Rate to Another Rate

A *rate* is a fraction with different units of measurement in the numerator and denominator. For example, 50 *miles* per *hour* written as 50 miles/hour and 3 *pounds* per *week* written as 3 pounds/week are rates. In dosage calculation, the bottom unit of measurement is frequently time (for example, *hours* or *minutes*). We sometimes want to change one rate into another rate. These problems are done in a manner similar to the method that was used to do the single unit of measurement problems.

### EXAMPLE 3.20

**Convert 5 feet per hour to an equivalent rate of speed in inches per hour.**

In this problem, there are two rates.

Think of the problem this way:

$$\frac{5\ feet}{hour} = \frac{?\ inches}{hour}$$

Notice that the given rate and the rate you are looking for both have the same denominator, *hour*. Therefore, the denominator does not have to be changed. But the given rate has *feet* in the numerator, and the rate you want has a different unit, *inches*, in the numerator. Therefore, the problem becomes

$$5\ feet = x\ inches$$

The proportion could be set up as

$$\frac{ft}{in} = \frac{ft'}{in'}$$

Because you know that 1 foot equals 12 inches, you can substitute to obtain

$$\frac{1\ ft}{12\ in} = \frac{5\ ft}{x\ in}$$

Eliminate the units of measurement and cross multiply

$$\frac{1}{12} = \frac{5}{x}$$

$$(5)(12) = (1)(x)$$

Simplify

$$60 = x$$

Therefore, 5 feet equals 60 inches, and *5 feet per hour* equals *60 inches per hour*.

## EXAMPLE 3.21

Convert *90 feet per hour* to an equivalent rate in *feet per minute*.

In this problem, there are two rates. Think of the problem this way:

$$\frac{90 \; feet}{1 \; hour} = ?\frac{ft}{min}$$

Notice that the given rate and the rate you are looking for both have the same numerator, *feet*. Therefore, the numerator does not have to be changed. But the given rate has *hour* in the denominator, and the rate you want has a different unit, *minute*, in the denominator.

This change can be accomplished by replacing 1 hour with 60 minutes in the rate $\frac{90\,ft}{1\,h}$ as follows:

$$\frac{90 \; ft}{1 \; h} = \frac{90 \; ft}{60 \; min} = \frac{90}{60} \; \frac{ft}{min}$$

Because $\frac{90}{60} = 1.5$

$$\frac{90}{60} \; \frac{ft}{min} = 1.5\frac{ft}{min}$$

So, *90 feet/hour* is equivalent to *1.5 feet per minute*.

## EXAMPLE 3.22

Convert $10\frac{1}{2}$ *feet/hour* to an equivalent rate in *inches/minute*.

In this problem there are two rates.

$$\frac{10\frac{1}{2} \; feet}{1 \; hour} = ?\frac{inches}{minute}$$

Notice that the given rate and the rate you are looking for both have different numerators and different denominators. Therefore, both must be changed. $10\frac{1}{2}$ feet must be changed to inches, and 1 hour must be changed to minutes.

First change $10\frac{1}{2}$ *feet* to *inches* using the proportion

$$\frac{feet}{inches} = \frac{feet'}{inches'}$$

Think of the problem as

$$10\tfrac{1}{2} \text{ feet} = x \text{ inches}$$
$$1 \text{ foot} = 12 \text{ inches}$$

Substituting into a proportion you get

$$\frac{1 \text{ foot}}{12 \text{ inches}} = \frac{10\tfrac{1}{2} \text{ feet}}{x \text{ inches}}$$

Eliminate the units of measurement and cross multiply

$$\frac{1}{12} = \frac{10\tfrac{1}{2}}{x}$$

$$(10\tfrac{1}{2})(12) = (1)(x)$$
$$126 = x$$

So, $10\tfrac{1}{2}$ feet equals 126 inches, and the problem becomes

$$\frac{126 \text{ inches}}{1 \text{ hour}} = ?\frac{\text{inches}}{\text{minute}}$$

Now you need to change 1 hour to minutes. You replace 1 hour by 60 minutes

$$\frac{126 \text{ inches}}{1 \text{ hour}} = \frac{126 \text{ inches}}{60 \text{ minutes}} = \frac{126}{60} \frac{\text{inches}}{\text{minute}}$$

but $\frac{126}{60} = 2.1$

So, $10\tfrac{1}{2}$ *feet/hour* to an equivalent 2.1 *inches/minute*.

## EXAMPLE 3.23

**Write 3.2 *inches/second* in *feet/minute*.**

*Method 1*: In this problem there are two rates. Think of the problem this way:

$$\frac{3.2 \text{ in}}{1 \text{ sec}} = ?\frac{\text{ft}}{\text{min}}$$

Notice that the given rate and the rate you want have different numerators and different denominators. Therefore, both must be changed. The inches must be changed to feet, and the seconds must be changed to minutes.

You can change the denominator (1 sec) to minutes by multiplying both numerator and denominator by 60 as follows:

$$\frac{3.2 \text{ in}}{1 \text{ sec}} \times \frac{60}{60} = \frac{192 \text{ in}}{60 \text{ sec}}$$

Replace 60 seconds with 1 minute

$$\frac{192 \text{ in}}{60 \text{ sec}} = \frac{192 \text{ in}}{1 \text{ min}}$$

Now the problem becomes

$$\frac{192\ in}{1\ min} = \frac{?\ feet}{min}$$

Now, only the numerator must be changed. Change 192 inches to feet using the proportion

$$\frac{feet}{inches} = \frac{feet'}{inches'}$$

Think of the problem as

$$192\ feet = x\ inches$$
$$1\ foot = 12\ inches$$

Substituting into a proportion you get

$$\frac{1\ foot}{12\ inches} = \frac{x\ feet}{192\ inches}$$

Eliminate the units of measurement and cross multiply

$$\frac{1}{12} = \frac{x}{192}$$

$$(x)(12) = (1)(192)$$
$$12x = 192$$

Divide by 12 and cancel

$$\frac{\cancel{12}x}{\cancel{12}} = \frac{192}{12}$$
$$x = 16$$

Therefore, 192 inches = 16 feet and and 3.2 inches/second equals 16 feet/minute.

*Method 2*: A quicker technique for doing Example 3.23 uses substitution to change the larger units of measurement (*ft and min*) to smaller units (*in and sec*), as follows:

$$\frac{3.2\ in}{sec} = \frac{x\ ft}{min}$$

Writing the larger units, *ft* as *1 ft* and *min* as *1 min*, the proportion can be written as

$$\frac{3.2\ in}{sec} = \frac{x(1\ ft)}{1\ min}$$

Now, substitute *12 in for 1 ft* and *60 sec for 1 min*.

$$\frac{3.2\ in}{1\ sec} = \frac{x(12\ in)}{60\ sec}$$

Because $x(12)$ equals $12\,x$, you have

$$\frac{3.2\ in}{1\ sec} = \frac{12x\ in}{60\ sec}$$

Because the units of measurement now match, they can be eliminated and cross multiplication yields:

$$12x = 192$$

As before, dividing both sides by 12 gives

$$x = 16$$

Therefore,

$$\frac{3.2 \; in}{sec} = \frac{16 \; ft}{min}$$

# Summary

In this chapter the technique of ratio and proportion was introduced.

- A ratio is a comparison of two numbers.
- A ratio can be written as a fraction.
- Ratios are equal if their fractional forms are equivalent fractions.
- Order matters: a ratio of *2 to 3* is not the same as a ratio of *3 to 2*.
- A rate compares two quantities that have different units of measurement.
- Rates often have a unit of time in the denominator.
- A proportion can be written as an equation with a ratio on each side of the equal sign.
- A proportion is true if the products of cross multiplication are equal.
- Two quantities are proportional if, whenever you double one of the quantities, you double the other.

- The steps in solving a proportion are:
  1. Identify the two units of measurement in the problem.
  2. Write a known equivalence between the units of measure.
  3. Let $x$ stand for the unit you are trying to find and write an equivalence involving $x$.
  4. Write a proportion using the two units of measurement.
  5. Substitute into the proportion.
  6. Eliminate the units.
  7. Cross multiply.
  8. Divide both sides of the equation by the coefficient of $x$ (unless the coefficient is 1).
  9. Cancel and simplify if possible.
  10. Check the answer by substituting and cross multiplying.

**Workspace**

# Practice Sets

The answers to *Try These for Practice* and *Exercises* are found in Appendix A. Ask your instructor for the answers to the *Additional Exercises*.

## Try These for Practice

Test your comprehension after reading the chapter.

1. How many minutes are in 4.5 hours? _____

2. An infant weighs 7 lb 3 oz. What is this weight in ounces? _____

3. How many hours are in $1\frac{1}{2}$ weeks? _____

4. Water is flowing from a hose at 0.1 quarts per minute. Find this rate of flow in quarts per hour. _____

5. A certain animal eats 2.5 ounces of food per day. At this rate, find the number of *pounds of food per week* the animal eats. _____

## Exercises

Reinforce your understanding in class or at home.

1. 1.5 min = _____ sec

2. $5\frac{1}{2}$ years = _____ months

3. $4\frac{1}{4}$ days = _____ h

4. 40 ounces = _____ lb

5. $\dfrac{3}{4}$ hour = _____ min

6. 51 mon = _____ yr

7. 3 qt = _____ pt

8. 3 lb = _____ oz

9. $\dfrac{12 \text{ inches}}{\text{second}}$ = _____ $\dfrac{\text{feet}}{\text{second}}$

10. $\dfrac{30 \text{ pints}}{\text{minute}}$ = _____ $\dfrac{\text{pints}}{\text{sec}}$

11. An infant weighs 8 pounds 10 ounces at birth. What is the weight in ounces? _____

12. What is the height in inches of a person who is 6 feet 4 inches tall? _____

13. If 3 feet = 1 yard, convert 4 yards to an equivalent distance in inches. _____

14. If a person measures 42 inches in height, what does the patient measure in feet? _____

15. What fraction of an hour is 2,700 seconds? _____

16. Change $6\dfrac{\text{pints}}{\text{h}}$ to an equivalent rate in $\dfrac{\text{quarts}}{\text{day}}$. _____

17. Change $6\dfrac{\text{quarts}}{\text{day}}$ to an equivalent rate in $\dfrac{\text{pints}}{\text{hour}}$. _____

18. Change 1,680 hours to weeks. _____

19. Write 1,209,600 seconds as an equivalent amount of time in weeks. _____

20. There are 24 cans of soda in a case. Each can contains 12 ounces of soda. Every 60 ounces of soda contains 1 cup of sugar. How many cups of sugar are in 5 cases of soda? _____

## Additional Exercises

Now, test yourself!

1. 540 sec = _____ min

2. 1.25 yr = _____ mon

3. 4 d = _____ h

4. 4 lb = _____ oz

5. $\frac{3}{4}$ min = _____ sec

6. $1\frac{2}{3}$ yr = _____ mon

**Workspace**

7. 480 in = _____ ft

8. 12 oz = _____ lb

9. $\dfrac{0.25 \text{ feet}}{\text{sec}}$ = _____ $\dfrac{\text{in}}{\text{sec}}$

10. $\dfrac{120 \text{ qt}}{\text{min}}$ = _____ $\dfrac{\text{qt}}{\text{sec}}$

11. An infant weighs 8 pounds at birth. What is the weight in ounces? _____

12. Convert $1\frac{1}{2}$ yards to feet if 3 feet equal 1 yard. _____

13. How many yards are in 90 inches? _____

14. What part of an hour is 50 minutes? _____

15. How many years are there in 30 months? _____

16. Change 2.25 hours to seconds. _____

17. An IV solution has been infusing for 55 minutes. How many seconds is that? _____

18. $12 \dfrac{\text{qt}}{\text{day}}$ = _____ $\dfrac{\text{pt}}{\text{h}}$

19. $0.24 \dfrac{\text{in}}{\text{sec}}$ = _____ $\dfrac{\text{ft}}{\text{min}}$

20. If \$0.25 is equivalent to 1 Yuan, how many Yuan are equivalent to \$500? _____

**MediaLink**
www.prenhall.com/giangrasso

Animated examples, interactive practice questions with animated solutions, and challenge tests for this chapter can be found on the Pearson Dosage Calculation Tutor that accompanies this text. Additional, unique, interactive resources and activities can be found on the Companion Web site.

# Unit

# 2 Systems of Measurement

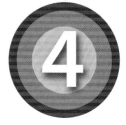

**Chapter**

# 4

# The Metric and Household Systems

## Learning Outcomes

20 mg = 1 mL

After completing this chapter, you will be able to

1. Identify the units of measurement in the metric and household systems.
2. Recognize the abbreviations for the units of measurement in the two systems.
3. State the equivalents for the units of volume.
4. State the equivalents for the units of weight.
5. State the equivalents for the units of length.
6. Convert from one unit to another within each of the two systems.

Historically, the United States has used three different systems to measure drugs: the apothecary, household, and metric systems.

The **apothecary** system is the oldest of the three systems, and it is very difficult to use. Because its use led to many medication errors, the Joint Commission and others have suggested that it be discontinued. Package inserts and other drug references no longer use the apothecary system for recommended medication dosages. Therefore, the apothecary system is not included in this chapter. However, students interested in the apothecary system will find it discussed in Appendix B.

The **household** system is designed so that dosages can be measured at home using ordinary containers found in the kitchen, such as cups and teaspoons. The household system is sometimes referred to as the English system.

The **metric** system is the most logically organized and easiest to use of all the systems of measurement. It was first adopted by France a few years after the French revolution of 1789. It is also referred to as the *International System of Units*. It can be abbreviated as SI, which are the first two initials of its French name, *Système International d'Unités*. The metric system will eventually replace all other systems of measurement used in healthcare.

In this chapter you will be introduced to the household and metric systems.

# The Household System

## Liquid Volume in the Household System

Occasionally, household measurements are used when prescribing liquid medication. Table 4.1 lists equivalent values, with their abbreviations, for units of liquid measurement in the household system.

| Table 4.1 **Household Equivalents of Liquid Volume** | | |
| --- | --- | --- |
| 1 quart (qt) | = | 2 pints (pt) |
| 1 pint (pt) | = | 2 measuring cups |
| 1 measuring cup | = | 8 ounces (oz) |
| 1 glass (usually) | = | 8 ounces (oz) |
| 1 ounce (oz) | = | 2 tablespoons (T) |
| 1 tablespoon (T) | = | 3 teaspoons (t) |

Now, you will apply the method of ratio and proportion you learned in Chapter 3 to problems in the household system.

### EXAMPLE 4.1

**A patient drank 24 oz of the laxative agent COLYTE. How many glasses did this patient drink?**

In this problem there are two quantities: *ounces* and *glasses*.
   Think of the problem this way:

$$8 \text{ ounces} = 1 \text{ glass} \quad \text{(known equivalent)}$$
$$24 \text{ ounces} = x \text{ glasses}$$

Because the number of ounces and the number of glasses are proportional, a proportion could be used to solve the problem. One way to set up the proportion is

$$\frac{oz}{glasses} = \frac{oz'}{glasses'}$$

Substituting, you obtain

$$\frac{8 \ oz}{1 \ glass} = \frac{24 \ oz}{x \ glasses}$$

Eliminate the units of measurement

$$\frac{8}{1} = \frac{24}{x}$$

Cross multiply

$$\frac{8}{1} = \frac{24}{x}$$

$$(24)(1) = (8)(x)$$

**ALERT**

Because the volume of ordinary household spoons, cups, and glasses may vary, medications should not be administered using ordinary household utensils.

**NOTE**

Whenever you set up a proportion, both fractions should have the units of measurement in corresponding positions. That is, the numerators should have matching units (*oz* in this case), and the denominator units (*glasses* in this case) should also match.

**ALERT**

Using ordinary tableware to measure medications may constitute a safety risk because ordinary tableware does not come in standard sizes. Therefore, patients and their families should be advised to use the measuring device provided with the medication rather than the kitchen tablespoon, for example.

Simplify

$$24 = 8x$$

Divide both sides of the equation by 8, the coefficient of $x$.

$$\frac{24}{8} = \frac{8x}{8}$$

Cancel

$$\frac{24}{8} = \frac{\cancel{8}x}{\cancel{8}}$$

Simplify

$$3 = x$$

The patient drank 3 glasses because 24 oz is approximately the same as 3 glasses.

**NOTE**

In the household system for quantities less than 1, either decimal numbers or fractions may be used. However, fractions are preferred. For example, $\frac{1}{2}$ qt is preferred over 0.5 qt.

### EXAMPLE 4.2

**A patient needs to drink $1\frac{1}{2}$ ounces of an elixir per day. How many teaspoons would be equivalent to this dosage?**

In this problem, there are two quantities: *ounces* and *teaspoons*.

Since you may not know the direct equivalence between ounces and teaspoons, you will first change $1\frac{1}{2}$ ounces to an equivalent number of tablespoons, and then change the resulting tablespoons to teaspoons. This problem, then, requires two steps.

**Step 1:** *Change $1\frac{1}{2}$ ounces to tablespoons*

$$1 \text{ ounce} = 2 \text{ tablespoons} \quad \text{(known equivalence)}$$
$$1\tfrac{1}{2} \text{ ounces} = x \text{ tablespoons}$$

One way to set up the proportion is

$$\frac{oz}{T} = \frac{oz'}{T'}$$

Substituting, you obtain

$$\frac{1\,oz}{2\,T} = \frac{1\frac{1}{2}\,oz}{x\,T}$$

Eliminate the units of measurement

$$\frac{1}{2} = \frac{1\frac{1}{2}}{x}$$

Cross multiply

$$\frac{1}{2} = \frac{1\frac{1}{2}}{x}$$

$$\left(1\tfrac{1}{2}\right)(2) = (1)(x)$$

$$3 = x$$

So, $1\frac{1}{2}$ oz is equivalent to 3 tablespoons.

**Step 2:** *Change 3 tablespoons to teaspoons*

  1 tablespoon = 3 teaspoons  (known equivalence)
  3 tablespoons = $x$ teaspoons

One way to set up the proportion is

$$\frac{t}{T} = \frac{t'}{T'}$$

Substituting, you obtain

$$\frac{3t}{1T} = \frac{xt}{3T}$$

Eliminate the units of measurement

$$\frac{3}{1} = \frac{x}{3}$$

Cross multiply

$$\frac{3}{1} = \frac{x}{3}$$

$$x = 9$$

So, $1\frac{1}{2}$ oz is equivalent to 9 teaspoons

## Weight in the Household System

The only units of weight used in the household system of medication administration are ounces (oz) and pounds (lb), as shown in Table 4.2.

| Table 4.2  **Household Equivalents of Weight** |
| --- |
| 1 pound (lb)  =  16 ounces (oz) |

**EXAMPLE 4.3**

**An infant weighs 5 lb 8 oz. What is the weight of the infant in ounces?**

First change the 5 lb to ounces.

**NOTE**

Teaspoon is sometimes abbreviated as *tsp*, and tablespoon is sometimes abbreviated as *tbs*.

**NOTE**

The unit *ounce*, when it is used to measure liquid volumes, is sometimes referred to as *fluid ounce*.

**NOTE**

Ounces used for weight should not be confused with ounces used for volume.

Think:

$$16 \text{ ounces} = 1 \text{ pound} \quad \text{(known equivalence)}$$
$$x \text{ ounces} = 5 \text{ pounds}$$

One way to set up the proportion is

$$\frac{oz}{lb} = \frac{oz'}{lb'}$$

Substituting, you obtain

$$\frac{16 \text{ } oz}{1 \text{ } lb} = \frac{x \text{ } oz}{5 \text{ } lb}$$

Eliminate the units of measurement and cross multiply

$$\frac{16}{1} = \frac{x}{5}$$

$$x = 80$$

Now, add the extra 8 ounces

$$80 \text{ } oz + 8 \text{ } oz = 88 \text{ } oz$$

So, the 5 lb 8 oz infant weighs 88 ounces.

# Length in the Household System

The only units of length used in the household system for medication administration are feet (ft) and inches (in), as shown in Table 4.3.

| Table 4.3 **Household Equivalents for Length** |
| --- |
| 1 foot (ft)  =  12 inches (in) |

## EXAMPLE 4.4

**A child is 3 ft 2 in tall. Find the child's height in inches.**

First, change the 3 feet to inches.
   Think of the problem this way:

$$1 \text{ ft} = 12 \text{ in} \quad \text{(known equivalent)}$$
$$3 \text{ ft} = x \text{ in}$$

Because the number of feet and the number of inches are proportional, a proportion could be used to solve the problem. One way to set up the proportion is

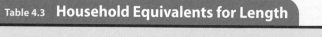

$$\frac{ft}{in} = \frac{ft'}{in'}$$

Substituting, you obtain

$$\frac{1\ ft}{12\ in} = \frac{3\ ft}{x\ in}$$

Eliminate the units of measurement

$$\frac{1}{12} = \frac{3}{x}$$

Cross multiply

$$\frac{1}{12} \underset{\longrightarrow}{=} \frac{3}{x}$$

$$(12)(3) = (1)(x)$$

Simplify

$$36 = x$$

So, 3 feet equal 36 inches. Now, add the extra 2 inches.

$$36\ in + 2\ in = 38\ in$$

So, the 3 ft 2 in child is 38 inches tall.

## Decimal-Based Systems

As seen in Chapter 1, our *place-value number system* is a decimal system, that is, it is based on the number 10. The *United States monetary system* and the *metric system* are also decimal systems.

The *U.S. monetary system* uses the dollar as its fundamental unit. All other denominations are decimal multiples or fractions of the dollar.

| hundred-dollar bill | ten-dollar bill | dollar bill | dime | penny |
|---|---|---|---|---|

An amount of money measured in one denomination can be easily converted to another denomination by merely moving the decimal point the appropriate number of places.

For example, to convert *60 dimes* to *pennies*, see in the chart that *dime* to *penny* is one jump to the *right*.

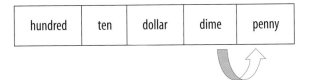

| hundred | ten | dollar | dime | penny |
|---|---|---|---|---|

So, move the decimal point in 60 dimes one place to the *right* as follows:

60 dimes = 60.0 dimes = 6 0 0 . pennies, or 600 pennies

To convert *80 dollars* to *ten dollar bills*, see in the chart that *dollar* to *ten* is one jump to the *left*.

| hundred | ten | dollar | dime | penny |
|---------|-----|--------|------|-------|

So, move the decimal point in 80 dollars one place to the *left,* as follows:

80 dollars = 80. dollars = 8 . 0 tens = 8 tens

To convert *4 hundreds* to *dimes*, see in the chart that *hundred* to *dime* is a jump of *3 places to the right.*

| hundred | ten | dollar | dime | penny |
|---------|-----|--------|------|-------|

So, move the decimal point in 4 hundreds *3 places to the right.*

4 hundreds = 4.000 hundreds = 4 0 0 0 . dimes or 4,000 dimes.

# The Metric System

**NOTE**

To help remember the important metric prefixes, various mnemonics may be employed. Two are: <u>K</u>ing <u>H</u>enry <u>D</u>oesn't <u>U</u>sually <u>D</u>rink <u>C</u>old <u>M</u>alted <u>M</u>ilk, or <u>K</u>ids <u>H</u>ate <u>D</u>rudgery <u>U</u>ntil <u>D</u>awn <u>C</u>alculating <u>M</u>any <u>M</u>etrics (<u>k</u>ilo, <u>h</u>ecto, <u>d</u>eka, <u>u</u>nit, <u>d</u>eci, <u>c</u>enti, <u>m</u>illi, <u>m</u>icro).

**NOTE**

Depending on the country, spellings may be *meter/metre, liter/litre,* or *deca/deka.*

The metric system is the most widely used general system of measurement in the world today, with the United States being the only exception among developed countries. However, in all countries, the metric system is the preferred system for prescribing medications.

Because the *metric system* is based on 10, converting quantities in this system is also simply a matter of shifting the decimal point. The simplicity of its decimal basis has encouraged the proliferation of the metric system.

At the heart of the *metric* system are the *fundamental* or *base units*. The **base units** needed for medical dosages are *gram (g), liter (L),* and *meter (m)*; these base units are used to measure weight, liquid volume, and length, respectively.

Decimal multiples of any of the base units are obtained by appending standard *metric prefixes* to the base unit. Table 4.4 shows both the base units and their **metric prefixes** with their abbreviations. Note that only the prefixes in blue are used in dosage calculation.

**Table 4.4  Format of the Metric System**

| Name | kilo | hecto | deka | BASE UNIT | deci | centi | milli | * | * | micro |
|------|------|-------|------|-----------|------|-------|-------|---|---|-------|
| Abbreviation | k | h | da | g, L, m | d | c | m | * | * | mc |
| Multiple of the Base | 1,000 | 100 | 10 | 1 | 0.1 | 0.01 | 0.001 | * | * | 0.000001 |

In the metric system, the prefixes indicate multiples of 10 times the base unit, or the base unit divided by multiples of 10. The meanings of the necessary prefixes are found in Table 4.5.

### Table 4.5  Metric Prefixes Used in Health Care

| Metric Prefixes | | | |
| --- | --- | --- | --- |
| kilo | means | one thousand | (1,000 times the base) |
| deci | means | one tenth | (0.1 times the base) |
| centi | means | one hundredth | (0.01 times the base) |
| milli | means | one thousandth | (0.001 times the base) |
| micro | means | one millionth | (0.000001 times the base) |

The metric prefixes are appended to the base units. For example,

$$1 \underline{kilo}gram = 1,000 \text{ grams}$$

and

$$1 \underline{centi}meter = 0.01 \text{ meter.}$$

Fractions, such as $\frac{1}{2}$, are not formally used in the metric system. For example, $3\frac{1}{2}$ grams is written as 3.5 grams.

## Liquid Volume in the Metric System

Drugs in liquid form are measured by volume. The volume of a liquid is the amount of space it occupies. In dosage calculations for liquid volumes only, *liters* and *milliliters* are used (see Table 4.6).

### Table 4.6  Metric Equivalents of Liquid Volume

| | | |
| --- | --- | --- |
| 1 cubic centimeter (cc or cm³) | = | 1 milliliter (mL) |
| 1,000 milliliters (mL) | = | 1 liter (L) |

**NOTE**

The abbreviation mL should be used instead of the abbreviation cc because "c" may be confused with "u" (units) or "cc" with "00" (double zero).

*Milliliters* are used for smaller amounts of fluids. The prefix milli means $\frac{1}{1,000}$, so

$$1 \text{ liter (L)} = 1,000 \text{ milliliters (mL)}$$

*Milliliters* are equivalent to *cubic centimeters* (cm³ or cc), so

$$1 \text{ mL} = 1 \text{ cm}^3 = 1 \text{ cc}$$

You must be able to convert from one unit of measurement to another within the metric system. With liquids in the metric system you need to make conversions only between *liters* and *milliliters*. Of course, you could make such conversions by using *ratio and proportion*. However, conversions involving metric-system units are easier to do by merely *moving the decimal point*. In Example 4.5, both of these methods will be compared.

**NOTE**

Deciliters (dL) may be encountered in lab reports. However, deciliters are not used in calculating medical dosages.

**NOTE**

In example 4.5 when converting 0.5 L to 500 mL, the unit of measurement got smaller, whereas the number got larger.

## EXAMPLE 4.5

**If the prescriber ordered 0.5 L of 5% dextrose in water, how many milliliters were ordered?**

**Method 1:**   *By ratio and proportion*

In this problem there are two quantities: *liters* and *milliliters*. Think of the problem like this:

$$1 \text{ L} = 1{,}000 \text{ mL} \quad \text{(known equivalence)}$$
$$0.5 \text{ L} = x \text{ mL}$$

One way to set up the proportion is

$$\frac{L}{mL} = \frac{L'}{mL'}$$

Substituting, you obtain

$$\frac{1 \text{ L}}{1{,}000 \text{ mL}} = \frac{0.5 \text{ L}}{x \text{ mL}}$$

Eliminate the units of measurement and cross multiply

$$\frac{1}{1{,}000} = \frac{0.5}{x}$$
$$500 = x$$

So, 500 mL were ordered.

**Method 2:**   *By moving the decimal point (preferred method)*

The metric system for liters has the following format, but only the units in blue are used in dosage calculations of liquid volume:

| kilo | hecto | deka | Base Unit | deci | centi | milli | * | * | micro |
|------|-------|------|-----------|------|-------|-------|---|---|-------|
| kL | hL | daL | liter (L) | dL | cL | mL | | | mcL |

Because for liquid volume the only units needed for medical dosage calculations are liter (L) and milliliter (mL), the jump will always be three places.

| Base Unit | deci | centi | milli |
|-----------|------|-------|-------|
| L | dL | cL | mL |

For this example, to convert *liters* to *milliliters* is a jump of *3 places to the right*, so, in the quantity 0.5 L, move the decimal point *3 places to the right*, as follows:

$$0.5 \text{ L} = 0.500 \text{ L} = 0\,5\,0\,0.\text{ mL} = 500.\text{ mL} = 500 \text{ mL}.$$

So, the prescriber ordered *500 milliliters* of 5% dextrose in water.

**NOTE**

Because moving the decimal place is easier than using ratio and proportion, throughout the textbook metric conversions will be accomplished by moving the decimal point.

**ALERT**

Write 0.5 L instead of $\frac{5}{10}$ L or $\frac{1}{2}$ L because in the metric system, quantities are written as decimal numbers instead of fractions.

NOTE

When converting 1,750 mL to 1.75 L, the unit of measurement got larger, whereas the number got smaller.

### EXAMPLE 4.6

**The patient is to receive *1,750 milliliters* of *0.9% NaCl IV q12h*. What is this volume in liters?**

For this example, to convert *1,750 milliliters* to *liters* is a jump of *3 places to the left,*

| liter | deci | centi | milli |
|-------|------|-------|-------|
| L     |      |       | mL    |

So, in 1,750 mL move the decimal point *3 places to the left* as follows:

$$1{,}750 \text{ mL} = 1{,}750. \text{ mL} = 1\,.\,7\,5\,0 \text{ L} = 1.750 \text{ L} = 1.75 \text{ L}$$

So, 1,750 mL of 0.9% NaCl is the same amount as 1.75 L of 0.9% NaCl.

## Weight in the Metric System

ALERT

The abbreviation for microgram, mcg, is preferred over the abbreviation $\mu g$ because $\mu g$ may be mistaken for the abbreviation for milligram, mg. This error would result in a dose that would be 1,000 times greater than the prescribed dose.

Drugs in dry form are generally measured by weight. In dosage calculations, *kilograms, grams, milligrams,* and *micrograms* (written in order of size) are used to measure weight. *Kilograms* are the largest of these units of measurement, and *micrograms* are the smallest (see Table 4.7).

**Table 4.7  Metric Equivalents of Weight**

| | | |
|---|---|---|
| 1 kilogram (kg) | = | 1,000 grams (g) |
| 1 gram(g) | = | 1,000 milligrams (mg) |
| 1 milligram (mg) | = | 1,000 micrograms (mcg) |

*Kilograms* are used for heavier weights. The prefix kilo means 1,000, so

$$1 \textbf{ kilo}\text{gram (kg)} = 1{,}000 \textit{ grams} \text{ (g)}$$

*Milligrams* are used for lighter weights, and *micrograms* are used for even lighter weights.

The prefix milli means $\frac{1}{1{,}000}$, and micro means $\frac{1}{1{,}000{,}000}$, so

$$1 \text{ gram (g)} = 1{,}000 \textbf{ milli}\text{grams (mg)}$$

$$1 \text{ milligram (mg)} = 1{,}000 \textbf{ micro}\text{grams (mcg)}$$

The metric system for weight (grams) features the following format. Only the units in blue are needed for dosage calculations:

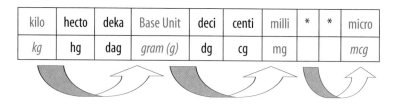

| kilo | hecto | deka | Base Unit | deci | centi | milli | * | * | micro |
|------|-------|------|-----------|------|-------|-------|---|---|-------|
| kg | hg | dag | gram (g) | dg | cg | mg | | | mcg |

For weight, the only units needed for medical dosage calculations are *kilogram (kg)*, *gram (g)*, *milligram (mg)*, and *microgram (mcg)*. Since these units are all 3 places apart, the jumps between them will always be three jumps. The following shortened version of the metric weight chart will be useful in the next few examples:

| kilogram | gram | milligram | microgram |
|----------|------|-----------|-----------|
| kg | g | mg | mcg |

3 jumps    3 jumps    3 jumps

**NOTE**

A dose is always expressed in the form of a number and a unit of measure. Both are important. For example:

150 mcg, 2.5 mg, 3 tablets, 1.5 mL, 0.5 L.

When you write your answer, be sure to include the appropriate unit of measurement.

## EXAMPLE 4.7

The order reads *125 mcg of Lanoxin (digoxin) PO* daily. How many milligrams of this cardiac medication would you administer to the patient?

$$125 \text{ mcg} = ? \text{ mg}$$

In this problem, you convert from mcg to mg. The movement from mcg to mg in the following chart is a movement of one column to the left.

Therefore, the conversion is accomplished by moving the decimal point three places to the left.

| Kilo- | Fundamental Unit | Milli- | Micro- |
|-------|------------------|--------|--------|
| kilogram (kg) | gram (g) | milligram (mg) | microgram (mcg) |

$$125 \text{ mcg} = 125. \text{ mcg} = .125 \text{ mg} = .125 \text{ mg} = 0.125 \text{ mg}$$

So, 125 mcg is the same amount as 0.125 mg, and you would administer 0.125 mg of digoxin.

## EXAMPLE 4.8

The order reads *Glucotrol (glipizide) 15 mg PO* daily ac breakfast. How many grams of this hypoglycemic agent would you administer?

$$15 \text{ mg} = ? \text{ g}$$

In this problem, you convert from mg to g. The movement from mg to g in the following chart is a movement of one column to the left. Therefore, the conversion is accomplished by moving the decimal point three places to the left.

| Kilo- | Fundamental Unit | Milli- | Micro- |
|-------|------------------|--------|--------|
| **kilo**gram (kg) | **gram**(g) | **milli**gram (mg) | **micro**gram (mcg) |

$$15 \text{ mg} = 15. \text{ mg} = .0\,1\,5 \text{ g} = .015 \text{ g} = 0.015 \text{ g}$$

So, 15 mg is the same amount as 0.015 g, and you would administer 0.015 g.

## EXAMPLE 4.9

Convert 4.5 kilograms to an equivalent amount in grams.

To convert kg to g, jump *3 places to the right*.

| kilogram | gram | milligram | Microgram |
|----------|------|-----------|-----------|
| kg | g | mg | mcg |

Move the decimal point *3 places to the right*.

$$4.5 \text{ kg} = 4.500 \text{ kg} = 4\,5\,0\,0. \text{ g} = 4{,}500 \text{ g}$$

So, 4.5 kilograms is equivalent to 4,500 grams.

## NOTE

"Gm" is an outdated abbreviation for gram, and "gr" is the apothecary abbreviation for grain. Both of these are obsolete, and can be easily confused with the correct abbreviation for gram, which is "g."

# Length in the Metric System

The metric system for meters has the following format, but only the units in blue are used in health care.

| kilo | hecto | deka | Base Unit | deci | centi | milli |
|------|-------|------|-----------|------|-------|-------|
| km | hm | dam | meter (m) | dm | cm | mm |

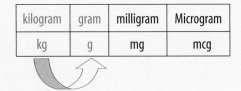

1 jump

**NOTE**

In metric conversions of liquid volumes and weights, the decimal point is always moved 3 places. However, in metric conversions of length (cm and mm) the decimal point is moved only one place.

**NOTE**

The basic metric units of meter, liter, and gram have the following relationship: 1 cubic centimeter of water has a volume of 1 milliliter and weighs 1 gram.

*Centimeters (cm)* and *millimeters (mm)* are the only metric units of length used in this textbook. A patient's height might be measured in *centimeters*, and the diameter of a tumor might be measured in *centimeters* or *millimeters*.

Because *centimeters* and *millimeters* are adjacent units, conversion between them will require a movement of one decimal place.

### EXAMPLE 4.10

**A wound has a length of 0.7 centimeters. What is the length of this wound in millimeters?**

$$0.7 \text{ cm} = ? \text{ mm}$$

To convert *centimeters* to *millimeters*, jump *1 place to the right*.

| meter | decimeter | centimeter | millimeter |
|-------|-----------|------------|------------|
| m | dm | cm | mm |

So, in 0.7 cm move the decimal point *1 place to the right*.

$$0.7 \text{ cm} = 0\,7.\text{ mm} = 7.\text{ mm} = 7 \text{ mm}$$

So, the wound has a length of 7 millimeters.

## Summary

In this chapter, the metric and household systems of measurement were introduced.

- The metric system is the dominant system used in health care.
- The apothecary system is being phased out.
- It is important to memorize the equivalences between the various units of measurement of the household and metric systems.
- It is important to memorize the abbreviations for the various units of measurement.
- To convert units of measure in the household system, use ratio and proportion.
- To convert units of measure in the metric system, use the shortcut method of moving the decimal point. Always jump 3 places except for cm-mm conversions, which use a 1 place jump.

- Remember, each jump is 3 places in this chart:

| kilogram | gram | milligram | microgram |
|----------|------|-----------|-----------|
| kg | g, L | mg, mL | mcg |

- Abbreviations for units of measurement are not followed by periods.
  Example: *40 mg and 5 t* (not 40 mg. and 5 t.).
- Abbreviations for units of measurement are not made plural by adding the letter s.
  Example: *70 mcg and 3 oz*
  (not 70 mcgs and 3 ozs).
- Insert a leading zero for decimal numbers less than 1.
  Example: *0.05 g and 0.34 mL*
  (not .05 g and .34 mL).

- Omit trailing zeros for decimal numbers.
  Example: *7.3 mL and 0.07 g*
          (not 7.30 mL and 0.070 g).
- Numbers greater than 999 need commas.
  Example: *2,500 mL and 20,000 mcg*
          (not 2500 mL and 20000 mcg).
- Leave space between the number and the unit of measurement.

- Example: *60 mL and 100 g*
          (not 60mL and 100g).
- Avoid the use of fractions with metric units of measurement.
  Example: *0.5 mL and 1.5 g*
          (not $\frac{1}{2}$ mL and $1\frac{1}{2}$ g).

# Practice Sets

Workspace

The answers to *Try These for Practice, Exercises,* and *Cumulative Review Exercises* are found in Appendix A. Ask your instructor for the answers to the *Additional Exercises.*

## Try These for Practice

Test your comprehension after reading the chapter.

1. You need to memorize all the metric and household equivalents. To test yourself, fill in the missing numbers in the following chart.

## Metric System

(a)  1 L            = _____ mL

(b)  1 mL           = _____ cc

(c)  1 L            = _____ cm$^3$

(d)  1 kg           = _____ g

(e)  1 g            = _____ mg

(f)  1 mg           = _____ mcg

(g)  1 cm           = _____ mm

## Household System

(h)  1 qt           = _____ pt

(i)  1 pt           = _____ cups

(j)  1 glass        = _____ oz

(k)  1 measuring cup = _____ oz

(l)  1 oz           = _____ T

(m)  1 T            = _____ t

(n)  1 ft           = _____ in

(o)  1 lb           = _____ oz

2. Use the label in ●**Figure 4.1** to determine the number of grams of OxyContin in 1 tablet of the drug.

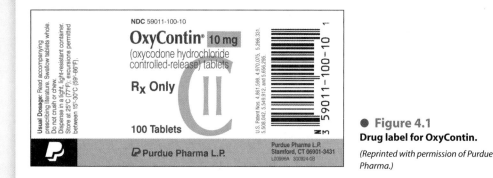

● **Figure 4.1**
**Drug label for OxyContin.**

*(Reprinted with permission of Purdue Pharma.)*

3. The prescriber ordered *methorexate 2.5 mg PO q12h*, for a patient with psoriasis. How many micrograms of this drug are administered in a day?

4. The urinary output of a patient with an indwelling Foley catheter is 1,800 mL. How many liters of urine are in the bag?

5. If a patient drank $1\frac{1}{2}$ quarts of water, how many pints of water did the patient drink?

## Exercises

Reinforce your understanding in class or at home.

1.  400 mg = _____ g

2.  0.003 g = _____ mg

3.  0.07 g = _____ mg

4.  3 L = _____ mL

5.  2,500 mL = _____ L

6.  600 mcg = _____ mg

7.  1.7 L = _____ mL

8.  $4\frac{1}{2}$ qt = _____ pt

9.  2.5 kg = _____ g

10. 4 T = _____ t

11. 5 T = _____ oz

12. 32 oz = _____ pt

13. Using the drug label in ●**Figure 4.2**, determine the number of micrograms of Depakote in one tablet.

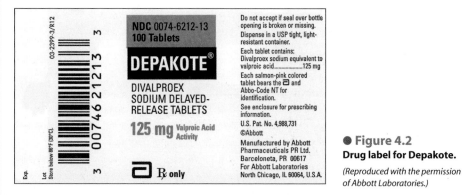

● **Figure 4.2**
**Drug label for Depakote.**

*(Reproduced with the permission of Abbott Laboratories.)*

14. The physician ordered a loading dose of *digoxin 520 mcg PO stat*. How many milligrams are in this dose?

15. According to the physician's order sheet in ● **Figure 4.3**, what is the dose in grams of the chlorpromazine?

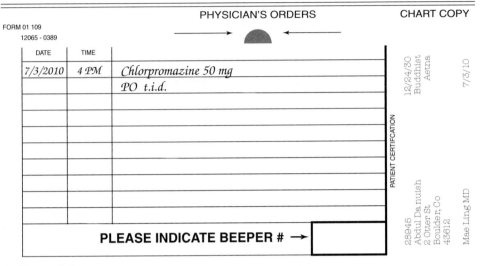

PHYSICIAN'S ORDERS                    CHART COPY

FORM 01 109
   12065 - 0389

| DATE | TIME | | |
|---|---|---|---|
| 7/3/2010 | 4 PM | Chlorpromazine 50 mg | |
| | | PO  t.i.d. | |

PLEASE INDICATE BEEPER #  →

PATIENT CERTIFCATION

12/24/30
Buddhist
Aetna

7/3/10

28945
Abdul Danush
2 Otter St
Boulder, Co
43612

Mae Ling MD

● **Figure 4.3**
**Physician's order sheet.**

16. A patient is drinking $\frac{1}{2}$ pint of orange juice every two hours. At this rate, how many quarts of orange juice will the patient drink in eight hours?

17. Use the label in ●**Figure 4.4** to determine the number of grams in one capsule of Norvir.

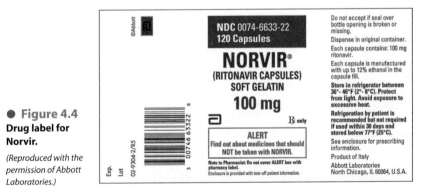

● **Figure 4.4**
**Drug label for Norvir.**

*(Reproduced with the permission of Abbott Laboratories.)*

NDC 0074-6633-22
120 Capsules

NORVIR®
(RITONAVIR CAPSULES)
SOFT GELATIN

100 mg

℞ only

ALERT
Find out about medicines that should
NOT be taken with NORVIR.

Do not accept if seal over
bottle opening is broken or
missing.

Dispense in original container.

Each capsule contains: 100 mg
ritonavir.

Each capsule is manufactured
with up to 12% ethanol in the
capsule fill.

Store in refrigerator between
36°- 46°F (2°- 8°C). Protect
from light. Avoid exposure to
excessive heat.

Refrigeration by patient is
recommended but not required
if used within 30 days and
stored below 77°F (25°C).

See enclosure for prescribing
information.

Product of Italy

Abbott Laboratories
North Chicago, IL 60064, U.S.A.

Note to Pharmacist: Do not cover ALERT box with
pharmacy label.
Enclosure is provided with tear-off patient information.

18. An infant weighs 3,400 grams. How much does the infant weigh in kilograms?

19. 2.1 cm = _____ mm

20. 5 ft = _____ in

## Additional Exercises

Now, test yourself!

1. 6.5 mg = _____ mcg    2. 0.05 g = _____ mg

3. 0.04 g = _____ mg    4. 4.75 L = _____ mL

5. 15 mm = _____ cm    6. 1 pt = _____ cups

7. 120 mL = _____ cc    8. 100,000 mcg = _____ mg

9. 2 qt = _____ pt    10. 6 T = _____ t

11. 8 pt = _____ qt    12. 0.26 kg = _____ g

13. The label in ● **Figure 4.5** indicates the quantity of Wellbutrin in one tablet. Change milligrams to grams.

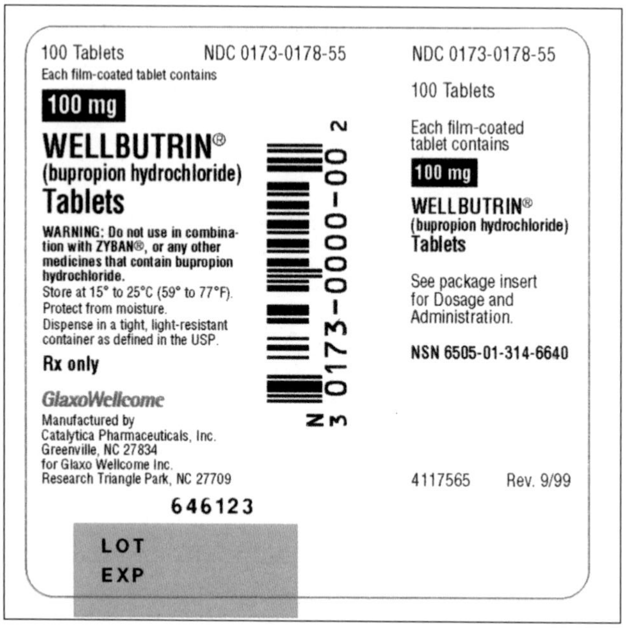

● **Figure 4.5**
**Drug label for Wellbutrin.**
*(Reproduced with permission of GlaxoSmithKline.)*

14. The physician ordered *ProBanthine 30 mg PO ac hs*. What is this dose in PO grams?

15. According to the physician's order sheet in ● **Figure 4.6**, what is the dose of Timentin in milligrams?

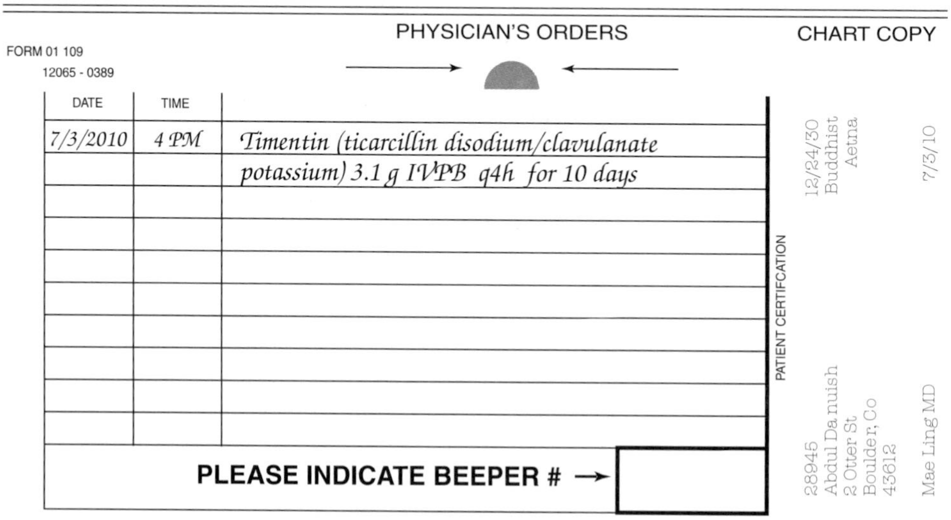

● **Figure 4.6**
**Physician's order sheet.**

16. The prescriber ordered the following:

*Orange juice $\frac{1}{2}$ pint PO q2h.*

How many ounces of orange juice should be given q2h?

17. A patient is receiving 1 tablet of Xanax. Read the label in ●**Figure 4.7.** How many grams of Xanax is the patient receiving?

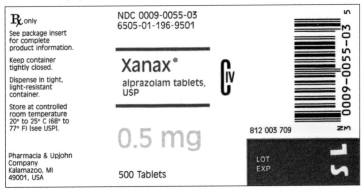

● **Figure 4.7**
**Drug label for Xanax.**

*(Reg. Trademark of Pfizer Inc. Reproduced with permission.)*

18. The label in ●**Figure 4.8** indicates the amount of Zantac in each tablet. Convert milligrams to grams.

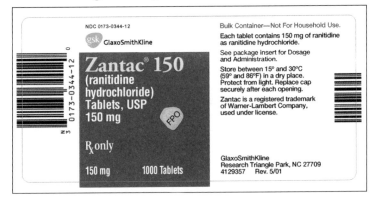

● **Figure 4.8**
**Drug label for Zantac.**

*(Reproduced with permission of GlaxoSmithKline.)*

19. An infant weighs 2.8 kg. How much does the infant weigh in grams?

20. Read the order on the physician's order sheet in ●**Figure 4.9.** Convert the dose to grams.

| | PHYSICIAN'S ORDERS | CHART COPY |
|---|---|---|

FORM 01 109
12065 - 0389

| DATE | TIME | |
|---|---|---|
| 8/4/2010 | 8AM | Cimetidine 400 mg PO b.i.d. |
| | | |
| | | |
| | | |
| | | |
| | | |
| | | |
| | | |
| | | |
| | | |

**PLEASE INDICATE BEEPER #** →

PATIENT CERTIFCATION

12/24/16
R.C.
Medicare

612408
Frank Kiernan
3 Elm St.
Bethpage, NY
11720

● **Figure 4.9**
**Physician's order sheet.**

**Workspace**

# Cumulative Review Exercises

Review your mastery of previous chapters.

1. 7.8 g = _____ mg

2. 0.25 mg = _____ mcg

3. 4.5 L = _____ mL

4. 12 T = _____ oz

5. 1,200 mL = _____ L

6. 7.6 kg = _____ g

7. Convert 750 mL to liters.

8. How many teaspoons are contained in 5 T?

9. The order reads Carafate 1 g PO q.i.d. Convert this dose to milligrams.

10. The patient must receive 250 mg of Cloxacillin PO q6h. Change to grams.

11. Change 0.65 mg to micrograms.

12. The physician ordered 2 T of Mylanta PO q2h. How many teaspoons of this antacid would you prepare?

13. The order is Colace 150 mg PO t.i.d. the label reads 150 mg/15 mL. How many milliliters would you prepare?

14. Change 250 mL to liters.

15. Change 0.032 g to milligrams.

**MediaLink**

www.prenhall.com/giangrasso

Animated examples, interactive practice questions with animated solutions, and challenge tests for this chapter can be found on the Pearson Dosage Calculation Tutor that accompanies this text. Additional, unique, interactive resources and activities can be found on the Companion Web site.

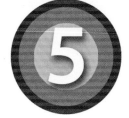

# Chapter

# Converting from One System of Measurement to Another

## Learning Outcomes

1 kilogram (kg) ≈ 2.2 pounds (lb)

After completing this chapter, you will be able to

1. State the equivalent units of weight between the metric and household systems.
2. State the equivalent units of volume between the metric and household systems.
3. State the equivalent units of length between the metric and household systems.
4. Convert a quantity from one system of measurement to its equivalent in another system of measurement.

**W**hen calculating drug dosages, you will sometimes need to convert a quantity expressed in one system of measurement to an equivalent quantity expressed in a different system of measurement. For example, you might need to convert a quantity measured in ounces to the same quantity measured in milliliters. This chapter will show you how to accomplish such conversions.

# Equivalents of Common Units of Measurement

To get started, you will need to learn some basic equivalent values of the various units in the different systems. Table 5.1 lists some common equivalent values for weight, volume, and length in the metric and household systems of measurement. Although these equivalents are considered standards, all of them are approximations.

A useful summary of the relationships that you should know among all the equivalents of liquid volume is provided in Table 5.2.

| Table 5.1 | Approximate Equivalents between Metric and Household Units of Volume, Weight, and Length | | |
|---|---|---|---|
| | **Metric** | | **Household** |
| Volume | 5 milliliters (mL) | ≈ | 1 teaspoon (t) |
| | 15 milliliters (mL) | ≈ | 1 tablespoon (T) |
| | 30 milliliters (mL) | ≈ | 1 ounce (oz) |
| | 240 milliliters (mL) | ≈ | 1 cup |
| | 500 milliliters (mL) | ≈ | 1 pint (pt) |
| | 1,000 milliliters (mL) | ≈ | 1 quart (qt) |
| Weight | 1 kilogram (kg) | ≈ | 2.2 pounds (lb) |
| Length | 2.5 centimeters (cm) | ≈ | 1 inch (in) |

| Table 5.2 | Summary Table of Equivalents Within and Approximate Equivalents Between Metric and Household Units of Volume | | |
|---|---|---|---|
| | 1 quart  =  2 pints  =  4 cups  =  32 ounces | ≈ | 1,000 mL  =  1L |
| | 1 pint  =  2 cups  =  16 ounces | ≈ | 500 mL |
| | 1 cup  =  8 ounces  =  16 tablespoons | ≈ | 240 mL |
| | 1 ounce  =  2 tablespoons  =  6 teaspoons | ≈ | 30 mL |
| | 1 tablespoon  =  3 teaspoons | ≈ | 15 mL |
| | 1 teaspoon | ≈ | 5 mL |

You can use ratio and proportion to convert from one system to another in exactly the same way you converted from one unit to another within the same system. ● Figure 5.1 depicts medication cups with units of measurement from various systems.

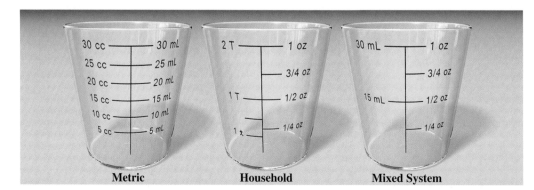

● **Figure 5.1**
**Medication cups showing equivalent units.**

Metric          Household          Mixed System

The surface, called the meniscus, of a liquid in a medication cup is not flat (● **Figure 5.2**). It is curved. Read the amount of liquid at the level of the bottom of the meniscus.

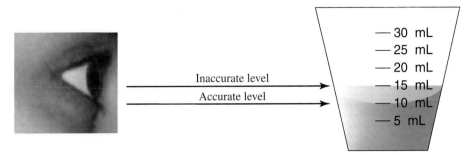

● **Figure 5.2**
**Medication cup filled to 10 mL.**

## Metric-Household Conversions

### EXAMPLE 5.1

**Convert 8 teaspoons to an equivalent volume measured in milliliters.**

$$8\,t = ?\,mL$$

In this problem, there are two quantities: *teaspoons* and *milliliters*.

Think of the problem this way:

$$8\,t = x\,mL$$
$$1\,t = 5\,mL \quad \text{(known equivalent)}$$

Because the number of teaspoons and the number of milliliters are proportional, a proportion could be used to solve the problem. One way to set up the proportion is

$$\frac{t}{mL} = \frac{t'}{mL'}$$

Substituting, you obtain

$$\frac{8t}{x\,mL} = \frac{1t}{5\,mL}$$

Eliminate the units of measurement

$$\frac{8}{x} = \frac{1}{5}$$

Cross multiply and simplify

$$\frac{8}{x} \diagdown \frac{1}{5}$$

$$(x)(1) = (8)(5)$$
$$x = 40$$

So, 8 teaspoons are equivalent to 40 milliliters.

**NOTE**

Although 1 t is approximately equal to 5 mL, in Example 5.1, for simplicity, the equal sign is used. This practice will be followed throughout the textbook.

### EXAMPLE 5.2

Change $1\frac{1}{2}$ pints to an equivalent number of milliliters.

$$1\frac{1}{2} \text{ pt } = ? \text{ mL}$$

Think of the problem this way:

$$1\frac{1}{2} \text{ pt } = x \text{ mL}$$

$$1 \text{ pt } = 500 \text{ mL} \quad \text{(known equivalent)}$$

One way to set up the proportion is

$$\frac{pt}{mL} = \frac{pt'}{mL'}$$

Substituting, you obtain

$$\frac{1\frac{1}{2}pt}{x \, mL} = \frac{1 \, pt}{500 \, mL}$$

Eliminate the units of measurement

$$\frac{1\frac{1}{2}}{x} = \frac{1}{500}$$

Cross multiply and simplify

$$\frac{1\frac{1}{2}}{x} = \frac{1}{500}$$

$$(x)(1) = \left(1\frac{1}{2}\right)(500)$$

$$x = 750$$

So, $1\frac{1}{2}$ pints is equivalent to 750 milliliters.

### EXAMPLE 5.3

**A patient is to receive 60 milliliters of a medication. How many ounces will the patient receive?**

Think of the problem this way:

$$60 \text{ mL } = x \text{ oz}$$

$$30 \text{ mL } = 1 \text{ oz} \quad \text{(known equivalent)}$$

One way to set up the proportion is

$$\frac{mL}{oz} = \frac{mL'}{oz'}$$

Substituting, you obtain

$$\frac{60\ mL}{x\ oz} = \frac{30\ mL}{1\ oz}$$

Eliminate the units of measurement

$$\frac{60}{x} = \frac{30}{1}$$

Cross multiply and simplify

$$\frac{60}{x} = \frac{30}{1}$$

$$(x)(30) = (1)(60)$$
$$30\,x = 60$$

Divide by 30 and cancel

$$\frac{\cancel{30}\,x}{\cancel{30}} = \frac{60}{30}$$
$$x = 2$$

So, the patient will receive 2 ounces of the medication.

> **NOTE**
>
> Example 5.3 could be done mentally by understanding that, because 1 ounce = 30 milliliters, then twice as many ounces (2 oz) will equal twice as many milliliters (60 mL). That is, 2 oz = 60 mL.

## EXAMPLE 5.4

**A medication cup contains 22.5 milliliters of a solution. How many tablespoons are in the medication cup?**

Think of the problem this way:

$$22.5\,mL = x\,T$$
$$15\,mL = 1\,T \quad \text{(known equivalent)}$$

One way to set up the proportion is

$$\frac{mL}{T} = \frac{mL'}{T'}$$

Substituting, you obtain

$$\frac{22.5\ mL}{x\ T} = \frac{15\ mL}{1\ T}$$

Eliminate the units of measurement, cross multiply, and simplify

$$\frac{22.5}{x} = \frac{15}{1}$$

$$(x)(15) = (1)(22.5)$$
$$15\,x = 22.5$$

Divide by 15 and cancel

$$\frac{\cancel{15}\,x}{\cancel{15}} = \frac{22.5}{15}$$

$$x = 1.5$$

So, the medication cup contains $1\frac{1}{2}$ tablespoons.

## EXAMPLE 5.5

**A patient weighs 150 pounds. What is the patient's weight measured in kilograms?**

Think of the problem this way:

$$150\,\text{lb} = x\,\text{kg}$$

$$2.2\,\text{lb} = 1\,\text{kg} \quad \text{(known equivalent)}$$

One way to set up the proportion is

$$\frac{lb}{kg} = \frac{lb'}{kg'}$$

Substituting, you obtain

$$\frac{150\ lb}{x\ kg} = \frac{2.2\ lb'}{1\ kg'}$$

Eliminate the units of measurement, cross multiply, and simplify

$$\frac{150}{x} = \frac{2.2}{1}$$

$$(x)(2.2) = (1)(150)$$

$$2.2\,x = 150$$

Divide by 2.2 and cancel

$$\frac{\cancel{2.2}\,x}{\cancel{2.2}} = \frac{150}{2.2}$$

$$x = 68.18$$

So, the patient weighs 68 kilograms.

## EXAMPLE 5.6

**An infant weighs 4 kilograms. What is the infant's weight measured in pounds and ounces?**

First change the weight to pounds.

Think of the problem this way:

$$4\,\text{kg} = x\,\text{lb}$$

$$1\,\text{kg} = 2.2\,\text{lb} \quad \text{(known equivalent)}$$

One way to set up the proportion is

$$\frac{lb}{kg} = \frac{lb'}{kg'}$$

Substituting, you obtain

$$\frac{x\ lb}{4\ kg} = \frac{2.2\ lb}{1\ kg}$$

Eliminate the units of measurement, cross multiply, and simplify

$$\frac{x}{4} = \frac{2.2}{1}$$

$$(4)(2.2) = (1)(x)$$
$$8.8 = x$$

The infant weighs 8.8 pounds (8 pounds + 0.8 pounds).
To change the 0.8 pound to ounces, think of the problem as

$$0.8\,lb = x\,oz$$
$$1\,lb = 16\,oz \quad \text{(known equivalent)}$$

One way to set up the proportion is

$$\frac{lb}{oz} = \frac{lb'}{oz'}$$

Substituting you obtain

$$\frac{0.8\ lb}{x\ oz} = \frac{1\ lb}{16\ oz}$$

Eliminate the units of measurement, cross multiply, and simplify

$$\frac{0.8}{x} = \frac{1}{16}$$

$$(1)(x) = (0.8)(16)$$
$$x = 12.8 \approx 13$$

The infant weighs 8 pounds 13 ounces.

## EXAMPLE 5.7

**A tumor has a diameter of 2 inches. What is the diameter of the tumor measured in millimeters?**

First use the equivalence 2.5 centimeters = 1 inch.
   Think of the problem this way:

$$2\,in = x\,cm$$
$$1\,in = 2.5\,cm \quad \text{(known equivalent)}$$

One way to set up the proportion is

$$\frac{in}{cm} = \frac{in'}{cm'}$$

Substituting, you obtain

$$\frac{2\ in}{x\ cm} = \frac{1\ in}{2.5\ cm}$$

Eliminate the units of measurement, cross multiply, and simplify

$$\frac{2}{x} = \frac{1}{2.5}$$

$$(x)(1) = (2)(2.5)$$
$$x = 5$$

So, the diameter of the tumor is 5 centimeters. Now change to millimeters.

$$5\ cm = ?\ mm$$

To convert *centimeters* to *millimeters*, is a jump of *1 place to the right.*

| meter | decimeter | centimeter | millimeter |
|-------|-----------|------------|------------|
| m     | dm        | cm         | mm         |

So, in 5 cm, move the decimal point *1 place to the right.*

$$5\ cm = 5.0\ cm = 5\ 0\ .\ mm = 50.\ mm = 50\ mm$$

So, the tumor has a diameter of 50 millimeters.

## EXAMPLE 5.8

**Adam is 6 feet 3 inches tall. What is his height in centimeters?**

$$6\ ft\ 3\ in \quad means \quad 6\ ft + 3\ in$$

First, determine Adam's height in inches. To do this, convert 6 feet to inches.

Think of the problem this way:

$$6\ ft = x\ in$$
$$1\ ft = 12\ in \quad (known\ equivalent)$$

One way to set up the proportion is

$$\frac{6\ ft}{x\ in} = \frac{1\ ft}{12\ in}$$

Eliminate the units of measurement, cross multiply, and simplify

$$\frac{6\ ft}{x\ in} = \frac{1\ ft}{12\ in}$$

$$(1)(x) = (6)(12)$$
$$x = 72$$

**NOTE**

In Example 5.8, the 6 feet could have been changed to 72 inches by understanding that because 1 foot = 12 inches, then 6 times as many feet (6 ft) will equal six times as many inches (72 in). That is, 6 ft = 72 in.

Now, add the extra 3 inches.

$$72\ in + 3\ in = 75\ in$$

Adam is 75 inches tall.

To change 75 inches to centimeters, think of the problem as

$$75\ in = x\ cm$$
$$1\ in = 2.5\ cm \quad \text{(known equivalent)}$$

One way to set up the proportion is

$$\frac{75\ in}{x\ cm} = \frac{1\ in}{2.5\ cm}$$

Eliminate the units of measurement, cross multiply, and simplify

$$\frac{75\ in}{x\ cm} = \frac{1\ in}{2.5\ cm}$$

$$(1)(x) = (75)(2.5)$$
$$x = 187.5 \approx 188$$

So, Adam is 188 centimeters tall.

## EXAMPLE 5.9

**Jennifer weighs 115 pounds 8 ounces. What is her weight in kilograms?**

$$115\ lb\ 8\ oz \quad \text{means} \quad 115\ lb + 8\ oz$$

First, determine Jennifer's weight in pounds. To do this, convert 8 ounces to pounds.

Think of the problem this way:

$$8\ oz = x\ lb$$
$$16\ oz = 1\ lb \quad \text{(known equivalent)}$$

One way to set up the proportion is

$$\frac{8\ oz}{x\ lb} = \frac{16\ oz}{1\ lb}$$

Eliminate the units of measurement, cross multiply, and simplify

$$\frac{8\ oz}{x\ lb} = \frac{16\ oz}{1\ lb}$$

$$(16)(x) = (8)(1)$$

$$16x = 8$$

Divide by the coefficient of $x$, cancel, and simplify

$$\frac{16x}{16} = \frac{8}{16}$$

$$x = \frac{1}{2}$$

Jennifer weighs $115\frac{1}{2}$ pounds.
Now, change 115.5 pounds to kilograms.
 To change 115.5 pounds to kilograms, think of the problem as

$$115.5\ \text{lb} = x\ \text{kg}$$

$$2.2\ \text{lb} = 1\ \text{kg} \quad \text{(known equivalent)}$$

One way to set up the proportion is

$$\frac{115.5\ lb}{x\ kg} = \frac{2.2\ lb}{1\ kg}$$

Eliminate the units of measurement, cross multiply, and simplify

$$\frac{115.5\ lb}{x\ kg} = \frac{2.2\ lb}{1\ kg}$$

$$(2.2)(x) = (115.5)(1)$$

$$2.2\ x = 115.5$$

Divide by the coefficient of $x$, cancel, and simplify

$$\frac{2.2\ x}{2.2} = \frac{115.5}{2.2}$$

$$x = 52.5$$

So, Jennifer weighs 52.5 kilograms.

> **NOTE**
>
> In Example 5.9, the 8 ounces could have been changed to $\frac{1}{2}$ pound mentally by understanding that because 16 ounces = 1 pound, then one-half as many ounces (8 oz) will equal one-half as many pounds ($\frac{1}{2}$ lb). That is, 8 oz = $\frac{1}{2}$ lb.

# Summary

In this chapter, quantities measured in one system of measurement were converted to equivalent quantities measured in a different system of measurement.

- It is important to memorize all the equivalences for volume, weight, and length between the metric and household systems of measurement.

- Ratio and proportion can be used to perform conversions between the metric and household systems.

- The equivalences between systems are not exact equivalences; they are approximate equivalences.

■ When performing conversions between two systems, your answers are not exact; they are approximate.

■ When performing conversions between two systems, answers may differ somewhat, depending on which approximate equivalences are used.

## Practice Sets

The answers to *Try These for Practice, Exercises,* and *Cumulative Review Exercises* are found in Appendix A. Ask your instructor for the answers to the *Additional Exercises.*

### Try These for Practice

Test your comprehension after reading the chapter.

1. In order to do the exercises at the end of this chapter, you need to memorize all the equivalents presented so far. To test yourself, fill in the missing numbers in the following chart.

### Metric System

(a)  1 L = _____ mL

(b)  1 kg = _____ g

(c)  1 g = _____ mg

(d)  1 mg = _____ mcg

(e)  1 cm = _____ mm

### Household System

(f)  1 qt = _____ pt

(g)  1 pt = _____ cups

(h)  1 cup = _____ oz

(i)  1 glass = _____ oz

(j)  1 oz = _____ T

(k)  1 T = _____ t

(l)  1 lb = _____ oz

(m)  1 ft = _____ in

### Mixed Systems

(n)  1 in ≈ _____ cm

(o)  1 kg ≈ _____ lb

(p)  1 t ≈ _____ mL

(q)  1 T ≈ _____ mL

(r)  1 oz ≈ _____ mL

(s)  1 cup ≈ _____ mL

(t)  1 glass ≈ _____ mL

(u)  1 pt ≈ _____ mL

(v)  1 qt ≈ _____ mL

(w)  1 oz = _____ T = _____ t ≈ _____ mL

(x)  1 qt = _____ pt = _____ cups = _____ oz ≈ _____ mL

2. A patient is receiving 5 mL of Indocin. Read the label in ● **Figure 5.3** to determine the number of grams the patient is receiving.

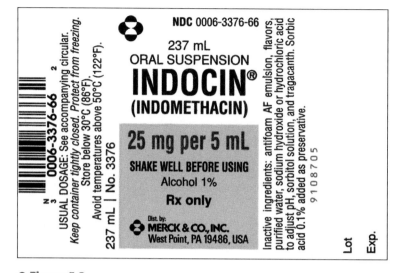

● **Figure 5.3**

**Drug label for Indocin.**

*(The labels for the products Indocin 25mg per 5mL are reproduced with permission of Merck & Co., Inc., copyright owner.)*

3. How many pounds is a person who weighs 50 kilograms?

4. Read the label in ● **Figure 5.4** and determine how many teaspoons of this antiviral drug would contain 50 milligrams of Retrovir.

5. A topical cream has been prescribed for a skin rash that covers an area of 4 cm by 5 cm. Change the dimensions of the rash to inches.

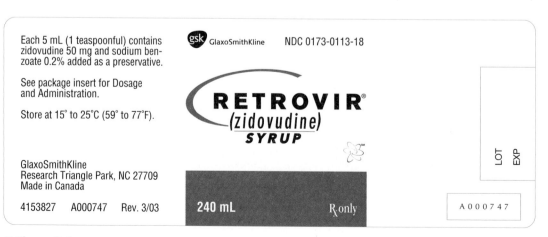

● **Figure 5.4**

**Drug label for Retrovir.**

*(Reproduced with permission of GlaxoSmithKline.)*

## Exercises

Reinforce your understanding in class or at home.

1. 4,500 mcg = _____ mg

2. 1.5 L = _____ mL

3. 4 t ≈ _____ mL

4. 15 mL ≈ _____ t

5. 45 kg ≈ _____ lb

6. 110 1b ≈ _____ kg

7. 48 oz = _____ pt

8. 3 oz = _____ T

9. 10 cm ≈ _____ in

10. 6 in ≈ _____ cm

11. A patient is 6 feet 2 inches tall. Find the height of the patient in centimeters.

12. Using the label in ●Figure 5.5, determine the number of ounces of the solution that would contain 10 mg of the antifungal drug fluconazole.

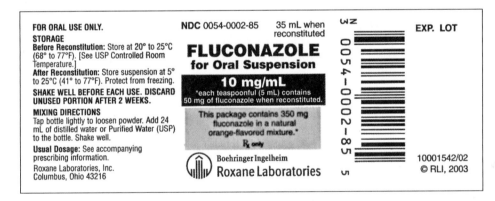

● Figure 5.5
**Drug label for fluconazole.**

*(Courtesy of Roxane Laboratories Inc.)*

13. A woman weighs 165 pounds. What is her weight in kilograms?

14. A patient takes 2 teaspoons of Robitussin (guaifenesin). How many milliliters of this cough suppressant did the patient take?

15. A nurse administers KCl 30 mL by mouth daily to Mrs. M. This patient is to be discharged, and she must continue to take the medication at home. How many tablespoons should she be advised to take daily?

16. Read the information in ●Figure 5.6 and determine the number of teaspoons of the bronchodilator metaproterenol you will administer if the label reads "10 mg/5 mL."

17. A patient drank 12 ounces of orange juice. How many milliliters did the patient drink?

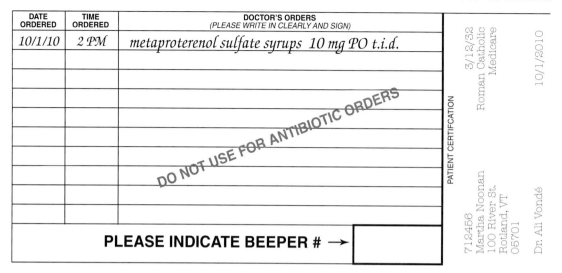

**UNIVERSITY HOSPITAL**

AUTHORIZATION IS HEPEBY GIVEN TO DISPENSE THE GENERIC OR CHEMICAL EQUIVALENT UNLESS OTHERWISE INDICATED BY THE WORDS — **NO SUBSTITUTE**

| DATE ORDERED | TIME ORDERED | DOCTOR'S ORDERS *(PLEASE WRITE IN CLEARLY AND SIGN)* |
|---|---|---|
| 10/1/10 | 2 PM | *metaproterenol sulfate syrups  10 mg PO t.i.d.* |
| | | |
| | | |
| | | |
| | | |
| | | |
| | | |
| | | |
| | | |

DO NOT USE FOR ANTIBIOTIC ORDERS

**PLEASE INDICATE BEEPER #** →

PATIENT CERTIFCATION

3/12/32
Roman Catholic
Medicare

10/1/2010

712456
Martha Noonan
100 River St.
Rotland, VT
05701

Dr. Ali Vondé

● **Figure 5.6**
**Physician's order sheet.**

Workspace

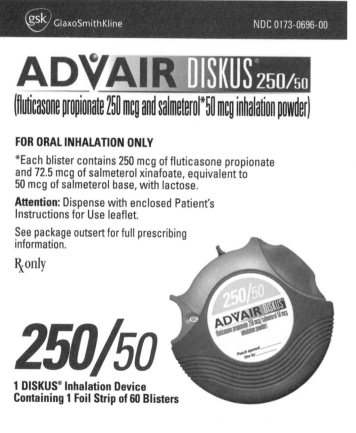

gsk GlaxoSmithKline                NDC 0173-0696-00

# ADVAIR DISKUS 250/50

(fluticasone propionate 250 mcg and salmeterol*50 mcg inhalation powder)

**FOR ORAL INHALATION ONLY**

*Each blister contains 250 mcg of fluticasone propionate
and 72.5 mcg of salmeterol xinafoate, equivalent to
50 mcg of salmeterol base, with lactose.

**Attention:** Dispense with enclosed Patient's
Instructions for Use leaflet.

See package outsert for full prescribing
information.

R only

## 250/50

**1 DISKUS® Inhalation Device
Containing 1 Foil Strip of 60 Blisters**

● **Figure 5.7**
**Drug label for Advair Diskus.**

*(Reproduced with permission of GlaxoSmithKline.)*

18. Use the label in ●**Figure 5.7** to determine the number of milligrams of fluticasone proprionate in one blister.

19. The label indicates that in the container there are 120 metered sprays, each of which contains 32 mcg of Rhinocort. Use this information to determine the total number of milligrams of this corticosteroid inhalant that are in the container.

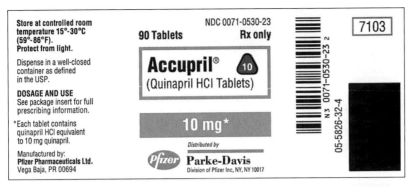

● **Figure 5.8**
**Drug label for Accupril.**

*(Reg. Trademark of Pfizer Inc. Reproduced with permission.)*

20. Read the label in ● **Figure 5.8** and determine the number of micrograms in 1 tablet of this antihypertensive drug.

# Additional Exercises

Now, test yourself!

1. Convert 3,200 micrograms to milligrams.

2. How many milligrams are contained in 250 grams?

3. 0.005 g = _____ mg

4. 0.004 mg = _____ mcg

5. 8 oz ≈ _____ mL

6. 0.7 mg = _____ g

7. 8.25 L = _____ mL

8. 10,700 mL = _____ L

9. A newborn is 50 cm long. The father wishes to know his infant's length in inches.

10. A person records his total fluid intake for one day as follows:

    Breakfast    8 oz coffee
                 4 oz pineapple juice
                 3 tablespoons of medication

    Lunch        8 oz water
                 12 oz broth
                 12 oz soda
                 6 oz gelatin dessert

    Dinner       12 oz water
                 1 pint tomato soup
                 16 oz tea
                 3 tablespoons of medication

    Calculate the total fluid intake for the day in liters.

11. Read the label in ● **Figure 5.9**. How many grams of codeine are contained in 5 milliliters?

12. A capsule of acetaminophen (Tylenol), an antipyretic drug, contains 0.5 gram. One capsule contains how many milligrams?

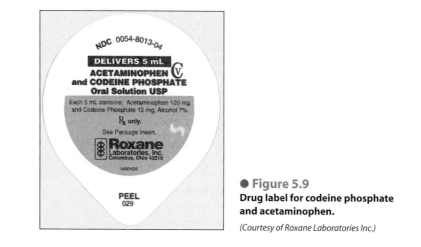

● **Figure 5.9**
**Drug label for codeine phosphate and acetaminophen.**

*(Courtesy of Roxane Laboratories Inc.)*

13. A prescriber ordered

*Biaxin (clarithromycin) 500 mg PO b.i.d.*

Using the label in ● **Figure 5.10**, determine the number of milliliters of this macrolide antibiotic drug you would give your patient.

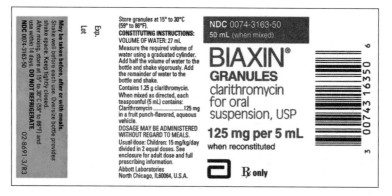

● **Figure 5.10**
**Drug label for Biaxin.**

*(Reproduced with permission of Abbott Laboratories.)*

14. How many teaspoons of the drug in ● **Figure 5.11** will contain 100 mg of the antibiotic Zyvox?

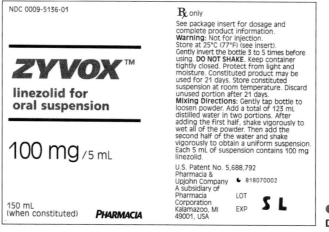

● **Figure 5.11**
**Drug label for Zyvox.**

15. Read the label in ●**Figure 5.12** to determine the number of grams in 1 tablet of the antibiotic ERY-TAB.

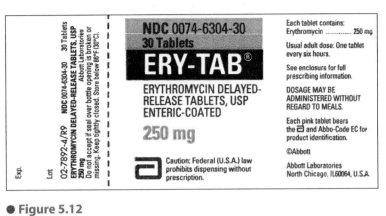

●**Figure 5.12**
**Drug label for Ery-Tab.**
*(Reproduced with permission of Abbott Laboratories.)*

16. The order is *Benadryl syrup (diphenhydramine HCl) 12.5 mg PO q6h.* The label reads 12.5 mg/5 mL. How many teaspoons of this antihistamine will you administer to your patient?

17. Read the label in ●**Figure 5.13** and determine the number of milligrams of this cardiac medication in one milliliter of this elixir.

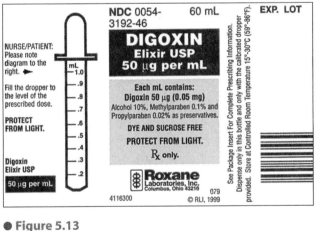

●**Figure 5.13**
**Drug label for Digoxin.**
*(Courtesy of Roxane Laboratories Inc.)*

18. Read the information on the physician's order sheet in ●**Figure 5.14**. How many micrograms of this antihypertensive drug will the patient receive in a day?

19. Read the label in ●**Figure 5.15** and determine the number of grams in 1 tablet of this oral hypoglycemic drug.

20. A postoperative patient has returned to the surgical unit after having received 5.3 liters of IV fluids during a procedure. How many milliliters of IV fluids did the patient receive?

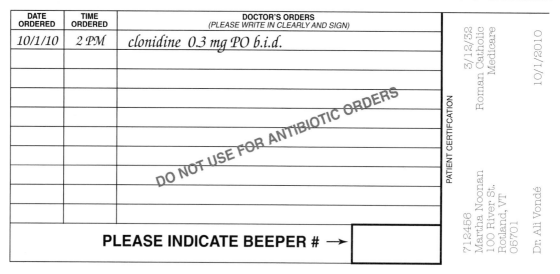

● **Figure 5.14**
**Physician's order sheet.**

Workspace

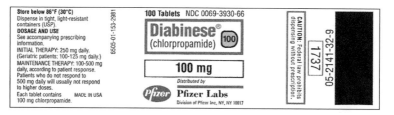

● **Figure 5.15**
**Drug label for Diabinese.**

*(Reg. Trademark of Pfizer Inc. Reproduced with permission.)*

# Cumulative Review Exercises

Review your mastery of previous chapters.

1.  Convert 0.125 milligrams to micrograms.

2.  0.009 g = _____ mg

3.  How many grams are contained in 5.65 kilograms?

4.  0.06 g = _____ mg

5.  7.75 L = _____ mL

6.  1,250 mL = _____ L

7.  Fill in the blanks:

    2.5 kg = _____ g = _____ mg = _____ mcg ≈ _____ lb = _____ oz

8.  In one day, a person drank 1 quart of water, $\frac{1}{2}$ pint of orange juice, and 2 cups of milk. How many milliliters of fluid did the person consume?

9. An infant's head circumference is 38 centimeters. What is this amount in inches?

10. The infant takes 4 ounces of formula every 3 hours (throughout both day and night). How many quarts of formula should the parents buy for a 1-week supply?

11. A patient drank two-thirds of a cup of water. How many milliliters of water did this patient drink?

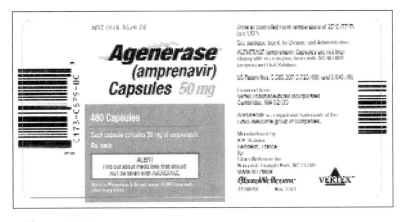

● Figure 5.16
**Drug label for Agenerase.**
*(Reproduced with permission of GlaxoSmithKline.)*

12. Read the label in ● **Figure 5.16**. How many grams of the antiretroviral drug Agenerase are contained in 3 capsules?

13. Read the label in ● **Figure 5.17**. Calculate the number of grams in 1 tablet of this antihistamine.

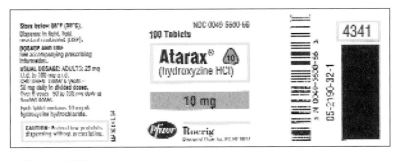

● Figure 5.17
**Drug label for Atarax.**
*(Reg. Trademark of Pfizer inc. Reproduced with permission.)*

14. The school nurse would like to administer $2\frac{1}{2}$ teaspoons of oral liquid Children's Tylenol to each child in a group of feverish students who come to her office. If the nurse has on hand only 15 ounces of the drug, how many doses can she administer?

**Workspace**

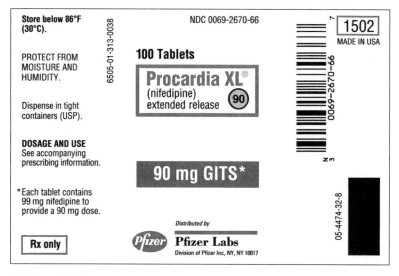

● **Figure 5.18**
**Drug label for Procardia XL.**

*(Reg. Trademark of Pfizer Inc. Reproduced with permission.)*

15. Read the label in ● **Figure 5.18** and determine the number of grams in 1 tablet of this antianginal drug.

**MediaLink**
www.prenhall.com/giangrasso

Animated examples, interactive practice questions with animated solutions, and challenge tests for this chapter can be found on the Pearson Dosage Calculation Tutor that accompanies this text. Additional, unique, interactive resources and activities can be found on the Companion Web site.

# Unit

# 3

# Oral and Parenteral Medications

# Chapter

## 6

# Oral Medication Doses

## Learning Outcomes

After completing this chapter, you will be able to

1. Calculate one-step problems for oral medications in solid and liquid form.
2. Calculate multi-step problems for oral medications in solid and liquid form.
3. Calculate doses for medications measured in milliequivalents.
4. Interpret drug labels in order to calculate doses for oral medication.
5. Calculate doses based on body weight.
6. Calculate body surface area (BSA) using a formula or a nomogram.
7. Calculate doses based on body surface area (BSA).

$\mathbf{I}$n this chapter you will learn how to calculate doses of oral medications in solid or liquid form. You will also be introduced to problems that use body weight or body surface area (BSA) to calculate dosages.

# One-Step Problems

In the calculations you have done in previous chapters, all the equivalents have come from standard tables, for example, 1t = 5 mL. In this chapter, the equivalent used will depend on the *strength of the drug* that is available; for example *1 tab = 15 mg*. In the following examples, the equivalent is found on the label of the drug container.

## Medication in Solid Form

Oral medications are the most common type of prescription. As discussed in Chapter 2, oral medications come in many forms (tablets, scored, enteric coated, capsules, caplets, and liquid), and drug manufacturers prepare oral medications in commonly prescribed dosages. Oral medications are usually supplied in different strengths.

Whenever possible, it is preferable to obtain the medication in the same strength as the dose ordered, or if that is not available, choose a strength that equals a multiple of the prescribed dose. For example, if the order requires 100 mg to be administered, tablets with a strength of 100 mg/tab would make dosage computation unnecessary, and 1 tablet would be administered. However, tablets with a strength of 50 mg/tab would make dosage computation simple (100 is 2 times 50), and 2 tablets would be administered.

In clinical settings, unit-dose medications are usually supplied by the pharmacist.

It is best to *administer the fewest number of tablets or capsules possible.* For example, if a prescriber orders *ampicillin 500 mg po q12h* and you have both the 250-mg and 500-mg capsules available, then you would administer one 500-mg capsule rather than two 250-mg capsules.

> **NOTE**
>
> If your calculations indicate a large number of tablets (or capsules) per dose, you should verify your calculations with another health professional. Also check the usual dosage of the medication with a pharmacist and/or a drug reference.

### EXAMPLE 6.1

**The order reads *Cymbalta (duloxetine HCl) 120 mg PO daily.***

Read the drug label shown in ● **Figure 6.1**. How many capsules of this antidepressant drug will you administer to the patient?

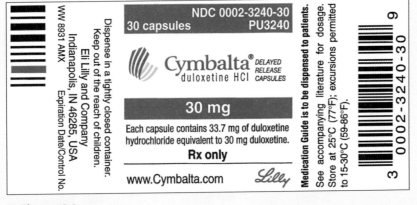

● **Figure 6.1**
**Drug label for Cymbalta.**

*(Copyright Eli Lilly and Company. Used with permission.)*

You want to change the prescribed dose of 120 mg to the number of capsules to be administered. The strength of the drug is 30 mg per cap.

Think of the problem this way:

$$120 \text{ mg} = x \text{ cap} \quad \text{(dose)}$$
$$30 \text{ mg} = 1 \text{ cap} \quad \text{(strength)}$$

One way to set up the proportion is

$$\frac{mg}{cap} = \frac{mg'}{cap'}$$

Substitute into the proportion

$$\frac{120 \; mg}{x \; cap} = \frac{30 \; mg}{1 \; cap}$$

Eliminate the units of measurement, cross multiply, and simplify

$$\frac{120}{x} = \frac{30}{1}$$

$$(30)(x) = (120)(1)$$
$$30x = 120$$

Divide both sides of the equation by 30, the coefficient of $x$.

$$\frac{30x}{30} = \frac{120}{30}$$

Simplify.

$$\frac{\cancel{30} x}{\cancel{30}} = \frac{120}{30}$$

$$x = 4$$

So, you would give 4 capsules by mouth once a day to the patient.

**NOTE**

Throughout this textbook, when calculating dosages to be administered to the patient, do your calculations for *one dose* of medication, unless otherwise directed.

## EXAMPLE 6.2

The prescriber orders *Geodon (ziprasidone) 40 mg PO b.i.d.* Read the drug label shown in ● Figure 6.2 and determine how many capsules you would give to the patient.

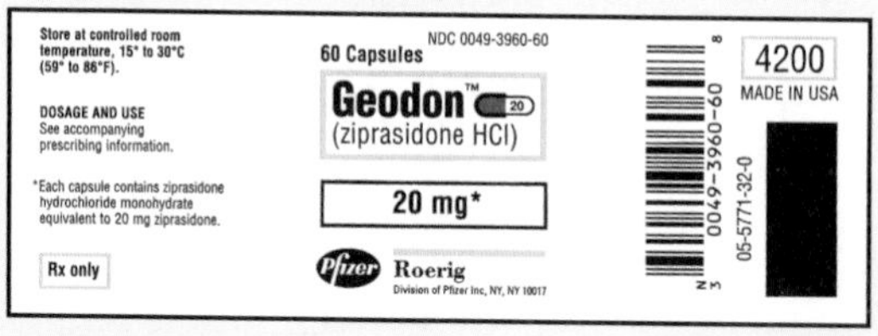

● **Figure 6.2**
**Drug label for Geodon.**

*(Reg. trademark of Pfizer Inc. Reproduced with permission.)*

You want to change the prescribed dose of 40 milligrams to the number of capsules to be administered. The strength of the drug is 20 mg per cap.

Think of the problem this way:

$$40 \text{ mg} = x \text{ cap} \quad \text{(dose)}$$
$$20 \text{ mg} = 1 \text{ cap} \quad \text{(strength)}$$

One way to set up the proportion is

$$\frac{mg}{cap} = \frac{mg'}{cap'}$$

Substitute into the proportion

$$\frac{40 \ mg}{x \ cap} = \frac{20 \ mg}{1 \ cap}$$

Eliminate the units of measurement, cross multiply, and simplify

$$\frac{40}{x} = \frac{20}{1}$$

$$(20)(x) = (40)(1)$$
$$20x = 40$$

Divide both sides of the equation by 20, the coefficient of $x$.

$$\frac{20x}{20} = \frac{40}{20}$$

Simplify.

$$\frac{20x}{20} = \frac{40}{20}$$
$$x = 2$$

So, you would give 2 capsules by mouth daily to the patient.

## EXAMPLE 6.3

Read the label in ● Figure 6.3. How many tablets of this narcotic analgesic will be needed for a dose containing 10 mg of hydrocodone bitartrate and 1,000 mg of acetaminophen?

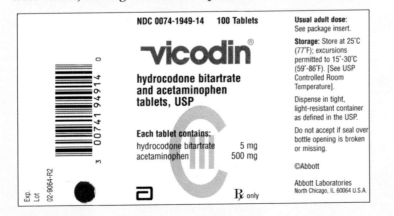

NDC 0074-1949-14     100 Tablets

**vicodin**®

**hydrocodone bitartrate and acetaminophen tablets, USP**

**Each tablet contains:**
hydrocodone bitartrate     5 mg
acetaminophen     500 mg

Usual adult dose:
See package insert.

**Storage:** Store at 25°C (77°F); excursions permitted to 15°-30°C (59°-86°F). [See USP Controlled Room Temperature].

Dispense in tight, light-resistant container as defined in the USP.

Do not accept if seal over bottle opening is broken or missing.

©Abbott

Abbott Laboratories
North Chicago, IL 60064 U.S.A.

℞ only

Exp.
Lot
02-9064-R2

● **Figure 6.3**
**Drug label for Vicodin.**

*(Reproduced with permission of Abbott Laboratories.)*

Vicodin is a combination drug (see Figures 2.24 and 2.25 in Chapter 2) composed of hydrocodone bitartrate and acetaminophen. Therefore, for computational purposes, you need address only the first listed drug (hydrocodone bitartrate). Because the dose requires 10 mg of hydrocodone bitartrate, convert the 10 mg to the appropriate number of tablets.

However, before doing any calculations, you should check to see if the ratios of the amounts of the two drugs in Vicodin are equivalent in both the *dose* and on the *label*.

The hydrocodone bitartrate-acetaminophen ratio in the *dose* is 10:1,000.

The hydrocodone bitartrate-acetaminophen ratio on the *label* is 5:500.

Set these two ratios equal to each other, and cross multiply as follows:

$$\frac{10}{1,000} = \frac{5}{500}$$

$$(5)(1,000) = (10)(500)$$
$$5,000 = 5,000$$

The ratios are equivalent because the products are equal, and you can now proceed with the calculations.

The strength of the drug is 10 mg (of hydrocodone Bitartrate) per tablet.

Think of the problem this way:

$$10 \text{ mg} = x \text{ tab} \quad \text{(dose)}$$
$$5 \text{ mg} = 1 \text{ tab} \quad \text{(strength)}$$

One way to set up the proportion is

$$\frac{mg}{tab} = \frac{mg'}{tab'}$$

Substitute into the proportion

$$\frac{10 \ mg}{x \ tab} = \frac{5 \ mg}{1 \ tab}$$

Eliminate the units of measurement, cross multiply, and simplify

$$\frac{10}{x} = \frac{5}{1}$$

$$(5)(x) = (10)(1)$$
$$5x = 10$$

Divide both sides of the equation by 5, the coefficient of $x$.

$$\frac{5x}{5} = \frac{10}{5}$$

Simplify.

$$\frac{5x}{5} = \frac{10}{5}$$
$$x = 2$$

So, 2 tablets are needed for the dose.

## EXAMPLE 6.4

The order is *Ery-Tab (erythromycin) 500 mg PO b.i.d.* The medication is available in two different strengths (● Figure 6.4). Determine how you would administer this dose using the fewest number of the available tablets.

**NOTE**

The chance of medication error increases as the number of tablets to be administered increases. Also, you need to consider the comfort of the patient who is required to swallow a large number of tablets. Many individuals do not like to take medication, and they may be reluctant to swallow large quantities of tablets.

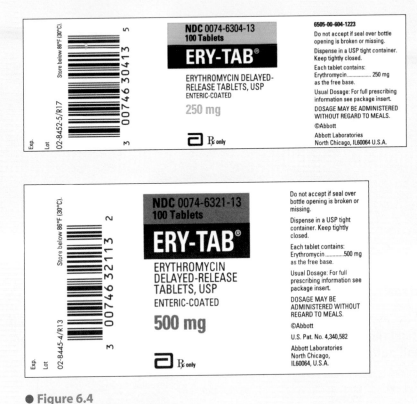

● **Figure 6.4**
**Ery-Tab labels of different strengths.**
*(Reproduced with permission of Abbott Laboratories.)*

If you select the *250 mg/tab strength*, you would need to administer *2 tablets* for the 500-mg dose.

If you select the *500 mg/tab strength*, you would need to administer *1 tablet* for the 500-mg dose.

Because you want to administer the fewest number of tablets, you would administer one 500-mg tablet.

## Medication in Liquid Form

Since pediatric and geriatric patients, as well as patients with neurological conditions, may be unable to swallow medication in tablet form, sometimes oral medications are ordered in liquid form. The label states how much drug is contained in a given amount of liquid.

For medications supplied in liquid form, you must calculate the volume of the liquid that contains the prescribed drug dosage. Medication cups, oral syringes, or calibrated droppers are used to measure the dose. See ● Figure 6.5.

**NOTE**

Some liquid oral medications are supplied with special calibrated droppers or oral syringes that are used *only* for these medications (e.g., digoxin and Lasix). Some medication cups do not accurately measure amounts less than 5 mL.

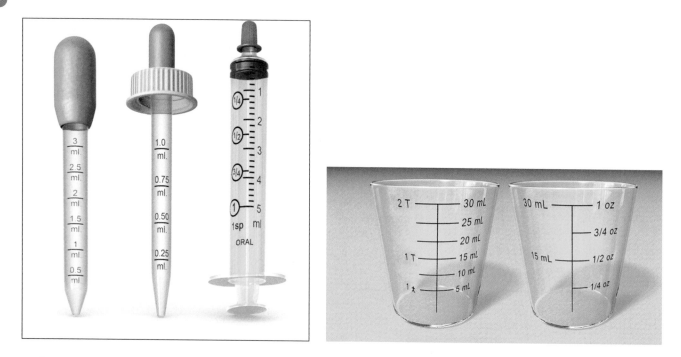

● **Figure 6.5**
**Measuring drugs in liquid form.**

## EXAMPLE 6.5

The prescriber orders *alprazolam oral solution 0.25 mg PO b.i.d.*
Read the label in ●Figure 6.6 and determine how many milliliters you
will administer.

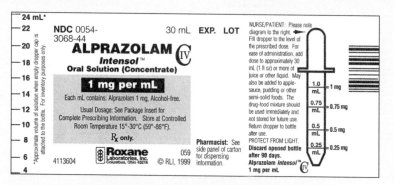

● **Figure 6.6**
**Drug label for alprazolam.**

*(Courtesy of Roxane Laboratories Inc.)*

You want to change the 0.25-mg dose prescribed to milliliters. The
strength of the drug is 1 mg (of alprazolam) per mL.

Think of the problem this way:

$$0.25 \text{ mg} = x \text{ mL} \quad \text{(dose)}$$
$$1 \text{ mg} = 1 \text{ mL} \quad \text{(strength)}$$

One way to set up the proportion is

$$\frac{mg}{mL} = \frac{mg'}{mL'}$$

Substitute into the proportion

$$\frac{0.25 \ mg}{x \ mL} = \frac{1 \ mg}{1 \ mL}$$

Eliminate the units of measurement, cross multiply, and simplify

$$\frac{0.25}{x} = \frac{1}{1}$$

$$(1)(x) = (0.25)(1)$$
$$x = 0.25$$

Because the label indicates that a calibrated dropper is included with this medication, this dropper should be used to administer 0.25 mL to the patient.

**NOTE**

The critical thinker would recognize that because the strength in Example 6.5 is 1 mg = 1 mL, this example does not require computation, that is, 0.25 mg = 0.25 mL.

## EXAMPLE 6.6

The physician orders *Lexapro (escitalopram oxalate) 10 mg PO once daily*. Read the label in ● Figure 6.7 and determine the number of milliliters you would administer to the patient.

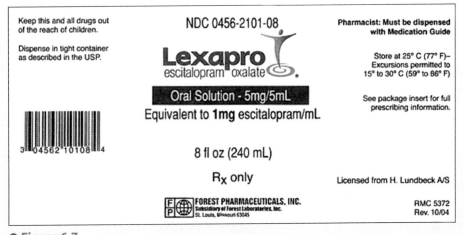

● **Figure 6.7**
**Drug label for Lexapro.**
*(Courtesy of Forest Pharmaceuticals, Inc.)*

You want to change the 10-mg dose to milliliters. The strength of the drug is 5 mg per 5 mL.

Think of the problem this way:

$$10 \ mg = x \ mL \quad \text{(dose)}$$
$$5 \ mg = 5 \ mL \quad \text{(strength)}$$

One way to set up the proportion is

$$\frac{mg}{mL} = \frac{mg'}{mL'}$$

Substitute into the proportion

$$\frac{10 \ mg}{x \ mL} = \frac{5 \ mg}{5 \ mL}$$

Eliminate the units of measurement, cross multiply, and simplify

$$\frac{10}{x} = \frac{5}{5}$$

$$(5)(x) = (10)(5)$$
$$5x = 50$$
$$x = 10$$

So, you would give 10 mL by mouth once a day to the patient. See ●Figure 6.8.

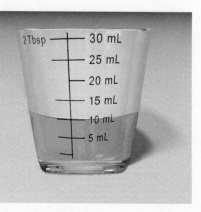

● **Figure 6.8**
**Medication cup with 10 mg (10 mL) of Lexapro.**

**NOTE**

In Example 6.6, the strength of 5 mg/5 mL is the same as 1 mg = 1 mL, as in Example 6.5. Therefore, this example also does not require computation, and 10 mg = 10 mL.

### EXAMPLE 6.7

The physician orders *Omnicef (cefdinir) 500 mg PO q12h*. Read the label in ● Figure 6.9. Determine the number of mL you would administer to the patient.

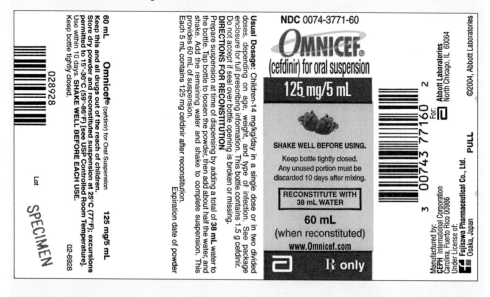

● **Figure 6.9**
**Drug label for Omnicef.**

*(Reproduced with permission of Abbott Laboratories.)*

You want to change the 500-mg dose prescribed to milliliters. The strength of the drug is 125 mg per 5 mL.

Think of the problem this way:

$$500 \text{ mg} = x \text{ mL} \quad \text{(dose)}$$
$$125 \text{ mg} = 5 \text{ mL} \quad \text{(strength)}$$

One way to set up the proportion is

$$\frac{mg}{mL} = \frac{mg'}{mL'}$$

Substitute into the proportion

$$\frac{500 \text{ mg}}{x \text{ mL}} = \frac{125 \text{ mg}}{5 \text{ mL}}$$

Eliminate the units of measurement, cross multiply, and simplify

$$\frac{500}{x} = \frac{125}{5}$$

$$(125)(x) = (500)(5)$$

$$125x = 2{,}500$$

$$x = \frac{2{,}500}{125}$$

$$x = 20$$

So, you would give 20 mL by mouth every 12 hours to the patient. See ● Figure 6.10.

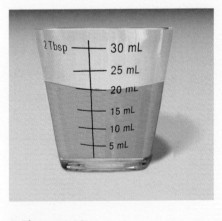

● **Figure 6.10**
**Medication cup with 500 mg (20 mL) of Omnicef.**

## Medications Measured in Milliequivalents

Some drugs are measured in **milliequivalents**, which are abbreviated as *mEq*. A milliequivalent is an expression of the number of grams of a drug contained in one milliliter of solution. Pharmaceutical companies label electrolytes (sodium chloride, potassium chloride, and calcium chloride, for example) in milligrams as well as in milliequivalents.

### EXAMPLE 6.8

Order: *potassium chloride 30 mEq PO daily*. Read the label in ● Figure 6.11 and determine how many tablets of this electrolyte supplement you should administer.

**potassium chloride**
extended-release tablets
## 10 mEq (750 mg)

● **Figure 6.11**
**Drug label for potassium chloride.**

In this problem, you want to change 30 mEq to tablets.
   The strength of the drug is 10 mEq per tablet.
   Think of the problem this way:

$$30 \text{ mEq} = x \text{ tab} \quad (\text{dose})$$
$$10 \text{ mEq} = 1 \text{ tab} \quad (\text{strength})$$

One way to set up the proportion is

$$\frac{mEq}{tab} = \frac{mEq'}{tab'}$$

Substitute into the proportion

$$\frac{30 \ mEq}{x \ tab} = \frac{10 \ mEq}{1 \ tab}$$

Eliminate the units of measurement, cross multiply, and simplify

$$\frac{30}{x} = \frac{10}{1}$$
$$10x = 30$$
$$x = 3$$

So, you would administer 3 tablets of potassium chloride by mouth once daily.

### EXAMPLE 6.9

The prescriber ordered *potassium chloride 10 mEq PO daily*. Read the label in ● Figure 6.12 and determine how many milliliters of this electrolyte supplement you should administer.

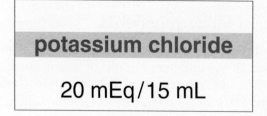

**potassium chloride**

## 20 mEq/15 mL

● **Figure 6.12**
**Drug label for potassium chloride.**

You want to change 10 mEq to milliliters. The strength of the drug is 20 mEq per 15 mL.

Think of the problem this way:

$$10 \text{ mEq} = x \text{ mL} \quad \text{(dose)}$$
$$20 \text{ mEq} = 15 \text{ mL} \quad \text{(strength)}$$

One way to set up the proportion is

$$\frac{mEq}{mL} = \frac{mEq'}{mL'}$$

Substitute into the proportion

$$\frac{10 \ mEq}{xmL} = \frac{20 \ mEq}{15 \ mL}$$

Eliminate the units of measurement, cross multiply, and simplify

$$\frac{10}{x} = \frac{20}{15}$$

$$20x = 150$$
$$x = 7.5$$

So, you should administer 7.5 mL of potassium chloride.

**ALERT**

Potassium chloride is a high alert drug. Follow the manufacturer's directions for diluting.

## Multistep Problems

Sometimes you will encounter problems that require more than one step to solve. These are called **multistep problems**. Recall that multistep problems were first examined in Chapter 3.

For example, suppose that you would like to know the number of tablets that would contain a dose of 0.0025 gram when the tablet strength is 1.25 mg per tablet.

You want to change 0.0025 g to tablets. The strength of the tablets is 1.25 mg per tab.

Think of the problem this way:

$$0.0025 \ \boxed{\text{g}} = x \text{ tab} \quad \text{(dose)}$$
$$1.25 \ \boxed{\text{mg}} = 1 \text{ tab} \quad \text{(strength)}$$

Notice that the g and mg do not match. Therefore, a conversion must be done before you can set up a proportion. In this case, change 0.0025 g to an equivalent amount of milligrams.

| kilogram | gram | milligram | microgram |
|----------|------|-----------|-----------|
| kg | g | mg | mcg |

Move the decimal point *3 places to the right.*

$$0.0025 \text{ g} = 0.\ 0\ 0\ 2\ 5 \text{ g} = 0002.5 \text{ mg} = 2.5 \text{ mg}$$

Now, think of the problem this way:

$$2.5 \text{ mg} = x \text{ tab} \quad \text{(dose)}$$
$$1.25 \text{ mg} = 1 \text{ tab} \quad \text{(strength)}$$

One way to set up the proportion is

$$\frac{2.5 \text{ mg}}{x \text{ tab}} = \frac{1.25 \text{ mg}}{1 \text{ tab}}$$

Eliminate the units of measurement, cross multiply, and simplify

$$\frac{2.5}{x} = \frac{1.25}{1}$$

$$1.25x = 2.5$$
$$x = 2$$

So, 2 tablets contain 0.0025 grams.

### EXAMPLE 6.10

**How many 300-mg aspirin tablets contain 0.9 g of aspirin?**

You want to change 0.9 g to tablets. The strength of the tablets is 300 mg per tab.

Think of the problem this way:

$$\begin{array}{c|c} 0.9 & g \\ \hline 300 & mg \end{array} = x \text{ tab} \quad \text{(dose)} \\ = 1 \text{ tab} \quad \text{(strength)}$$

Notice that the g and mg do not match. Therefore, a conversion must be done before you can set up a proportion. In this case, change 0.09 g to an equivalent amount of milligrams.

| kilogram | gram | milligram | microgram |
|----------|------|-----------|-----------|
| kg | g | mg | mcg |

Move the decimal point *3 places to the right.*

$$0.9 \text{ g} = 0.900 \text{ g} = 0.\,9\,0\,0 \text{ g} = 0900. \text{ mg} = 900 \text{ mg}$$

Now, think of the problem this way:

$$900 \text{ mg} = x \text{ tab} \quad \text{(dose)}$$
$$300 \text{ mg} = 1 \text{ tab} \quad \text{(strength)}$$

One way to set up the proportion is

$$\frac{900 \text{ mg}}{x \text{ tab}} = \frac{300 \text{ mg}}{1 \text{ tab}}$$

Eliminate the units of measurement, cross multiply, and simplify

$$\frac{900}{x} = \frac{300}{1}$$

$$300x = 900$$

$$x = 3$$

So, 3 tablets contain 0.9 grams of aspirin.

## EXAMPLE 6.11

Read the label in ● Figure 6.13 to determine the number of Diflucan tablets that would contain a dose of 0.4 g.

| Store below 86°F (30°C). | 6505-01-319-8248 | NDC 0049-3420-30 | | 1201 |
|---|---|---|---|---|
| **DOSAGE AND USE** See accompanying prescribing information. | | **30 Tablets** **DIFLUCAN®** ⟨100⟩ (Fluconazole Tablets) | 3 N 0049-3420-30  05-4671-32-4 | |
| Each tablet contains 100 mg fluconazole. | | **100 mg** | | |
| MADE IN USA | | | | |
| **Rx only** | | *Pfizer* **Roerig** Division of Pfizer Inc, NY, NY 10017 | | |

● **Figure 6.13**
**Drug label for Diflucan.**
*(Reg. trademark of Pfizer Inc. Reproduced with permission.)*

You want to change 0.4 g to tablets. The strength of the tablets is 100 mg per tab.

Think of the problem this way:

$$0.4 \boxed{\text{g}} = x \text{ tab} \quad \text{(dose)}$$

$$100 \boxed{\text{mg}} = 1 \text{ tab} \quad \text{(strength)}$$

Notice that the g and mg do not match. Therefore, a conversion must be done before you can set up a proportion. In this case change 0.0025 g to an equivalent amount of milligrams.

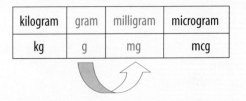

| kilogram | gram | milligram | microgram |
|---|---|---|---|
| kg | g | mg | mcg |

Move the decimal point *3 places to the right.*

$$0.4 \text{ g} = 0.400 \text{ g} = 0.\,4\,0\,0 \text{ g} = 0400. \text{ mg} = 400 \text{ mg}$$

Now, think of the problem this way:

$$400 \text{ mg} = x \text{ tab} \quad \text{(dose)}$$
$$100 \text{ mg} = 1 \text{ tab} \quad \text{(strength)}$$

One way to set up the proportion is

$$\frac{400 \; mg}{x \; tab} = \frac{100 \; mg}{1 \; tab}$$

Eliminate the units of measurement, cross multiply, and simplify

$$\frac{400}{x} = \frac{100}{1}$$

$$100x = 400$$
$$x = 4$$

So, 4 tablets contain 0.4 grams.

**NOTE**

Although Example 6.12 would be simpler using milligrams, we will do the calculation using micrograms in order to practice complex problems. For safety purposes, drug manufacturers often place both microgram and milligram concentrations on drug labels.

## EXAMPLE 6.12

The order is *Tikosyn (dofetilide) 0.5 mg PO b.i.d.* Read the label shown in ● Figure 6.14. Calculate how many capsules of this antiarrhythmic drug should be given to the patient. Although there are two strengths on the label (mcg and mg), calculate the problem using microgram strength.

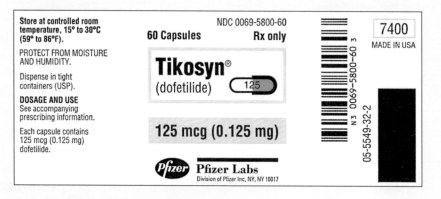

● **Figure 6.14**
**Drug label for Tikosyn.**
*(Reg. trademark of Pfizer Inc. Reproduced with permission.)*

You want to change 0.5 mg to capsules. The strength of the capsules is 125 mcg per cap.
Think of the problem this way:

$$0.5 \; \boxed{\text{mg}} = x \text{ cap} \quad \text{(dose)}$$

$$125 \; \boxed{\text{mcg}} = 1 \text{ cap} \quad \text{(strength)}$$

Notice that the mg and mcg do not match. Therefore, a conversion must be done before you can set up a proportion. In this case, change 0.5 mg to an equivalent amount of micrograms.

| kilogram | gram | milligram | microgram |
|----------|------|-----------|-----------|
| kg | g | mg | mcg |

Move the decimal point *3 places to the right.*

0.5 mg = 0.500 mg = **0. 5 0 0 mg** = 0500. mcg = 500 mcg

Now, think of the problem this way:

$$500 \text{ mcg} = x \text{ cap} \quad \text{(dose)}$$
$$125 \text{ mcg} = 1 \text{ cap} \quad \text{(strength)}$$

One way to set up the proportion is

$$\frac{500 \; mcg}{x \; cap} = \frac{125 \; mcg}{1 \; cap}$$

Eliminate the units of measurement, cross multiply, and simplify

$$\frac{500}{x} = \frac{125}{1}$$

$$125x = 500$$
$$x = 4$$

So, you should give 4 capsules by mouth twice a day to the patient.


## EXAMPLE 6.13

**The order is *Daypro (oxaprozin) 1.8 g PO once daily each morning*. The drug is supplied as 600 mg per caplet. How many caplets of this anti-inflammatory drug should be given the patient?**

You want to change 1.8 g to caplets. The strength of the caplets is 600 mg per cap.

Think of the problem this way:

$$1.8 \;|\; g \;| = x \text{ cab} \quad \text{(dose)}$$
$$600 \;|\; mg \;| = 1 \text{ cab} \quad \text{(strength)}$$

Notice that the g and mg do not match. Therefore, a conversion must be done before you can set up a proportion. In this case, change 1.8 g to an equivalent amount of milligrams.

| kilogram | gram | milligram | microgram |
|----------|------|-----------|-----------|
| kg | g | mg | mcg |

Move the decimal point *3 places to the right*.

$$1.8 \text{ g} = 1.800 \text{ g} = \textbf{1. 8 0 0 g} = \textbf{1800. mg} = 1,800 \text{ mg}$$

Now, think of the problem this way:

$$1,800 \text{ mg} = x \text{ cap} \quad \text{(dose)}$$
$$600 \text{ mg} = 1 \text{ cap} \quad \text{(strength)}$$

One way to set up the proportion is

$$\frac{1800 \; mg}{x \; cap} = \frac{600 \; mg}{1 \; cap}$$

Eliminate the units of measurement, cross multiply, and simplify

$$\frac{1800}{x} = \frac{600}{1}$$

$$600x = 1,800$$
$$x = 3$$

So, you should give 3 caplets by mouth to the patient once a day in the morning.

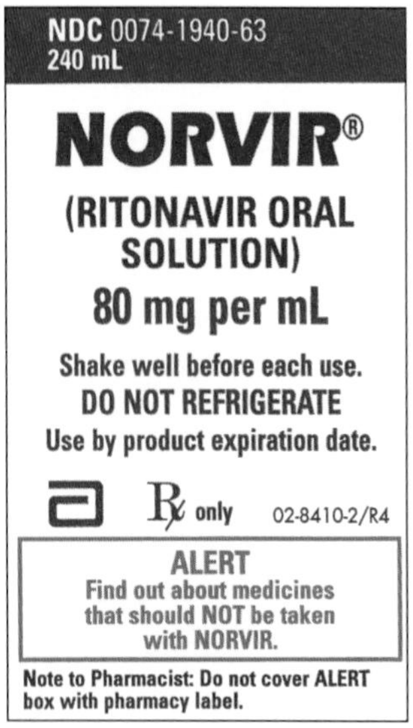

NDC 0074-1940-63
240 mL

# NORVIR®

**(RITONAVIR ORAL SOLUTION)**

**80 mg per mL**

Shake well before each use.
**DO NOT REFRIGERATE**
Use by product expiration date.

ᵃ  ℞ only    02-8410-2/R4

**ALERT**
Find out about medicines
that should NOT be taken
with NORVIR.

Note to Pharmacist: Do not cover ALERT
box with pharmacy label.

● **Figure 6.15**
**Drug label for Norvir.**

*(Reproduced with permission of Abbott Laboratories.)*

## EXAMPLE 6.14

The physician orders *Norvir (ritonavir) 0.6 g PO q12 hours*. Read the label in ● Figure 6.15 and determine the number of mL of this protease inhibitor your patient would receive.

You want to change 0.6 g to milliliters. The strength of the Norvir is 80 mg per mL.

Think of the problem this way:

$$0.6 \;\boxed{\text{g}} = x \text{ mL} \quad \text{(dose)}$$
$$80 \;\boxed{\text{mg}} = 1 \text{ mL} \quad \text{(strength)}$$

Notice that the g and mg do not match. Therefore, a conversion must be done before you can set up a proportion. In this case, change 0.6 g to an equivalent amount of milligrams.

| kilogram | gram | milligram | microgram |
|----------|------|-----------|-----------|
| kg | g | mg | mcg |

Move the decimal point *3 places to the right*.

$$0.6 \text{ g} = 0.600 \text{ g} = \textbf{0. 6 0 0 g} = \textbf{600. mg} = 600 \text{ mg}$$

Now, think of the problem this way:

$$600 \text{ mg} = x \text{ mL} \quad \text{(dose)}$$
$$80 \text{ mg} = 1 \text{ mL} \quad \text{(strength)}$$

One way to set up the proportion is

$$\frac{600 \, mg}{x \, mL} = \frac{80 \, mg}{1 \, mL}$$

Eliminate the units of measurement, cross multiply, and simplify

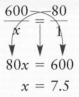

$$80x = 600$$
$$x = 7.5$$

So, you would give 7.5 mL by mouth to the patient every 12 hours.

### EXAMPLE 6.15

The order is *Indocin (indomethacin) 75 mg PO daily in 3 divided doses*. Read the label in ●Figure 6.16 and determine number of teaspoons of this anti-inflammatory drug you should administer.

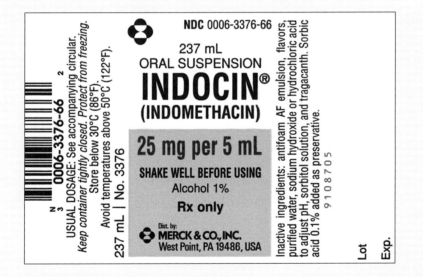

● **Figure 6.16**
**Drug label for Indocin.**

*(The labels for the products Indocin 25mg per 5mL are reproduced with permission of Merck & Co., Inc., copyright owner.)*

You want to change 75 mg to teaspoons. The strength of the Indocin is 25 mg/5 mL.

Think of the problem this way:

$$75 \text{ mg} = x \boxed{\text{ t }} \quad \text{(daily dose)}$$
$$25 \text{ mg} = 5 \boxed{\text{ mL}} \quad \text{(strength)}$$

**NOTE**

In Example 6.15, the order states "in three divided doses." This instructs the practitioner to separate the total daily dose into 3 equal parts over a 24-hour period. To ensure even distribution of the medication, the frequency of the doses should also be regular and consistent, so the drug is administered every 8 hours.

Notice that the t and mL do not match. Therefore, a conversion must be done before you can set up a proportion. In this case change 5 mL to an equivalent amount of teaspoons. You know that 5 mL = 1 t.

Now, think of the problem this way:

$$75 \text{ mg} = x \text{ t} \quad \text{(daily dose)}$$
$$25 \text{ mg} = 1 \text{ t} \quad \text{(strength)}$$

One way to set up the proportion is

$$\frac{75 \text{ } mg}{x \text{ } t} = \frac{25 \text{ } mg}{1 \text{ } t}$$
$$25x = 75$$
$$x = 3$$

So, the order is for 3 teaspoons daily.

Because the order specifies "3 divided doses," the 3 t must be divided into 3 equal amounts over 24 hours. Therefore, each dose would be 1 teaspoon (25 mg), and you would give 1 teaspoon of Indocin by mouth to the patient every 8 hours.

# Calculating Dosage by Body Weight

Sometimes the amount of medication is prescribed based on the patient's body weight. A patient who weighs more will receive a larger dose of the drug, and a patient who weighs less will receive a smaller dose of the drug.

Because the amount of drug is proportional to patient weight, a ratio and proportion method can be used to determine the amount of drug to administer to the patient. To save time, however, a shortcut method can also be used in which the weight of the patient is multiplied by the order to determine the amount of drug to administer. Although both methods are compared in Example 6.16, throughout the remainder of this book, the shortcut method will be used.

**NOTE**

The expression 15 mg/kg means that the patient is to receive 15 milligrams of the drug for each kilogram of body weight. Therefore, you will use the equivalent 15 mg (of drug) = 1 kg (of body weight).

### EXAMPLE 6.16

**The prescriber orders 15 milligrams per kilogram of a drug for a patient who weighs 80 kilograms. How many milligrams of this drug should the patient receive?**

*Using ratio and proportion:*

You want to "change" the body weight of the patient (80 kg) to milligrams of drug. The order is 15 mg/kg.

Think of the problem this way:

$$80 \text{ kg (body weight)} = x \text{ mg (drug)} \quad \text{(dose)}$$
$$1 \text{ kg (body weight)} = 15 \text{ mg (drug)} \quad \text{(order)}$$

One way to set up the proportion is

$$\frac{80\ kg}{x\ mg} = \frac{1\ kg}{15\ mg}$$

$$x = 1,200$$

*Using the shortcut:*

To determine the dose, simply multiply the *size of the patient* by the *order* as follows:

$$80\ kg \times \frac{15\ mg}{kg} = 1,200\ mg$$

Notice that you can cancel the *kg* units of measurement.

Therefore, the patient should receive 1,200 mg of the drug.

## EXAMPLE 6.17

The prescriber orders *Klonopin (clonazepam) 0.05 mg/kg PO daily in three divided doses* for a patient who weighs 60 kilograms. If each tablet contains 1 mg, how many tablets of this anticonvulsant drug should the patient receive per day? How many tablets would the patient receive per dose?

| | |
|---|---|
| Body weight: | 60 kg |
| Order: | 0.05 mg/kg |
| Strength: | 1 tab = 1 mg |
| Find: | ? tab |

When drugs are prescribed based on body weight, you generally start the problem with the weight of the patient.

The patient's weight is 60 kg and the order is for 0.05 mg/kg. Multiply the *size of the patient* by the *order* to determine how many milligrams of Klonopin to give the patient.

$$60\ kg \times \frac{0.05\ mg}{kg} = 3\ mg$$

So, the patient should receive 3 mg of Klonopin.

Now, convert the 3 mg of Klonopin to tablets. Since the strength of the tablets is 1 mg/tab, 3 mg would be contained in 3 tablets.

The patient should receive 3 tablets of Klonopin by mouth per day in 3 divided doses, and therefore the patient should receive 1 tablet every 8 hours.

**EXAMPLE 6.18**

The physician orders *Biaxin (clarithromycin) 7.5 milligrams per kilogram PO q12h*. If the drug strength is 250 milligrams per 5 mL, how many mL of this antibiotic drug should be administered to a patient who weighs 70 kilograms?

| | |
|---|---|
| Body weight: | 70 kg |
| Order: | 7.5 mg/kg |
| Strength: | 250 mg/5 mL |
| Find: | ? mL |

The patient's weight is 70 kg and the order is for 7.5 mg/kg. Multiply the *size of the patient* by the *order* to determine how many milligrams of Biaxin to give the patient.

$$70 \, kg \times \frac{7.5 \, mg}{kg} = 525 \, mg$$

So, the patient must receive 525 mg of Biaxin.

Now, convert the 525 mg of Biaxin to milliliters. The strength of the solution is 250 mg/5 mL.

Think of the problem this way:

$$525 \, mg = x \, mL \quad (dose)$$
$$250 \, mg = 5 \, mL \quad (strength)$$

One way to set up the proportion is

$$\frac{525 \, mg}{x \, mL} = \frac{250 \, mg}{5 \, mL}$$

$$250x = 2,626$$
$$x = 10.5$$

The patient should receive 10.5 mL of Biaxin by mouth every 12 hours.

# Calculating Dosage by Body Surface Area

In some cases, **body surface area (BSA)** may be used rather than weight in determining appropriate drug dosages. This is particularly true when calculating dosages for children, those receiving cancer therapy, burn patients, and patients requiring critical care. A patient's BSA can be estimated by using formulas or nomograms.

## BSA Formulas

Body surface area can be approximated by formula using either a hand-held calculator or an online Web site. BSA, which is measured in square meters ($m^2$), can be determined by using either of the following two mathematical formulas:

**NOTE**

Use a search engine, such as Google, to search the Web for "Body Surface Area Calculators" to obtain links to online BSA calculators.

**Formula for metric units:**

$$BSA = \sqrt{\frac{\text{weight in kilograms} \times \text{height in centimeters}}{3{,}600}}$$

**Formula for household units:**

$$BSA = \sqrt{\frac{\text{weight in pounds} \times \text{height in inches}}{3{,}131}}$$

### EXAMPLE 6.19

**Find the BSA of an adult who is 183 cm tall and weighs 92 kg.**

Because this example has metric units (kilograms and centimeters), we use the following formula:

$$BSA = \sqrt{\frac{\text{weight in kilograms} \times \text{height in centimeters}}{3{,}600}}$$

$$= \sqrt{\frac{92 \times 183}{3{,}600}}$$

At this point we need a calculator with a square-root key.

$$= \sqrt{4.6767}$$
$$= 2.16256$$

Therefore, the BSA of this adult is 2.16 m².

### EXAMPLE 6.20

**What is the BSA of a man who is 4 feet 10 inches tall and weighs 142 pounds?**

First you convert 4 feet 10 inches to 58 inches.

Because the example has household units (pounds and inches), we use the following formula:

$$BSA = \sqrt{\frac{\text{weight in pounds} \times \text{height in inches}}{3{,}131}}$$

$$= \sqrt{\frac{142 \times 58}{3{,}131}}$$

$$= \sqrt{2.6305}$$

$$= 1.62187$$

Therefore, the BSA of this adult is 1.62 m².

## Nomograms

BSA can also be approximated by using a chart called a nomogram (● **Figure 6.17**). The nomogram includes height, weight, and body surface area. If a straight line is drawn on the nomogram from the patient's height (left column) to the patient's weight (right column), the line will cross the center column at

**NOTE**

In Example 6.19, the metric formula for BSA was used, and in Example 6.20, the household formula for BSA was used. However, each formula provided the BSA measured in square meters (m²). In this book, we will round off BSA to two decimal places.

**NOTE**

Whether formulas or nomograms are used to obtain body surface area, the results are only approximations. This explains why we obtained both 2.16 m² (using the formula) and 2.20 m² (using the nomogram) as the BSA for the same patient in Example 6.19. This also occurred in Example 6.20, where the BSA was 1.62 m² (using the formula) and 1.59 m² (using the nomogram).

the approximate BSA of the patient. Before handheld calculators were used, the nomogram was the best tool available for determining BSA. Since electronic technology has been incorporated into most healthcare settings to ensure more accurate measurements, nomograms are becoming obsolete.

In Example 6.19 we used the formula to calculate the BSA of an 183 cm, 92 kg patient to be 2.16 m². Now let's use the adult nomogram to do the same problem. In ●Figure **6.18**, you can see that the line from 183 cm to 92 kg intersects the BSA column at about 2.20 m².

In Example 6.20, by using the formula we calculated the BSA of a 4 ft 10 in, 142 lb patient to be 1.62 m². If we use the adult nomogram to determine the BSA (●Figure **6.19**), we get 1.59 m².

## EXAMPLE 6.21

**The physician orders 40 mg/m² of a drug PO once daily. How many milligrams of the drug would you administer to an adult patient weighing 88 kg with a height of 150 cm?**

The first step is to determine the BSA of the patient. This can be done by formula or nomogram.

Using the formula, you get

$$BSA = \sqrt{\frac{88 \times 150}{3,600}}$$
$$= \sqrt{3.6667}$$
$$= 1.91 \text{ m}^2$$

Using the adult nomogram, you get 1.81 m². So, you can use either 1.91 m² or 1.81 m² as the BSA. If you choose to use 1.81 m², you want to convert BSA to dosage in mg.

BSA:      1.81 m²
Order:    40 mg/m²
Find:     ? mg

The patient's BSA is 1.81 *m²*, and the order is for 40 *mg/m²*. Multiply the *size of the patient* by the *order* to determine how many milligrams of the drug to give the patient.

$$1.81 \text{ m}^2 \times \frac{40 \text{ mg}}{\text{m}^2} = 72.4 \text{ mg}$$

If you use the BSA of 1.91 m², the calculations are similar.

$$1.91 \text{ m}^2 \times \frac{40 \text{ mg}}{\text{m}^2} = 76.4 \text{ mg}$$

So, if you use 1.81 m², you would administer 72.4 mg. However if you use 1.91 m², you would administer 76.4 mg of the drug to the patient.

**ALERT**

Before a medication is administered, it is the responsibility of the healthcare practitioner administering the medication to check the *safe dosage and administration range* for the drug in the *Physicians' Desk Reference* (PDR), in a designated drug book, or with the pharmacist.

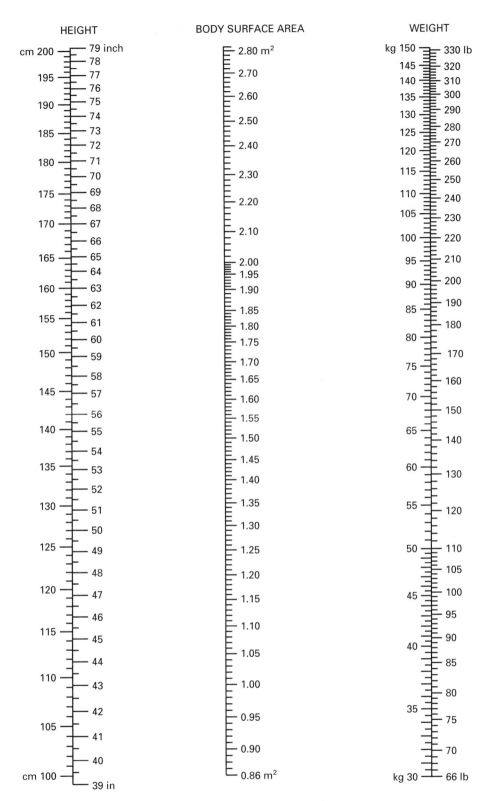

● Figure 6.17
Adult nomogram.

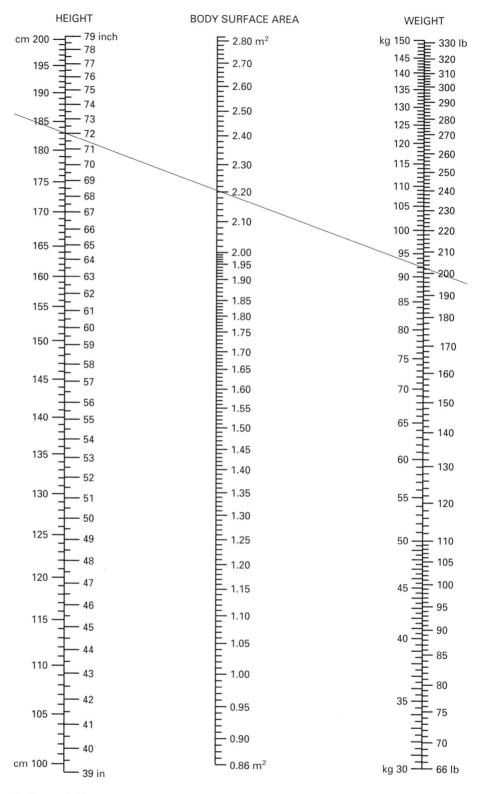

**● Figure 6.18**
**Nomogram for Example 6.19.**

HEIGHT                BODY SURFACE AREA              WEIGHT

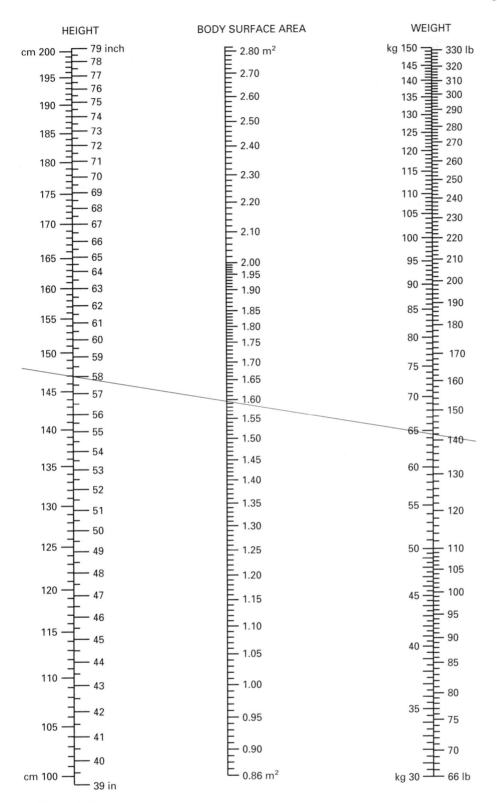

● **Figure 6.19**
**Nomogram for Example 6.20.**

**EXAMPLE 6.22**

The prescriber ordered 30 mg/m² of a drug PO stat for a patient who has a BSA of 1.65 m². The "safe dose range" for this drug is 20 to 40 mg per day. Calculate the prescribed dose in milligrams and determine if it is within the safe range.

| | |
|---|---|
| BSA: | 1.65 m² |
| Order: | 30 mg/m² |
| Find: | ? mg |

The patient's BSA is 1.65 $m^2$, and the order is for 30 $mg/m^2$. Multiply the *size of the patient* by the *order* to determine how many milligrams of the drug to give the patient.

$$1.65 \, \cancel{m^2} \times \frac{30 \text{ mg}}{\cancel{m^2}} = 49.5 \text{ mg}$$

The safe dose range is 20–40 mg per day.

So, the dose prescribed, 49.5 mg, is higher than the upper limit (40 mg) of the daily "safe dose range." Therefore, the prescribed dose is not safe, and you may not administer this drug. You must consult with the prescriber.

**EXAMPLE 6.23**

A drug is ordered at 3.3 mg/m² PO q12h for three doses. How many scored 5 mg tablets of this drug would you administer to patient with a BSA of 2.29 m²?

| | |
|---|---|
| BSA: | 2.29 m² |
| Order: | 3.3 mg/m² |
| Strength: | 1 tab = 5 mg |
| Find: | ? tab |

The patient's BSA is 2.29 $m^2$, and the order is for 3.3 $mg/m^2$. First, multiply the *size of the patient* by the *order* to determine how many milligrams of the drug to give the patient.

$$2.29 \, \cancel{m^2} \times \frac{3.3 \, mg}{\cancel{m^2}} \approx 7.56 \, mg$$

So, the patient must receive 7.56 mg of the drug.

Now, convert the 7.56 mg of the drug to tablets. The strength is 5 mg/tab.

Think of the problem this way:

$$7.56 \text{ mg} = x \text{ tab} \quad \text{(dose)}$$
$$5 \text{ mg} = 1 \text{ tab} \quad \text{(strength)}$$

One way to set up the proportion is

$$\frac{7.56 \, mg}{x \, tab} = \frac{5 \, mg}{1 \, tab}$$

$$5x = 7.56$$
$$x \approx 1.5 \text{ tab}$$

The patient should receive $1\frac{1}{2}$ scored tablets of the drug by mouth every 12 hours for 3 doses.

## Summary

In this chapter, you learned the computations necessary to calculate dosages of oral medications in liquid and solid form. You also learned about the equipment used to accurately measure liquid medication.

- It is crucial to ensure that every medication administered is within the recommended safe dosage range.

### Calculating doses for oral medications in solid and liquid form

- The label states the strength of the drug (e.g., 10 mg/tab, 15 mg/mL).
- Sometimes oral medications are ordered in liquid form for special populations such as pediatrics, geriatrics, and patients with neurological conditions.
- Some medication cups cannot accurately measure volumes less than 5 mL.
- Special calibrated droppers or oral syringes that are supplied with some liquid oral medications may be used to administer *only those medications*.
- Some drugs, such as electrolytes, are measured in milliequivalents (mEq).

### Calculating doses based on body weight

- Dosages based on body weight are generally measured in milligrams per kilogram (mg/kg).
- Start calculations with the weight of the patient.
- Multiply the size of the patient (kg) by the order to obtain the dosage.
- Medications may be prescribed by body weight in special populations such as pediatrics and geriatrics.

### Calculating doses based on body surface area

- Body surface area (BSA) is measured in square meters ($m^2$).
- Start calculations with the BSA of the patient.
- Multiply the size of the patient ($m^2$) by the order to obtain the dosage.
- BSA is determined by using either a formula or a nomogram.
- BSA may be utilized to determine dosages for special patient populations such as those receiving cancer therapy, burn therapy, and for patients requiring critical care.

# Case Study 6.1

Read the Case Study and answer the questions. The answers are found in Appendix A.

Mr. M. is a 68-year-old male patient with a past medical history of diabetes mellitus Type II and severe ischemic cardiomyopathy. He reported that for 6 weeks he had been experiencing shortness of breath and fatigue with moderate activity, difficulty sleeping at night, and has a weight gain of 5 lbs, even though he described his appetite as poor. There is no evidence of smoking or illegal drug use. Upon examination, the practitioner noted periorbital edema and bilateral 4+ pitting edema in both lower extremities. His present weight is 154 lb and his vital signs are BP 160/100, T 98.4, P 104, and R 28. Mr. M. was admitted for intravenous support and aggressive diuresis.

His orders are as follows:

- Complete CBC and SMA18
- Coronary angiogram; ECG; stress perfusion scan; chest X-ray
- Low-salt diet (2 g/day)
- Lasix (furosemide) 80 mg PO stat
- Lasix (furosemide) 60 mg PO q12h to begin 12 hours after the stat dose
- Digoxin 0.25 mg PO once daily
- Micro-K 10 Extencaps (potassium chloride) 20 mEq PO daily
- Diabinese (chlorpropamide) 125 mg PO each morning with breakfast
- Colace (docusate sodium) 100 mg PO t.i.d.
- Ativan (lorazepam) 3 mg PO HS
- Fluid restriction 1,500 mL/24 h
- Strict intake and output
- Foley catheter to bedside drainage

1. The patient drank 650 mL of $H_2O$, 150 mL of cranberry juice, and 200 mL of ginger ale during the 7 A.M. to 7 P.M. shift. How many mL of fluid may the patient be given over the next 12 hours?

2. At 8 P.M., Mr. M.'s wife fed him $1\frac{1}{2}$ cups of an organic brand of chicken broth, which contains 390 mg salt in each 1 cup serving.
   (a) How many mL of chicken broth did the patient receive?
   (b) How many grams of salt did he consume?
   (c) How much more salt should Mr. M. consume for the remainder of the day?

3. The diuretic drug Lasix (furosemide) is available in 20 mg tablets.
   (a) How many tablets will you administer for the stat dose?
   (b) How many tablets will the patient have received within the first 20 hours?

4. How many milliequivalents of the electrolyte supplement micro-K will the patient have received after 5 days of therapy?

5. Colace (docusate sodium), a stool-softening drug, is supplied as an oral liquid, 20 mg/5 mL.
   (a) How many times a day does the patient receive this medication?
   (b) How many mL would the patient receive in two days?

6. The available strength of Ativan (lorazepam) is 1 mg/tab. How many tablets of this sedative contain the prescribed dose?

7. The cardiac drug digoxin is supplied in the following strengths: 50 mcg, 100 mcg, and 200 mcg tablets. Which combination of tablets would yield the least number of tablets that would deliver the prescribed dose?

8. Mr. M. remains hospitalized for one week.
   (a) How many milligrams of Diabinese (chlorpropamide) would he have received by the end of the first seven days?
   (b) The Diabinese is available in 250 mg scored tablets. How many tablets would Mr. M. have received by the end of the seven days?

# Practice Reading Labels

Using the following labels, identify the strength of the medication and calculate the doses indicated. The answers are found in Appendix A.

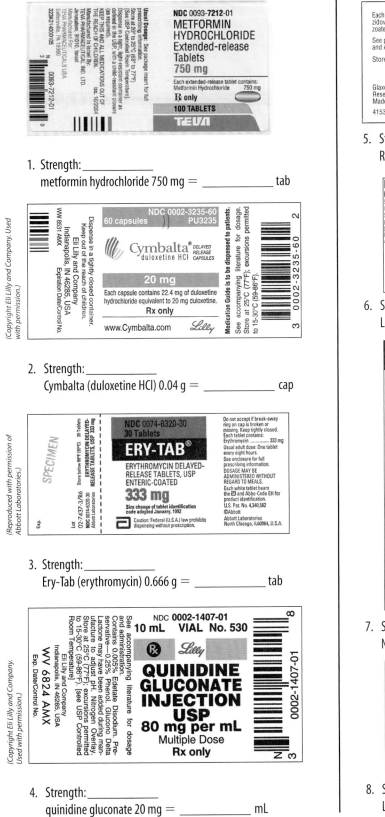

(Copyright Eli Lilly and Company. Used with permission.)

(Reproduced with permission of Abbott Laboratories.)

(Copyright Eli Lilly and Company. Used with permission.)

1. Strength: _____
   metformin hydrochloride 750 mg = _____ tab

2. Strength: _____
   Cymbalta (duloxetine HCl) 0.04 g = _____ cap

3. Strength: _____
   Ery-Tab (erythromycin) 0.666 g = _____ tab

4. Strength: _____
   quinidine gluconate 20 mg = _____ mL

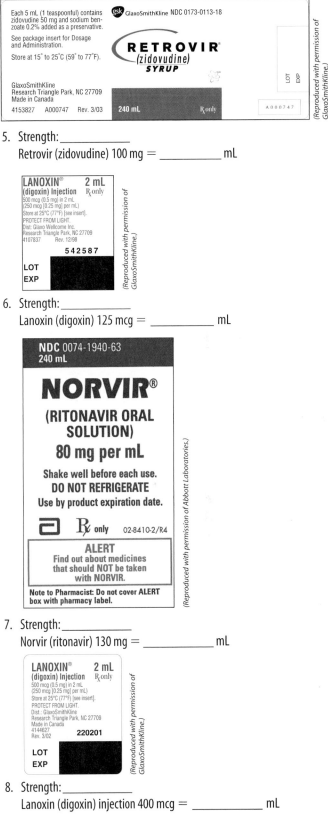

(Reproduced with permission of GlaxoSmithKline.)

(Reproduced with permission of GlaxoSmithKline.)

(Reproduced with permission of Abbott Laboratories.)

(Reproduced with permission of GlaxoSmithKline.)

5. Strength: _____
   Retrovir (zidovudine) 100 mg = _____ mL

6. Strength: _____
   Lanoxin (digoxin) 125 mcg = _____ mL

7. Strength: _____
   Norvir (ritonavir) 130 mg = _____ mL

8. Strength: _____
   Lanoxin (digoxin) injection 400 mcg = _____ mL

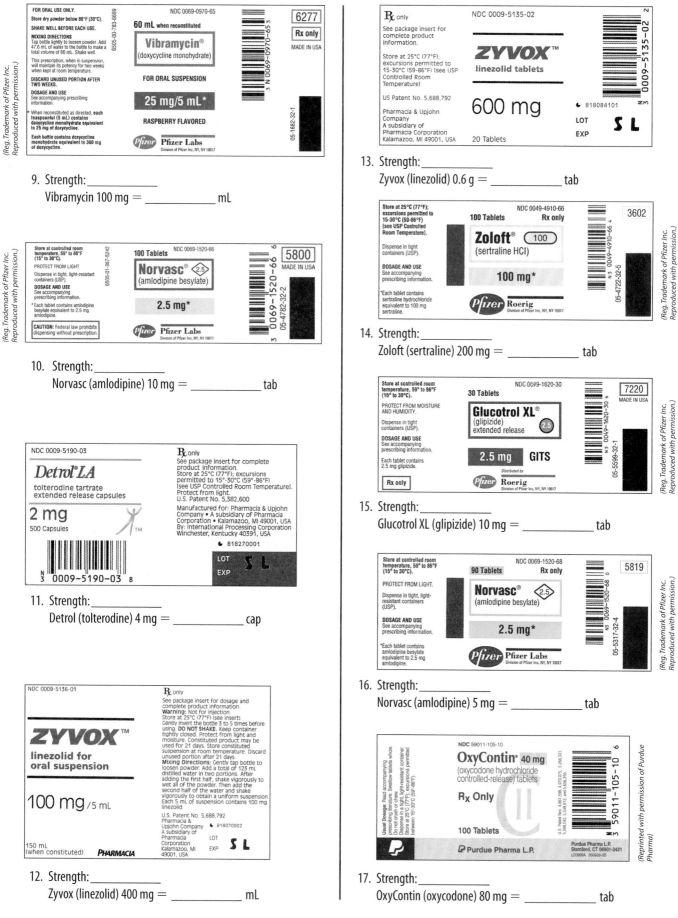

(Reg. Trademark of Pfizer Inc. Reproduced with permission.)

FOR ORAL USE ONLY.
Store dry powder below 86°F (30°C).
SHAKE WELL BEFORE EACH USE.
MIXING DIRECTIONS
Tap bottle lightly to loosen powder. Add 47.6 mL of water to the bottle to make a total volume of 60 mL. Shake well.
This prescription, when in suspension, will maintain its potency for two weeks when kept at room temperature.
DISCARD UNUSED PORTION AFTER TWO WEEKS.
DOSAGE AND USE
See accompanying prescribing information.
* When reconstituted as directed, each teaspoonful (5 mL) contains doxycycline monohydrate equivalent to 25 mg of doxycycline.
Each bottle contains doxycycline monohydrate equivalent to 300 mg of doxycycline.

NDC 0069-0970-65
**60 mL** when reconstituted
**Vibramycin®**
(doxycycline monohydrate)
FOR ORAL SUSPENSION
**25 mg/5 mL***
RASPBERRY FLAVORED
*Pfizer* **Pfizer Labs**
Division of Pfizer Inc, NY, NY 10017

6277
**Rx only**
MADE IN USA

9. Strength:_____
   Vibramycin 100 mg = _____ mL

Store at controlled room temperature, 59° to 86°F (15° to 30°C).
PROTECT FROM LIGHT.
Dispense in tight, light-resistant containers (USP).
DOSAGE AND USE
See accompanying prescribing information.
* Each tablet contains amlodipine besylate equivalent to 2.5 mg amlodipine.
CAUTION: Federal law prohibits dispensing without prescription.

100 Tablets   NDC 0069-1520-66
**Norvasc®** ⟨2.5⟩
(amlodipine besylate)
**2.5 mg***
*Pfizer* **Pfizer Labs**
Division of Pfizer Inc, NY, NY 10017

5800
MADE IN USA

10. Strength:_____
    Norvasc (amlodipine) 10 mg = _____ tab

NDC 0009-5190-03
*Detrol® LA*
tolterodine tartrate
extended release capsules
**2 mg**
500 Capsules

**R** only
See package insert for complete product information.
Store at 25°C (77°F); excursions permitted to 15°-30°C (59°-86°F) [see USP Controlled Room Temperature].
Protect from light.
U.S. Patent No. 5,382,600
Manufactured for: Pharmacia & Upjohn Company • A subsidiary of Pharmacia Corporation • Kalamazoo, MI 49001, USA
By: International Processing Corporation Winchester, Kentucky 40391, USA
☾ 818270001
LOT
EXP

11. Strength:_____
    Detrol (tolterodine) 4 mg = _____ cap

NDC 0009-5136-01
**ZYVOX™**
linezolid for
oral suspension
**100 mg** /5 mL
150 mL
(when constituted)   **PHARMACIA**

**R** only
See package insert for dosage and complete product information.
**Warning:** Not for injection.
Store at 25°C (77°F) (see insert).
Gently invert the bottle 3 to 5 times before using. **DO NOT SHAKE.** Keep container tightly closed. Protect from light and moisture. Constituted product may be used for 21 days. Store constituted suspension at room temperature. Discard unused portion after 21 days.
**Mixing Directions:** Gently tap bottle to loosen powder. Add a total of 123 mL distilled water in two portions. After adding the first half, shake vigorously to wet all of the powder. Then add the second half of the water and shake vigorously to obtain a uniform suspension. Each 5 mL of suspension contains 100 mg linezolid.
U.S. Patent No. 5,688,792
Pharmacia & Upjohn Company
A subsidiary of Pharmacia Corporation Kalamazoo, MI 49001, USA
☾ 818070002
LOT
EXP

12. Strength:_____
    Zyvox (linezolid) 400 mg = _____ mL

**R** only
See package insert for complete product information.
Store at 25°C (77°F); excursions permitted to 15-30°C (59-86°F) [see USP Controlled Room Temperature]
US Patent No. 5,688,792
Pharmacia & Upjohn Company
A subsidiary of Pharmacia Corporation Kalamazoo, MI 49001, USA

NDC 0009-5135-02
**ZYVOX™**
linezolid tablets
**600 mg**
20 Tablets

☾ 818084101
LOT
EXP
**S L**

13. Strength:_____
    Zyvox (linezolid) 0.6 g = _____ tab

Store at 25°C (77°F); excursions permitted to 15-30°C (59-86°F) [see USP Controlled Room Temperature].
Dispense in tight containers (USP).
DOSAGE AND USE
See accompanying prescribing information.
*Each tablet contains sertraline hydrochloride equivalent to 100 mg sertraline.

NDC 0049-4910-66
100 Tablets    **Rx only**
**Zoloft®** ⟨100⟩
(sertraline HCl)
**100 mg***
*Pfizer* **Roerig**
Division of Pfizer Inc, NY, NY 10017

3602

(Reg. Trademark of Pfizer Inc. Reproduced with permission.)

14. Strength:_____
    Zoloft (sertraline) 200 mg = _____ tab

Store at controlled room temperature, 59° to 86°F (15° to 30°C).
PROTECT FROM MOISTURE AND HUMIDITY.
Dispense in tight containers (USP).
DOSAGE AND USE
See accompanying prescribing information.
Each tablet contains 2.5 mg glipizide.
**Rx only**

NDC 0049-1620-30
30 Tablets
**Glucotrol XL®**
(glipizide)
extended release    ⟨2.5⟩
**2.5 mg**  **GITS**
Distributed by
*Pfizer* **Roerig**
Division of Pfizer Inc, NY, NY 10017

7220
MADE IN USA

(Reg. Trademark of Pfizer Inc. Reproduced with permission.)

15. Strength:_____
    Glucotrol XL (glipizide) 10 mg = _____ tab

Store at controlled room temperature, 59° to 86°F (15° to 30°C).
PROTECT FROM LIGHT.
Dispense in tight, light-resistant containers (USP).
DOSAGE AND USE
See accompanying prescribing information.
*Each tablet contains amlodipine besylate equivalent to 2.5 mg amlodipine.

NDC 0069-1520-68
90 Tablets    **Rx only**
**Norvasc®** ⟨2.5⟩
(amlodipine besylate)
**2.5 mg***
*Pfizer* **Pfizer Labs**
Division of Pfizer Inc, NY, NY 10017

5819

(Reg. Trademark of Pfizer Inc. Reproduced with permission.)

16. Strength:_____
    Norvasc (amlodipine) 5 mg = _____ tab

Usual Dosage: Read accompanying prescribing literature. Swallow tablets whole. Do not crush or chew.
Dispense in a tight, light-resistant container. Store at 25°C (77°F); excursions permitted between 15-30°C (59-86°F).
U.S. Patent Nos. 4,861,598, 4,970,075, 5,266,331, 5,508,042, 5,549,912, and 5,656,295.

NDC 59011-105-10
**OxyContin®** **40 mg**
(oxycodone hydrochloride controlled-release) tablets
**R**ₓ **Only**
100 Tablets
**P** **Purdue Pharma L.P.**
Purdue Pharma L.P.
Stamford, CT 06901-3431
L00999A 300928-00

(Reprinted with permission of Purdue Pharma)

17. Strength:_____
    OxyContin (oxycodone) 80 mg = _____ tab

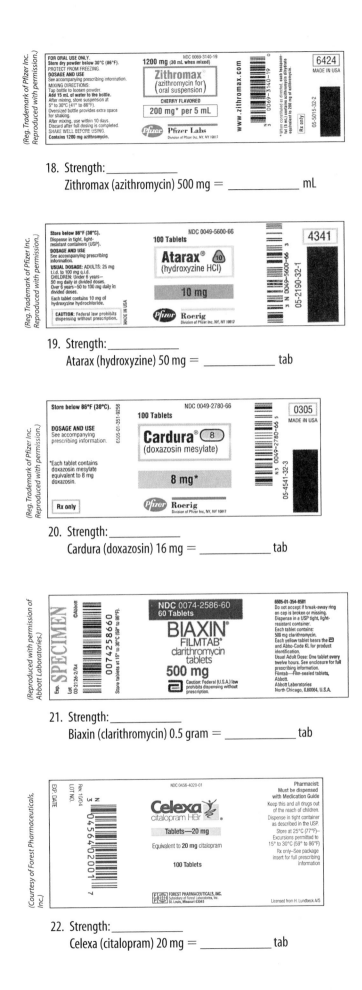

18. Strength:_____

    Zithromax (azithromycin) 500 mg = _____ mL

19. Strength:_____

    Atarax (hydroxyzine) 50 mg = _____ tab

20. Strength:_____

    Cardura (doxazosin) 16 mg = _____ tab

21. Strength:_____

    Biaxin (clarithromycin) 0.5 gram = _____ tab

22. Strength:_____

    Celexa (citalopram) 20 mg = _____ tab

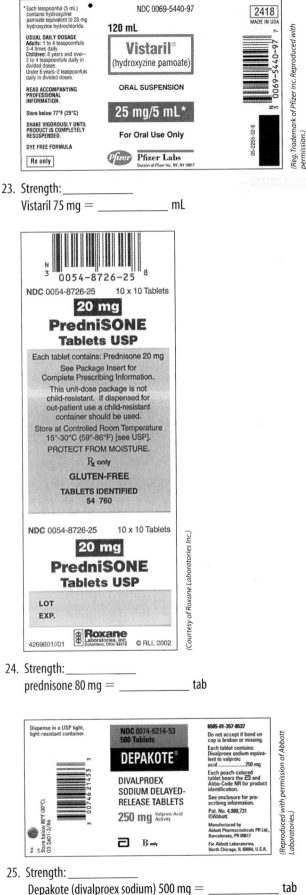

23. Strength:_____

    Vistaril 75 mg = _____ mL

24. Strength:_____

    prednisone 80 mg = _____ tab

25. Strength:_____

    Depakote (divalproex sodium) 500 mg = _____ tab

# Practice Sets

The answers to *Try These for Practice, Exercises,* and *Cumulative Review Exercises* are found in Appendix A. Ask your instructor for the answers to the *Additional Exercises.*

## Try These for Practice

Test your comprehension after reading the chapter.

1.  The order is *Accupril (quinapril HCl) 30 mg PO b.i.d.*

    (a)  Read the Label in ● **Figure 6.20** to determine how many tablets of this antihypertensive drug you will administer.
    (b)  Express the daily dose in grams.

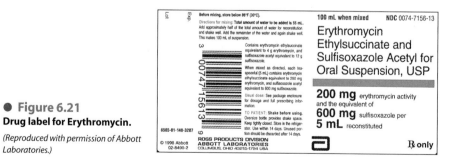

● **Figure 6.20**
**Drug label for Accupril.**

*(Reg. trademark of Pfizer Inc. Reproduced with permission.)*

2.  The physician orders *Trexall (methotrexate) 25 mg/m² PO twice per week* to treat leukemia. How many milligrams would you administer in one week if the patient is 150 centimeters tall and weighs 70 kg?

3.  The physician ordered *E.E.S (erythromycin ethylsuccinate) 400 mg PO q6h*. Read the label in ● **Figure 6.21**. How many mL of this antibacterial drug will the patient receive in 24 hours?

● **Figure 6.21**
**Drug label for Erythromycin.**

*(Reproduced with permission of Abbott Laboratories.)*

4.  A physician's order reads: *Lyrica (pregabalin) 50 mg PO t.i.d.* The bottle contains 25-mg capsules. How many capsules of this anticonvulsive medication would you administer in 24 hours?

5. The physician orders *Mellaril (thioridazine HCl) 80 mg PO t.i.d.* for a patient with schizophrenia. If you have 10, 15, and 50 mg nonscored tablets to choose from, which combination of tablets would contain the exact dosage with the smallest number of tablets?

## Exercises

Reinforce your understanding in class or at home.

1. *Paxil (paroxetine HCl) 50 mg PO daily* has been ordered for your patient. Only 10-mg, 20-mg, and 30-mg strength tablets are available. Which combination of tablets contains the exact dosage using the smallest number of tablets?

2. The physician prescribes *500 mcg of Baraclude (entecavir) per day* via NG (nasogastric tube) for a patient with chronic hepatitis B virus infection. The oral solution contains 0.05 mg of entecavir per milliliter. How many mL of this antiviral medication would you deliver?

3. Order: *Prilosec (omeprazole) 40 mg PO once daily for 4 weeks*. The available strength is 10 mg per capsule. Determine the number of capsules of this antacid drug that you would administer to the patient over the entire treatment period.

4. The prescriber ordered *Precose (acarbose) 75 mg PO t.i.d. with meals*. The medication is available in 25 mg tablets. How many tablets of this α glucosidase inhibitor (antidiabetic agent) will you give your patient in 24 hours?

5. *Toprol-XL (metoprolol succinate) extended release tablets 200 mg PO daily* has been prescribed for a patient. The label reads 200 mg per tablet. Calculate the number of tablets of this antihypertensive drug the patient would have received after 7 days.

6. *Keftab (cephalexin) 50 mg/kg PO in two equally divided doses* is prescribed for an elderly patient who weighs 40 kilograms. If each tablet contains 500 mg, how many tablets of this cephalosporin antibiotic will the patient receive per dose?

7. *Zyvox (linezolid) 600 mg PO q12h* has been prescribed for an elderly patient who is diagnosed with pneumonia. Read the label in ● **Figure 6.22**.

   (a) Calculate the number of milliliters of this antibacterial suspension you would administer.
   (b) Indicate the dose on the medication cup shown in Figure 6.22.

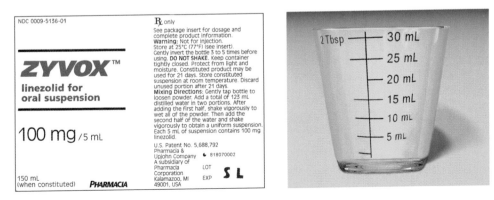

● **Figure 6.22**
**Drug label for Zyvox and medication cup.**

8. A patient is scheduled to receive 0.015 g of a drug by mouth every morning. The drug is available as 7.5 mg tablets. How many tablets would you administer?

9. A patient who is diagnosed with rheumatoid arthritis is ordered *Voltaren (diclofenac sodium) 50 mg PO t.i.d.* Your drug reference book states that the dose should not exceed 225 mg daily. Is the prescribed dose safe?

10. An elderly patient who has depression is ordered *Aventyl (nortriptyline HCl) 25 mg PO t.i.d.* The label reads Aventyl Oral Solution 10 mg/ 5mL. How many mL will you administer?

11. *Antivert (meclizine HCl) 25 mg PO once daily for three days* has been ordered for a patient who has a history of motion sickness who is planning extensive traveling. Read the information on the label in ● **Figure 6.23** and calculate the number of scored tablets that the patient will receive when the prescription is completed at the end of the three days.

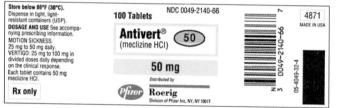

● **Figure 6.23**
**Drug label for Antivert.**
*(Reg. trademark of Pfizer Inc. Reproduced with permission.)*

12. The physician orders *7.5 mg of Tranxene SD (clorazepate dipotassium) PO t.i.d.* for an elderly patient who is diagnosed with extreme anxiety. This drug is available in 15 mg scored tablets. How many tablets would the patient receive in 24 hours?

13. A patient develops a mild skin reaction to a transfusion of a unit of packed red blood cells and is given 75 milligrams of Benadryl (diphenhydramine HCl) PO stat. The only drug strength available is 25 mg capsules. How many capsules will you give?

14. The physician orders two Tylenol #3 (codeine 30 mg, acetaminophen 300 mg) PO every 6 hours. How many milligrams of acetaminophen will the patient receive in 24 hours?

15. The physician orders *Detrol LA (tolterodine tartrate) 4 mg PO daily* for a patient with an overactive bladder. Read the label in ● **Figure 6.24** and determine how many capsules you will give this patient.

NDC 0009-5190-03

*Detrol* LA

tolterodine tartrate
extended release capsules

**2 mg**

500 Capsules

TM

N 3  0009-5190-03  8

Rx only
See package insert for complete product information.
Store at 25°C (77°F); excursions permitted to 15°-30°C (59°-86°F) [see USP Controlled Room Temperature]. Protect from light.
U.S. Patent No. 5,382,600
Manufactured for: Pharmacia & Upjohn Company • A subsidiary of Pharmacia Corporation • Kalamazoo, MI 49001, USA
By: International Processing Corporation Winchester, Kentucky 40391, USA

818270001

LOT

EXP

● **Figure 6.24**
**Drug label for Detrol LA.**

16. A patient who has difficulty sleeping is medicated for insomnia with 0.25 g PO at bedtime. The drug is available as 500 mg per scored tablet. How many tablets will you administer to your patient?

17. The physician orders *Coumadin (warfarin sodium) 6.5 mg PO* every other day from Monday through Sunday. How many milligrams of Coumadin will your patient receive in the week?

18. A physician is treating a patient for H. influenzae. He writes the following prescription:

    *Vantin (cefpodoxime proxetil) 200 mg PO q12h for 14 days*

    Read the label in ● **Figure 6.25**.

    (a) Calculate the number of milliliters you will give this patient.
    (b) Indicate the dose on the medication cup in Figure 6.25.

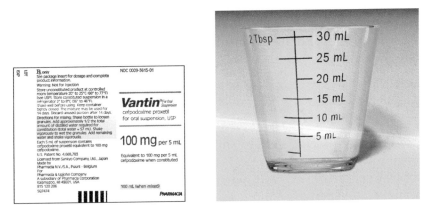

● **Figure 6.25**
**Drug label for Vantin and medication cup.**

19. The physician orders *Deltasone (prednisone) 60 mg/m$^2$ PO daily* as part of the treatment protocol for a patient with leukemia.

    (a) How many milligrams of this steroid drug would you administer if the patient is 5 feet 6 inches tall and weighs 140 pounds?
    (b) The drug is supplied in 50 mg per tablet. How many tablets will you administer?

20. The antibiotic, Zithromax (azithromycin), is ordered to treat a patient who has a diagnosis of chronic obstructive pulmonary disease (COPD). The order is:

    *Zithromax (azithromycin) 500 mg PO as a single dose on day one, followed by 250 mg once daily on days 2 through 5*

    How many milligrams will the patient receive by the completion of the prescription?

## Additional Exercises

Now, test yourself!

1. A drug (40 mg PO daily) has been ordered for your client. Each tablet contains 0.02 grams. How many tablets of this drug will you prepare?

2. The physician ordered a drug (0.55 mg/kg PO). The patient weighs 32 kilograms. The drug is supplied with a strength of 30 mg/mL. Calculate the number of milliliters you would administer.

3. *Glucophage (metformin) 850 mg PO ac breakfast and dinner* has been prescribed for your client.

   The maximum recommended dose is 1,000–2,500 mg per day.

   (a) Is the prescribed dose safe?
   (b) What is the patient's daily dose, expressed in grams?

4. Prescriber's order:

   *Micronase (glyburide) 5 mg PO with breakfast*

   Each tablet contains 2.5 mg. How many tablets will you prepare?

5. *Ditropan XL (oxybutynin chloride) 20 mg per day PO for 5 days* has been prescribed for a patient. Each tablet contains 5 mg. How many tablets of this anticholinergic medication will the patient receive by the end of the treatment?

6. *Norvasc (amlodipine) 5 mg PO once daily for 7 days* has been ordered for a patient with angina. Each tablet contains 0.0025 grams. How many tablets will you administer to this patient for the week?

7. *Vasotec (enalapril maleate) 7.5 mg PO daily* is ordered. The following strengths are available: 2.5 mg, 5 mg, 10 mg, and 20 mg tablets. Which combination of tablets will contain the prescribed dose of this ACE-inhibiting antihypertensive drug using the fewest number of tablets?

8. *Alprazolam 0.5 mg PO t.i.d.* has been prescribed for your client. Read the information on the label in ● **Figure 6.26**.

   (a) How many milliliters of this antianxiety drug will you administer to your patient?
   (b) Draw an arrow on the dropper on the label in Figure 6.26 that indicates the dose to be administered.

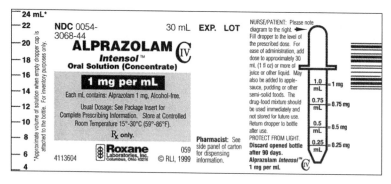

● **Figure 6.26**
**Drug label for Alprazolam Intensol.**

*(Courtesy of Roxane Laboratories Inc.)*

9. A patient is to receive 0.01 g PO qhs of a drug. Each tablet contains 0.005 g. How many tablets will you administer to your patient?

10. Order:

    *Coumadin (warfarin sodium) 2.5 mg PO Monday, Wednesday, and Friday and 1 mg PO Tuesday, Thursday, Saturday, and Sunday*

    How many milligrams of Coumadin will your patient receive in one week?

11. A drug (0.5 g PO stat) has been ordered for your patient. Each tablet contains 0.25 gram. How many tablets of this drug will you give to your patient?

12. *Decadron (dexamethasone) 3 mg PO q12h* has been ordered for a patient. The drug is supplied in 1.5 mg tablets. Calculate the number of tablets of this steroid that the patient will receive in 24 hours.

13. Physician's order:

    *furosemide 80 mg PO daily*

    The drug is supplied in 20 mg tablets. What would the patient's daily dose be if it were expressed in grams?

14. Physician's order:

    *Pavabid (papaverine) 50 mg PO q8h*

    Your drug reference book states that a patient may receive 100–300 mg 3–5 times per day. Is the prescribed dose safe?

15. Prescriber's order:

    *Motrin (ibuprofen) 600 mg PO q8h for five days only*

    Each caplet contains 200 mg. How many caplets will you give this patient in the 5 days?

16. The antigout medication *colchicine 1.2 mg PO q1h for 8 doses* has been ordered. Each tablet contains 0.6 mg.

    (a) How many milligrams of colchicine will the patient receive in 8 hours?
    (b) How many tablets will the patient receive in 8 hours?

17. Physician's order:

    *Cytovene (ganciclovir) 500 mg PO q3h while awake*

    The drug is available in 250 mg capsules. How many capsules will you administer?

18. The physician ordered Retrovir (zidovudine) PO, an antiviral drug used for the treatment of CMV retinitis. The order is 160 mg/m$^2$ every 8 hours. The patient weighs 60 kg and is 140 cm in height. How many milligrams of this drug will you give the patient per day? (Use the formula for BSA.)

19. Physician's order: *Cytoxan (cyclophosphamide) 3 mg/kg PO twice weekly.* The client weighs 148 lb. The drug is supplied in 50 mg tablets. How many tablets will you prepare?

20. Physician's order: *prednisone 40 mg PO q12h for 5 days* for a patient with acute asthma. The drug is supplied in 20 mg tablets. How many tablets will you give this patient?

# Cumulative Review Exercises

Review your mastery of previous chapters.

1. Prescriber's order: *digoxin 0.4 mg PO stat, then give 0.3 mg PO q6h.*

   You have available the following strengths: 0.05 mg, 0.1 mg, and 0.2 mg capsules.

   (a) Which combination of capsules will you give for the stat dose?
   (b) Which combination of capsules will you give for the subsequent doses?
   (c) How many milligrams of digoxin will the patient receive per day *after* the first day?

2. *Lorabid (loracarbef) 400 mg PO q12h.* The label reads 200 mg in 5 mL. How many mL will you give your patient? _____

3. What is the dose in grams of an order for 500 mg of azithromycin? _____

4. 0.4 g = _____ mg

5. 2.5 liters = _____ milliliters

6. 7 lb 11 oz ≈ _____ g

7. 1 pint = _____ cups

8. The order reads 267 mg/m$^2$ of a drug PO. The patient weighs 72 kg and is 70 in tall. The label reads 50 mg/mL. How many mL will you administer to this patient? Use the nomogram to estimate the BSA.

9. A physician orders *Tylenol (acetaminophen) 650 mg PO q8h.* The label reads as follows: Each capsule contains 325 mg. How many capsules will you give this patient?

10. The order reads *Tenormin (atenolol) 100 mg PO daily.* You have 25-mg, 50-mg, and 100-mg tablets available. Which tablet or combination of tablets would you administer (using the smallest number of tablets for the patient to swallow)?

11. The physician orders *Parlodel (bromocriptine mesylate) 7.5 mg PO b.i.d.* with meals. Each tablet contains 2.5 mg. How many tablets of this anti-Parkinsonian drug will you prepare?

12. A patient must receive 60 mEq of potassium chloride PO stat. Each tablet is labeled 20 mEq/tab. How many tablets will you prepare?

13. 200 mg = _____ g

14. A patient must receive *Videx (didanosine) 2.2 mg/kg PO stat.* The patient weighs 90 kg. How many tablets will the patient receive if each tablet contains 100 mg?

15. 1 t ≈ _____ mL

**MediaLink**
www.prenhall.com/giangrasso

Animated examples, interactive practice questions with animated solutions, and challenge tests for this chapter can be found on the Pearson Dosage Calculation Tutor that accompanies this text. Additional, unique, interactive resources and activities can be found on the Companion Web site.

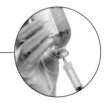
# Syringes

## Learning Outcomes

After completing this chapter, you will be able to

1. Identify the parts of a syringe and needle.
2. Identify various types of syringes.
3. Read and measure dosages on syringes.
4. Select the appropriate syringe to administer prescribed doses.
5. Read the calibrations on syringes of various sizes.
6. Measure single insulin dosages.
7. Measure combined insulin dosages.

In this chapter, you will learn how to use various types of syringes to measure medication dosages. You will also discuss the difference between the types of insulin and how to measure single insulin dosages and combined insulin dosages.

**Syringes** are made of plastic or glass, designed for one-time use, and are packaged either separately or together with needles of appropriate sizes. After use, syringes must be discarded in special puncture-resistant containers. See ● **Figure 7.1**.

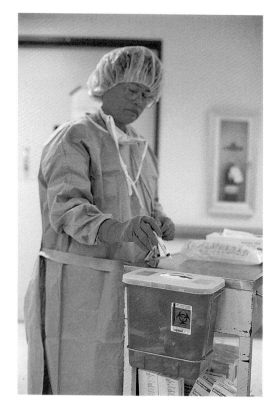

● **Figure 7.1**
**Puncture-resistant container for needles,
syringes, and other "sharps."**

## Parts of a Syringe

A syringe consists of a barrel, plunger, and tip.

- **Barrel:** a hollow cylinder that holds the medication. It has calibrations (markings) on the outer surface.
- **Plunger:** fits in the barrel and is moved back and forth. Pulling back on the plunger draws medication or air into the syringe. Pushing in the plunger forces air or medication out of the syringe.
- **Tip:** the end of the syringe that holds the needle. The needle slips onto the tip or can be twisted and locked in place (Luer-Lok™).

The inside of the barrel, plunger, and tip must always be sterile.

### Needles

**ALERT**

The patient's size, the type of tissue being injected, and the viscosity of the medication will determine the size of the needle to be used. The inside of the barrel, plunger, tip of the syringe, and the needle should never come in contact with anything unsterile.

Needles are made of stainless steel and come in various lengths and diameters. They are packaged with a protective cover that keeps them from being contaminated. The parts of a needle are the **hub**, which attaches to the syringe, the **shaft**, the long part of the needle that is embedded in the hub, and the **bevel**, the slanted portion of the tip. The **length** of the needle is the distance from the point to the hub. Needles most commonly used in medication administration range from $\frac{3}{8}$ inch to 2 inches. The **gauge** of the needle refers to the thickness of the inside of the needle and varies from 18 to 28 (the larger the gauge, the thinner the needle). The parts of a needle are shown in ● **Figure 7.2**.

### Parts of a 10 mL Luer-Lok™ Hypodermic Syringe and Needle

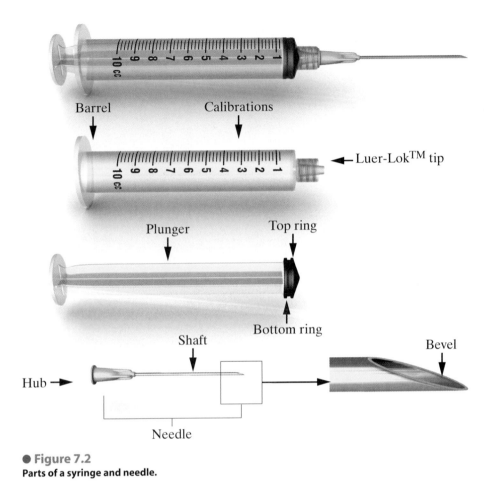

● **Figure 7.2**
**Parts of a syringe and needle.**

# Types of Syringes

The two major types of syringes are hypodermic and oral. In 1853, Drs. Charles Pravaz and Alexander Wood were the first to develop a syringe with a needle that was fine enough to pierce the skin. This is known as a **hypodermic syringe**. (Use of oral syringes will be discussed in Chapter 12.)

**Hypodermic syringes** are calibrated (marked) in cubic centimeters (cc), milliliters (mL), or units. Practitioners often refer to syringes by the volume of cubic centimeters they contain, for example, a 3 cc syringe. Although many syringes are still labeled in cubic centimeters, manufacturers are now phasing in syringes labeled in milliliters. In this text, we will generally use mL instead of cc.

The smaller capacity syringes (0.5, 1, 2, $2\frac{1}{2}$, and 3 mL) are used most often for intradermal, subcutaneous, or intramuscular injections of medication. The larger sizes (5, 6, 10, and 12 mL) are commonly used to draw blood or prepare medications for intravenous administration. Syringes 20 mL and larger are used to inject large volumes of solutions. A representative sample of commonly used syringes is shown in ● **Figure 7.3.**

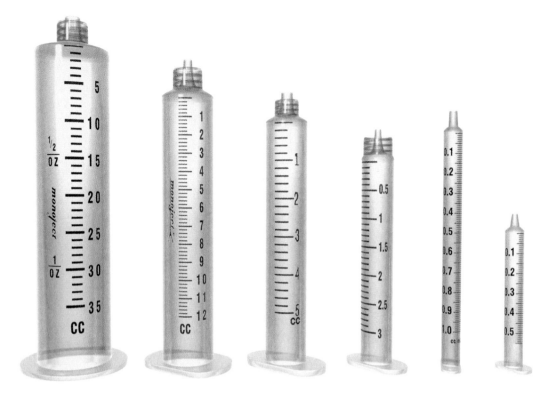

● **Figure 7.3**
**A sample of commonly used hypodermic syringes (35 cc, 12 cc, 5 cc, 3 mL, 1 mL, and 0.5 mL).**

A 35 cc syringe is shown in ● **Figure 7.4**. Each line on the barrel represents 1 mL, and the longer lines represent 5 mL.

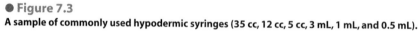

● **Figure 7.4**
**35 cc syringe.**

A 12 cc syringe is shown in ● **Figure 7.5**. Each line on the barrel represents 0.2 mL, and the longer lines represent 1 mL.

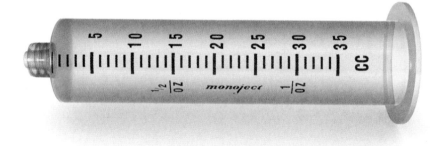

● **Figure 7.5**
**12 cc syringe.**

A 5 cc syringe is shown in ● **Figure 7.6**. Each line on the barrel represents 0.2 mL, and the longer lines represent 1 mL.

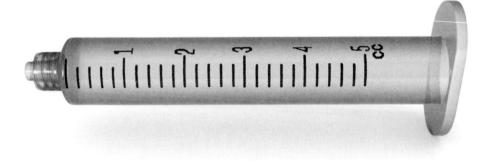

● **Figure 7.6**
**5 cc syringe.**

In ● **Figure 7.7**, a 3 cc/mL syringe is shown. There are 10 spaces between the largest markings. This indicates that the syringe is measured in tenths of a milliliter. So, each of the lines is 0.1 mL. The longer lines indicate half and full milliliter measures. The liquid volume in a syringe is read from the *top ring*, **not** the bottom ring or the raised section in the middle of the plunger. Therefore, this syringe contains 0.9 mL.

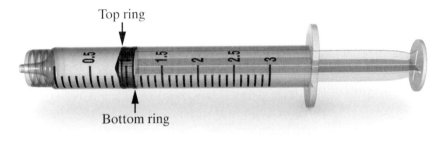

● **Figure 7.7**
**Partially filled 3 cc/mL syringe.**

## EXAMPLE 7.1

**How much liquid is in the 12 mL syringe partially shown in ● Figure 7.8?**

The top ring of the plunger is at the second line after the 5 mL line. Because each line measures 0.2 mL, the second line measures 0.4 mL. Therefore, the amount in the syringe is 5.4 mL.

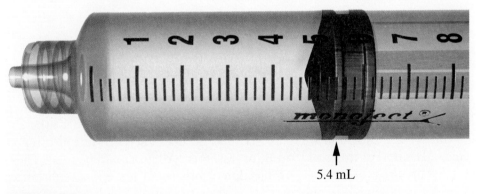

● **Figure 7.8**
**A partially filled 12 mL syringe.**

## EXAMPLE 7.2

**How much liquid is in the 5 cc syringe shown in ● Figure 7.9?**

The top ring of the plunger is at the third line after 4 mL. Because each line measures 0.2 mL, the third line measures 0.6 mL. Therefore, the amount of liquid in the syringe is 4.6 mL.

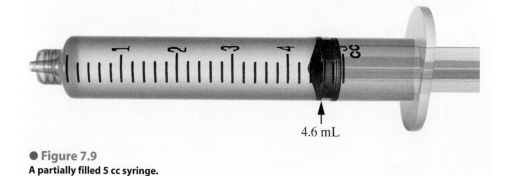

4.6 mL

● **Figure 7.9**
**A partially filled 5 cc syringe.**

## EXAMPLE 7.3

**How much liquid is in the 3 mL syringe in ● Figure 7.10?**

The top ring of the plunger is at the second line after 1 mL. Because each line measures 0.1 mL, the two lines measure 0.2 mL. Therefore, the amount in the syringe is 1.2 mL.

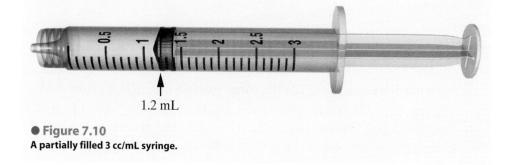

1.2 mL

● **Figure 7.10**
**A partially filled 3 cc/mL syringe.**

## ALERT

The calibrations on the 1 mL syringe are very small and close together. Use caution when drawing up medication in this syringe.

When small volumes of 1 milliliter or less are required, a low-volume syringe provides the greatest accuracy. The 1 mL syringe, also called a tuberculin syringe, shown in ● **Figure 7.11** is calibrated in hundredths of a milliliter. Because there are 100 lines on the syringe, each line represents 0.01 mL. The 0.5 mL syringe shown in ● **Figure 7.12** has 50 lines and each line also represents 0.01 mL. For doses of 0.5 mL or less, this syringe should be used. These syringes are used for intradermal injection of very small amounts of substances in tests for tuberculosis, allergies, as well as for intramuscular injections of small quantities of medication.

0.52 mL

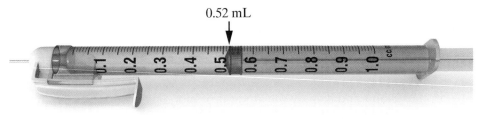

● Figure 7.11
A partially filled 1 mL tuberculin syringe.

The top ring of the plunger in Figure 7.11 is at the second line after 0.5 mL. Therefore, the amount in the syringe is 0.52 mL.

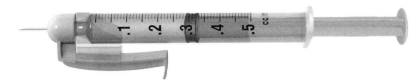

● Figure 7.12
A partially filled 0.5 mL syringe.

The top ring of the plunger in Figure 7.12 is at the first line before 0.3 mL (0.30 mL). Therefore, the syringe contains 0.29 mL.

### EXAMPLE 7.4

How much liquid is shown in the portion of the 1 mL tuberculin syringe shown in ● Figure 7.13?

0.36 mL

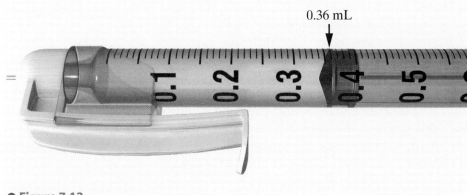

● Figure 7.13
A portion of a partially filled 1 mL syringe.

The top ring of the plunger is 6 lines after the 0.3 mL calibration. Because each line represents 0.01 mL, the amount of liquid in the syringe is 0.36 mL.

**NOTE**

Because 0.5 mL and 1 mL tuberculin syringes can accurately measure amounts to hundredths of a milliliter, the volume of fluid to be measured in these syringes is rounded off to the nearest hundredth; for example, 0.358 mL is rounded off to 0.36 mL. The 3 mL syringe can accurately measure amounts to tenths of a milliliter. The volume of fluid to be measured in this syringe is rounded off to the nearest tenth of a milliliter; for example, 2.358 mL is rounded off to 2.4 mL.

**Insulin syringes** are used for the subcutaneous injection of insulin and are calibrated in *units* rather than *milliliters*. Insulin is a hormone used to treat patients who have insulin-dependent diabetes mellitus (IDDM). Insulin dosage is determined by the patient's daily blood-glucose readings, frequently referred to as a "fingerstick." A blood-glucose monitor is small and can quickly analyze a drop of blood and display the amount of blood glucose measured in milligrams per deciliter (mg/dL). See ● **Figure 7.14**.

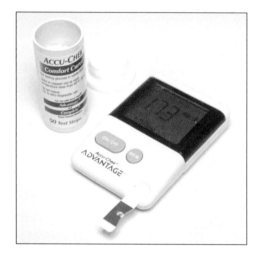

● Figure 7.14
**Blood-Glucose Monitor.**

Insulin is supplied as a premixed liquid measured in standardized units of potency rather than by weight or volume. These standardized units are called **USP** *units*, which are often shortened to *units*. The most commonly prepared concentration of insulin is 100 units per milliliter, which is referred to as *units 100 insulin* and is abbreviated as U-100. Although a 500 unit concentration of insulin (U-500) is also available, it is used only for the rare patient who is markedly insulin-resistant. U-40 insulin is used in some countries; however in the United States, insulin is standardized to U-100. For the rest of this text, we will refer to U-100 insulin only.

Insulin syringes have three different capacities: the standard 100 unit capacity, and the **Lo-Dose** 50 unit or 30 unit capacities. The plunger of the insulin syringe is flat, and the liquid volume is measured from the top ring.

● **Figure 7.15** shows a *single-scale standard* 100 unit insulin syringe calibrated in 2 unit increments. Any odd number of units (e.g., 23, 35) is measured between the even calibrations. These calibrations and spaces are very small, so this is not the syringe of choice for a person with impaired vision.

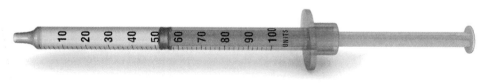

● Figure 7.15
**A single-scale standard 100 unit insulin syringe with 52 units of insulin.**

The dual-scale version of this syringe is easier to read. ● **Figure 7.16** shows a *dual-scale* 100 unit insulin syringe, also calibrated in 2 unit increments. However, it has a scale with *even* numbers on one side and a scale with *odd* numbers on the opposite side. Both the even and odd sides are shown. Even numbered doses are measured using the "even" side of the syringe, while odd numbered doses are measured using the "odd" side.

Each line on the barrel represents 2 units.

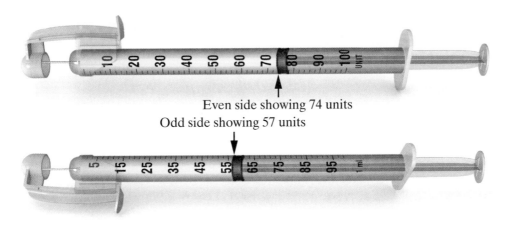

Even side showing 74 units
Odd side showing 57 units

● **Figure 7.16**
**Two views of the same dual-scale standard 100 unit insulin syringe.**

For small doses of insulin (50 units or fewer) Lo-Dose insulin syringes more accurately measure these doses, and should be used. A 50 unit Lo-Dose insulin syringe, shown in ● **Figure 7.17**, is a single-scale syringe with 50 units. It is calibrated in 1 unit increments.

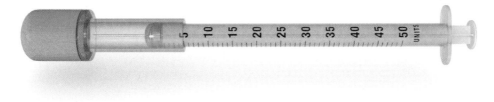

● **Figure 7.17**
**A 50 unit Lo-Dose insulin syringe.**

A 30 unit Lo-Dose insulin syringe, shown in ● **Figure 7.18**, is a syringe with 30 units. It is calibrated in 1 unit increments and is used when the dose is less than 30 units.

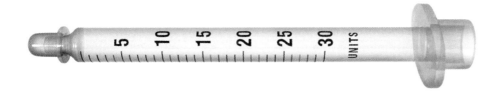

● **Figure 7.18**
**A 30 unit Lo-Dose insulin syringe.**

## NOTE

Insulin is always ordered in units, the medication is supplied in 100 units/mL, and the syringes are calibrated for 100 units/mL. Therefore, no calculations are required to prepare insulin that is administered subcutaneously.

*The insulin syringe is to be used in the measurement and administration of U-100 insulin* **only**. *It must not be used to measure other medications that are also measured in units, such as heparin or Pitocin.*

# Measuring Insulin Doses

## Measuring a Single Dose of Insulin in an Insulin Syringe

Insulin is available in 100 units/mL multidose vials. The major route of administration of insulin is by subcutaneous injection. *Insulin is never given intramuscularly.* It can also be administered with an insulin pen that contains a cartridge filled with insulin or with a CSII pump (Continuous Subcutaneous Insulin Infusion). The CSII pump is used to administer a programmed dose of a rapid-acting 100 units insulin at a set rate of units per hour.

The *source* (animal or human) and *type* (rapid, short, intermediate, or long-acting) are indicated on the insulin label. Today, the most commonly used *source* is human insulin. Insulin from a human source is designated on the label as recombinant DNA (rDNA origin). The *type* of insulin relates to both the *onset and duration of action.* It is indicated by the uppercase bold letter that follows the trade name on the label, for example, Humulin **R (Regular)**, Humulin **L (Lente)**, Humulin **N (NPH)**, and Humulin **U (Ultralente)**. These letters are important visual identifiers when selecting the insulin type. ● **Figure 7.19**.

**ALERT**

Select the appropriate syringe and be very attentive to the calibrations when measuring insulin dosages. Both the single- and dual-scale standard 100 unit insulin syringes are calibrated in 2 unit increments. The Lo-Dose syringes are calibrated in 1 unit increments.

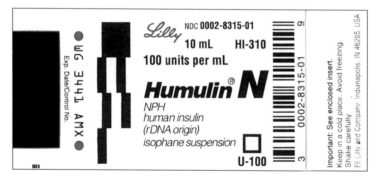

● **Figure 7.19**
**Drug label for Humulin N insulin.**

*(Copyright Eli Lilly and Company. Used with permission.)*

**ALERT**

Insulin should be at room temperature when administered, and one source or brand of insulin should not be substituted for another without medical supervision.

Healthcare providers must be familiar with the various **types of insulin**, as summarized in Table 7.1.

They are classified according to how fast they begin to work, when they reach maximum effect, and how long their effects last:

- **onset of action:** the length of time before insulin reaches the bloodstream and begins to lower blood glucose,

- **peak of action:** the time period when the insulin is the most effective in lowering blood glucose,

- **duration of action:** the period of time that the insulin continues to lower blood glucose.

| Table 7.1 **Types of Insulin** | | | | |
|---|---|---|---|---|
| **Types of insulin** | **Names of insulin** | **How fast they act** (*Onset*) | **When the action peaks** (*Peak*) | **How long they last** (*Duration*) |
| Rapid-acting | Humalog (insulin lispro) Novolog (insulin aspart) Apidra (insulin glulisine) Exubera (insulin human (rDNA origin) inhalation | 5 to 15 minutes 10 to 20 minutes | 30 to 90 minutes 1 to 3 hours | 5 hours 5 to 8 hours |
| Short-acting | Humulin R (regular insulin), Novolin Semilente | 30 to 60 minutes | 2 to 3 hours | 5 to 8 hours |
| Intermediate-acting | NPH insulin (N) Lente insulin (L) | 2 to 4 hours | 4 to 10 hours | 10 to 16 hours |
| Long-acting | Ultralente (U) | 6 to 14 hours | 10 to 18 hours | 24 to 36 hours |
| Very long-acting | Lantus (insulin glargine) Levemir (insulin detemir) | 2 to 4 hour 3 to 8 hours | None | 20 to 24 hours 5 to 23 hours |
| Pre-mixed | Novolog 70/30 (70% insulin aspart protamine suspension/30% insulin aspart) | 5–15 min. | Dual | 10–16 hours |
| | Humalog 50/50 (50% insulin lispro protamine suspension/50% insulin lispro) | 5–15 min. | Dual | 10–16 hours |
| | Humalog 75/25 (75% insulin lispro protamine suspension/25% insulin lispro) | 5–15 min. | Dual | 10–16 hours |
| | 70% NPH/30% regular | 30–60 min. | Dual | 10–16 hours |

*This table was adapted from AACE Diabetes Mellitus Guidelines, Endocr Pract. 2007.*

The types of insulin are *Rapid-acting, Short-acting, Intermediate-acting, Long-acting, Very long-acting, and Pre-mixed*. Table 7.1 summarizes this information. Each person responds differently to insulin. A physician will determine which insulin schedule is best for the particular patient.

## Measuring Insulin with an Insulin Pen

An insulin pen is an insulin delivery system that looks like a pen, uses an insulin cartridge, and has disposable needles. While insulin pens have been used throughout the world for some time, they are now beginning to be used more frequently in the United States. Compared to the traditional syringe and vial, a pen device is easier to use, provides greater dose accuracy, and is more satisfactory to patients.

Some pens are disposed of after one use, while others have replaceable insulin cartridges. All pens use needles that minimize the discomfort of injection because they are extremely short and very thin.

The parts of an insulin pen are shown in ● **Figure 7.20**. The dose knob is used to "dial" the desired dose of insulin. The dose is visible in the dose window.

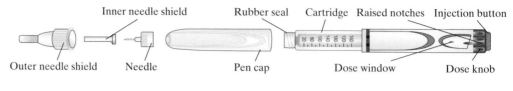

Inner needle shield    Rubber seal    Cartridge    Raised notches    Injection button

Outer needle shield    Needle    Pen cap    Dose window    Dose knob

● **Figure 7.20**
**Parts of an insulin pen.**

Once the pen has been "primed" (cleared of any air in the cartridge) and the dose set, the insulin is injected by pressing on the injection button. Because preparing a dose with a pen involves dialing a mechanical device and not looking at the side of a syringe, insulin users with reduced visual acuity can be more assured of accurate dosing. Some pens have a "memory," which records the date, time, and amount of doses administered.

**ALERT**

Insulin is a *high-alert medication*. Be sure to check your institution's policy regarding administration. For example, some agencies may require insulin doses to be checked by two nurses.

# Insulin Pumps

An insulin pump, shown in ● **Figure 7.21**, is a beeper-like, external, battery-powered device that delivers rapid-acting insulin continuously for 24 hours a day through a **cannula** (a small hollow tube) inserted under the skin. The pump contains an insulin cartridge that is attached to tubing with a cannula or needle on the end. The needle is inserted under the skin of the abdomen, and it can remain in place for two to three days. The insulin is delivered through this "infusion set." This eliminates the need for multiple daily injections of insulin.

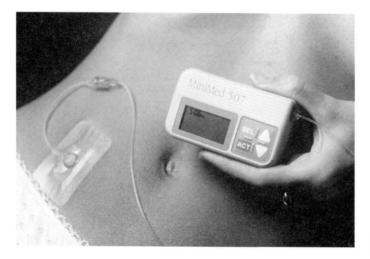

● **Figure 7.21**
**An insulin pump.**

The pump can be programmed to deliver a basal rate and/or a bolus dose. **Basal** insulin is delivered continuously over 24 hours to keep blood glucose levels in range between meals and overnight. The basal rate can be programmed to deliver different rates at different times. **Bolus** doses can be delivered at mealtimes to provide control for additional food intake. The insulin pump is currently the closest device on the market to an artificial pancreas.

## EXAMPLE 7.5

What is the dose of insulin in the single-scale 100 unit insulin syringe shown in ● Figure 7.22?

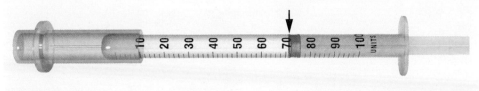

● **Figure 7.22**
**A single-scale 100 unit insulin syringe.**

The top ring of the plunger is one line after 70. Because each line represents 2 units, the dose is 72 units of insulin.

## EXAMPLE 7.6

What is the dose of insulin in the dual-scale 100 unit insulin syringe shown in ● Figure 7.23?

### 100 Unit Dual-scale Syringe

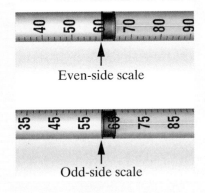

● **Figure 7.23**
**Two views of a dual-scale insulin syringe.**

The top ring of the plunger is slightly more than 2 lines after 55 on the odd side. Notice how difficult it would be to determine where 60 units would measure using the odd side of the syringe. However, on the even side, the plunger falls exactly on the 60. So, the dose is 60 units.

## EXAMPLE 7.7

What is the dose of insulin in the 50 unit insulin syringe shown in ● Figure 7.24?

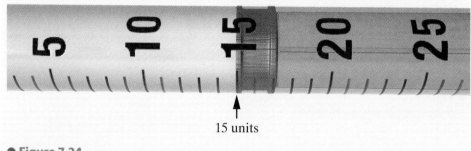

15 units

● **Figure 7.24**
**A 50 unit insulin syringe.**

The top ring of the plunger is at 15. Because each line represents 1 unit, the dose is 15 units.

## EXAMPLE 7.8

What is the dose of insulin in the 30 unit insulin syringe shown in ● Figure 7.25?

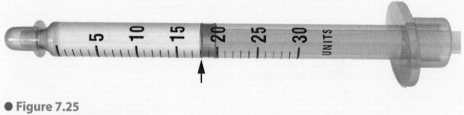

● **Figure 7.25**
**A 30 unit Lo-Dose insulin syringe.**

The top ring of the plunger is three lines after 15. Because each line represents one unit, the dose is 18 units of insulin.

## EXAMPLE 7.9

The physician prescribed 8 units of Humulin R insulin subcutaneously stat. Read the label in ● Figure 7.26 to determine the source of the insulin and place an arrow at the appropriate level of measurement on the insulin syringe in ● Figure 7.27.

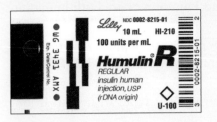

● **Figure 7.26**
**Drug label for Humulin R.**

*(Copyright Eli Lilly and Company. Used with permission.)*

The source of the insulin is human (rDNA origin), and the arrow should be placed three lines after 5, as shown in Figure 7.27.

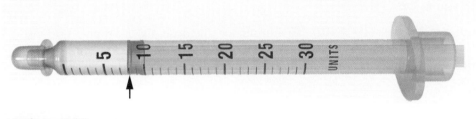

● **Figure 7.27**
**Insulin syringe for Example 7.9.**

## Measuring Two Types of Insulin in One Syringe

Individuals who have IDDM often must have two types of insulin administered at the same time. In order to reduce the number of injections, it is common practice to combine two insulins (usually a rapid-acting with either an intermediate- or a long-acting) in a single syringe. The important points to remember are these:

- The *total volume* in the syringe is the *sum of the two insulin* amounts.

- The smallest capacity syringe containing the dose should be used to measure the insulins because the enlarged scale is easier to read and therefore more accurate.

- The *amount of air equal to the amount of insulin to be withdrawn* from each vial must be injected into each vial.

- You must inject the air into the intermediate- or long-acting insulin before you inject the air into the regular insulin.

- The *regular* (rapid-acting) insulin is drawn up *first*; this prevents contamination of the regular insulin with the intermediate or long-acting insulin.

- The intermediate-acting or long-acting insulins can precipitate; therefore, they must be mixed well before drawing up and administered without delay.

■ Only insulins from the same source should be mixed together, for example, Humulin R and Humulin N are both human insulin and can be mixed.

■ If you draw up too much of the intermediate or long-acting insulin, you must discard the entire medication and start over.

The steps of preparing two types of insulin in one syringe are shown in Example 7.10.

## EXAMPLE 7.10

The prescriber ordered 10 units Humulin R insulin and 30 units Humulin N insulin subcutaneously, 30 minutes before breakfast. Explain how you would prepare to administer this in one injection. ● Figures 7.28 and ● 7.29.

The total amount of insulin is 40 units (10 + 30). To administer this dose, use a 50 unit Lo-Dose syringe. Inject 30 units of air into the Humulin **N** vial and 10 units of air into the Humulin **R** vial. Withdraw 10 units of the Humulin **R** first and then withdraw 30 units of the Humulin **N**.

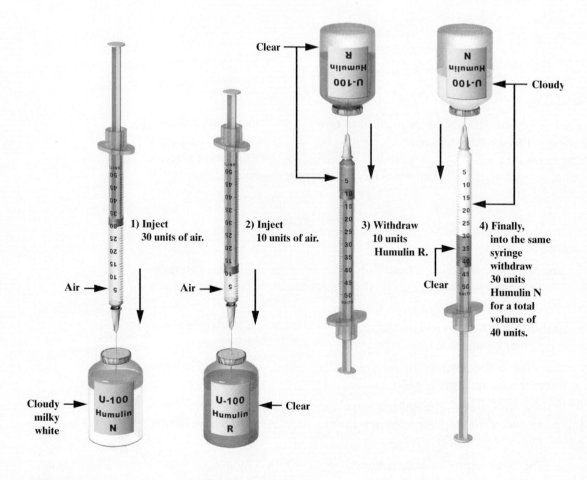

● **Figure 7.28**
**Mixing two types of insulin in one syringe.**

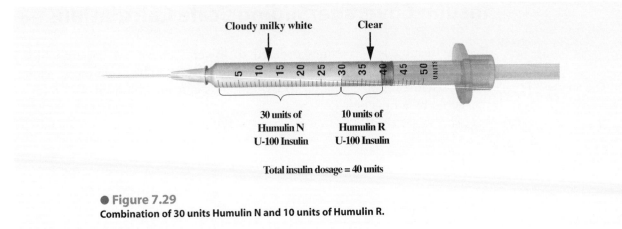

Cloudy milky white          Clear

30 units of
Humulin N
U-100 Insulin

10 units of
Humulin R
U-100 Insulin

Total insulin dosage = 40 units

● Figure 7.29
**Combination of 30 units Humulin N and 10 units of Humulin R.**

## Measuring Premixed Insulin

Using premixed insulin (see Table 7.1) eliminates errors that may occur when mixing two types of insulin in one syringe (Figure 7.28).

**NOTE**

When you are mixing two types of insulin, think: "Clear, then Cloudy."

### EXAMPLE 7.11

Order: Give 35 units of Humulin 70/30 insulin subcutaneously 30 minutes before breakfast. Use the label shown in ● Figure 7.30 and place an arrow at the appropriate calibration on the syringe.

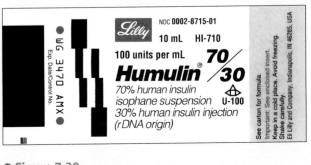

NDC 0002-8715-01
10 mL   HI-710
100 units per mL  **70/30**
**Humulin**®
70% human insulin
isophane suspension   U-100
30% human insulin injection
(rDNA origin)

● Figure 7.30
**Drug label for Humulin 70/30.**
*(Copyright Eli Lilly and Company. Used with permission.)*

In the syringe in ● **Figure 7.31**, the top ring of the plunger is at the 35 unit line.

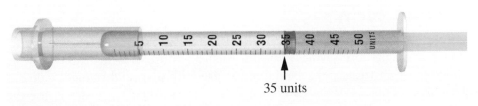

35 units

● Figure 7.31
**A 50 unit Lo-Dose insulin syringe measuring 35 units.**

# Insulin Coverage/Sliding Scale Calculations

Regular insulin is sometimes ordered to lower ("cover") a patient's blood sugar level. The prescriber may order regular insulin to be given on a "sliding scale" schedule that is related to the patient's current blood glucose level as measured by a fingerstick.

### EXAMPLE 7.12

Order: *fingersticks Q.I.D., ac breakfast, lunch, dinner, and at bedtime. Give regular insulin as follows:*

| | |
|---|---|
| *glucose less than 150 mg/dL* | *— no insulin* |
| *glucose of 150–200 mg/dL* | *— 2 units* |
| *glucose of 201–250 mg/dL* | *— 3 units* |
| *glucose of 251–300 mg/dL* | *— 5 units* |
| *glucose of more than 300 mg/dL* | *— give 6 units and contact the prescriber stat* |

Use the "sliding scale" to determine how much insulin you will give the patient if the glucose level before lunchtime is:

(a)  125 mg/dL

(b)  278 mg/dL

(c)  350 mg/dL

(a)  You need to compare the patient's level with the information provided in the sliding scale. Since 125 mg/dL is less than 150 mg/dL, you would not administer any insulin.

(b)  Since 278 mg/dL is between 251 and 300 mg/dL, you need to administer 5 units of regular insulin immediately.

(c)  Since 350 mg/dL is more than 300 mg/dL, you would give 6 units of regular insulin and contact the prescriber stat.

**ALERT**

More than 15 units of regular insulin for coverage is usually too much. Contact the physician.

**NOTE**

Currently, there is evidence that the routine use of the "sliding scale" should be discontinued because of an unacceptably high rate of hyper- and hypoglycemia and iatrogenic diabetic ketoacidosis in hospitalized patients with type 1 diabetes. Be sure to know your current hospital policies and protocols.

# Prefilled Syringes

A prefilled, single-dose syringe contains the usual dose of a medication. Some prefilled glass cartridges are available for use with a special plunger called a Tubex or Carpuject syringe (● **Figure 7.32**). If a medication order is for the exact amount of drug in the prefilled syringe, the possibility of measurement error by the person administering the drug is decreased.

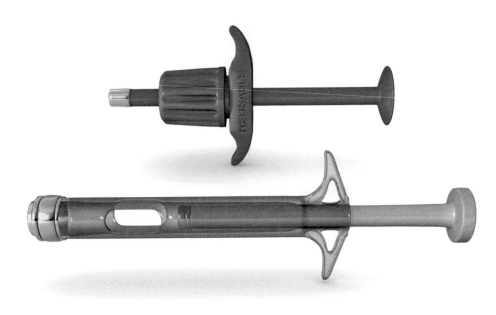

● **Figure 7.32**
**Carpuject and Tubex prefilled cartridge holders.**

## EXAMPLE 7.13

The prefilled syringe cartridge shown in ● Figure 7.33 is calibrated so that each line measures 0.1 mL and it has a capacity of 2.5 mL. How many milliliters are indicated by the arrow shown in Figure 7.33?

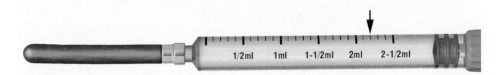

● **Figure 7.33**
**Prefilled cartridges (Tubex or Carpuject).**

The cartridge has a total capacity of 2.5 mL, and the arrow is at 2.2 mL.

## EXAMPLE 7.14

How much medication is in the prepackaged cartridge shown in ● Figure 7.34?

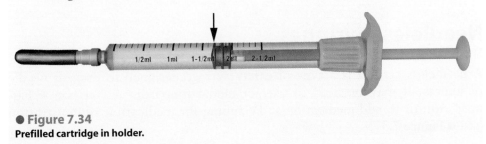

● **Figure 7.34**
**Prefilled cartridge in holder.**

The top of the plunger is at two lines after the 1.5 mL line. Because each line measures 0.1 mL, the two lines measure 0.2 mL. Therefore, there are 1.7 mL of medication in this prefilled cartridge.

## Safety Syringes

In order to prevent the transmission of blood-borne infections from contaminated needles, many syringes are now manufactured with various types of safety devices. For example, a syringe may contain a protective sheath that can be used to protect the needle's sterility. This sheath is then pulled forward and locked into place to provide a permanent needle shield for disposal following injection. Others may have a needle that automatically retracts into the barrel after injection. Each of these devices reduces the chance of needle stick injury. ● **Figure 7.35** shows examples of safety syringes.

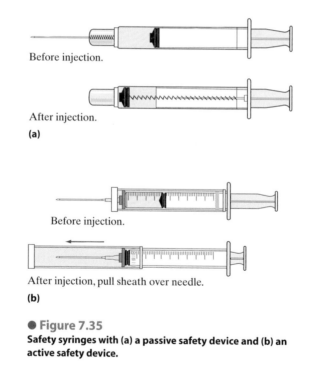

Before injection.

After injection.

**(a)**

Before injection.

After injection, pull sheath over needle.

**(b)**

● Figure 7.35
Safety syringes with (a) a passive safety device and (b) an active safety device.

## Needleless Syringes

A needleless syringe is a type of safety syringe designed to prevent needle punctures. It may be used to extract medication from a vial (see ● **Figure 7.36**), or to add medication to IV tubing for medication administration (see ● **Figure 7.37**).

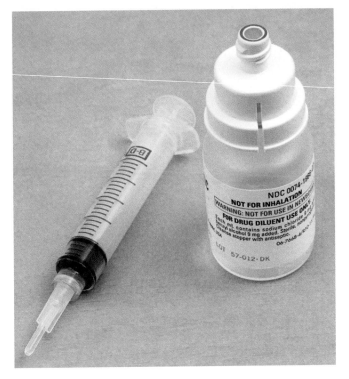

● Figure 7.36
A needleless syringe and vial.

● Figure 7.37
A needleless syringe and IV tubing.

# Summary

In this chapter, the various types of syringes were discussed. You learned how to measure the amount of liquid in various syringes. The types of insulin, how to measure a single dose, and how to mix two insulins in one syringe were explained. Prefilled, single-dose, and safety syringes were also presented.

- Milliliters (mL), rather than cubic centimeters (cc), are the preferred unit of measure for volume.
- All syringe calibrations must be read at the top ring of the plunger.
- Large-capacity hypodermic syringes (5, 12, 20, 35 mL) are calibrated in increments from 0.2 mL to 1 mL.
- Small-capacity hypodermic syringes (2, $2\frac{1}{2}$, 3 mL) are calibrated in tenths of a milliter (0.1 mL).
- The 0.5 mL and 1 mL hypodermic (tuberculin) syringes are calibrated in hundredths of a milliliter. They are the preferred syringes for use in measuring a dose of 1 millimeter or less.
- The calibrations on hypodermic syringes differ; therefore, be very careful when measuring medications in syringes.
- Insulin syringes are designed for measuring and administering U-100 insulin. They are calibrated for 100 units per mL.

- Standard insulin syringes have a capacity of 100 units.
- Lo-Dose insulin syringes are used for measuring small amounts of insulin. They have a capacity of 50 units or 30 units.
- For greater accuracy, use the smallest capacity syringe possible to measure and administer doses. However, avoid filling a syringe to its capacity.
- When measuring two types of insulin in the same syringe, Regular insulin is always drawn up in the syringe first. Think: first clear, then cloudy.
- The total volume when mixing insulins is the sum of the two insulin amounts.
- Insulin syringes are for measuring and administering insulin only. Tuberculin syringes are used to measure and administer other medications that are less than 1 mL. Confusion of the two can cause a medication error.
- The prefilled single-dose syringe cartridge is to be used once and then discarded.
- Syringes intended for injections should not be used to measure or administer oral medications.
- Use safety syringes to prevent needle stick injuries.

# Case Study 7.1

Read the Case Study and answer the questions. The answers are found in Appendix A.

A 55-year-old female with a medical history of obesity, hypertension, hyperlipidemia, and diabetes mellitus comes to the emergency department complaining of anorexia, nausea, vomiting, fever, chills, and severe sharp right upper quadrant pain that radiates to her back and right shoulder. She states that her pain is 9 (on a 0–10 pain scale). Vital signs are: T 100.2 °F, BP 148/94; P 104; R 24. The diagnostic workup confirms gallstones and she is admitted for a cholecystectomy (removal of gall bladder).

**Pre-Op Orders:**

- NPO
- V/S q4h

- Demerol (meperidine hydrochloride) 75 mg IM stat
- IV D5/RL @ 125 mL/h
- Insert NG (nasogastric) tube to low suction
- Pre-op meds: Demerol (meperidine hydrochloride) 75 mg and Phenergan (promethazine) 25 mg IM 30 minutes before surgery
- Cefuroxime 1.5 g IV 30 minutes before surgery

**Post-Op Orders:**

- Discontinue NG tube
- NPO
- V/S q4h

- IV D5/RL @ 125 mL/h
- Compazine (prochlorperazine) 4 mg IM q4h prn nausea
- Demerol (meperidine hydrochloride) 75 mg and Vistaril (hydroxyzine) 25 mg IM q3h prn pain
- Merrem (meropenem) 1g IVPB q8h

1. The label on the meperidine for the stat dose reads 100 mg/mL.
   (a) Draw a line indicating the stat dose on each of the following syringes below.
   (b) Which syringe will most accurately measure this dose?

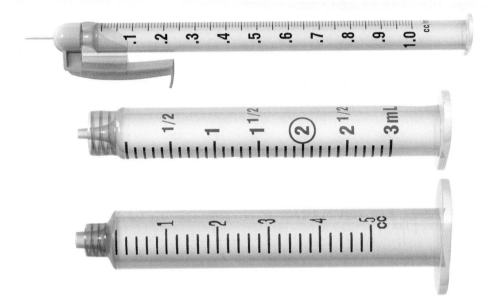

2. Calculate the pre-op dose of the Phenergan and Demerol to be administered 30 minutes before surgery. Phenergan is available in 25 mg/mL vials. Demerol is available in 2.5 mL capacity prefilled syringes, each containing 1 mL of Demerol. The Demerol prefilled syringes have strengths of 10 mg/mL, 25 mg/mL, 50 mg/mL, 75 mg/mL, and 100 mg/mL.
   (a) Which prepackaged syringe of Demerol will you use?
   (b) How many milliliters of Phenergan will you prepare?
   (c) Indicate, on the appropriate syringe below, the dose of each of these drugs that you will administer.

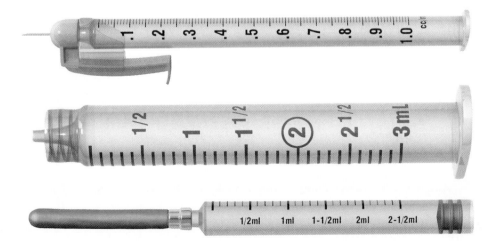

3. The label on the cefuroxime vial states: "add 9 mL of diluent to the 1.5 g vial." Draw a line on the appropriate syringe below indicating the amount of diluent you will add to the vial.

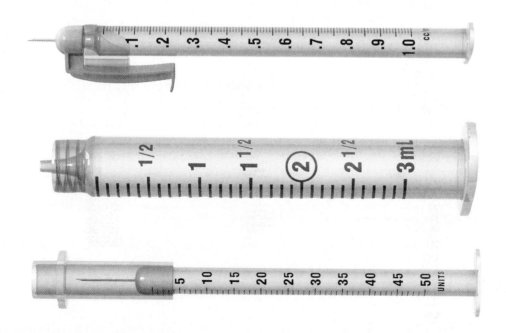

4. The patient is complaining of severe nausea. The Compazine vial is labeled 5 mg/mL. Draw a line on the appropriate syringe below indicating the dose of Compazine.

5. The patient is complaining of severe incisional pain of 10 (on a 0–10 pain scale) and has had no pain medication since her surgery. Calculate the dose of the Demerol and Vistaril order. The Vistaril is available in a concentration of 25 mg/mL. The Demerol is available as 100 mg/mL.
   (a) How many milliliters of Vistaril will you use?
   (b) How many milliliters of Demerol do you need?
   (c) How will you prepare these medications so that you can give the patient a single injection?
   (d) Indicate on the appropriate syringe below the number of milliliters you will administer.

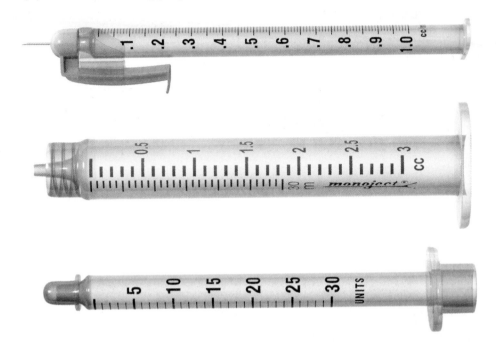

6. The label on the Merrem states 50 mg/mL.
   (a) How many mL will you need?
   (b) Draw a line on the appropriate syringe below indicating the dose of Merrem.

7. The patient has progressed to a regular diet and is ordered Humulin N 13 units and Humulin R 6 units subcutaneous 30 minutes ac breakfast, and Humulin N 5 units and Humulin R 5 units subcutaneous 30 minutes ac dinner.
   (a) How many units will the patient receive before breakfast?
   (b) Indicate on the appropriate syringe below the number of units of each insulin required before breakfast.

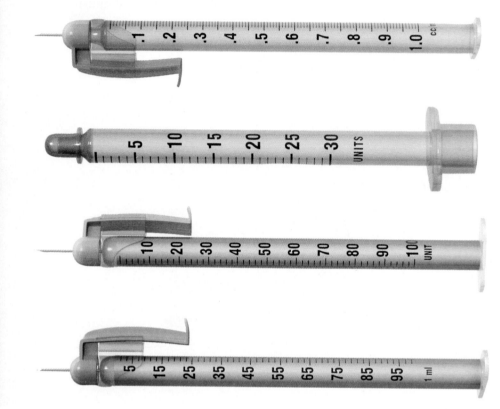

## Practice Sets

**Workspace**

The answers to *Try These for Practice, Exercises,* and *Cumulative Review Exercises* are found in Appendix A. Ask your instructor for the answers to the *Additional Exercises.*

### Try These for Practice

Test your comprehension after reading the chapter.

In Problems 1 through 4, identify the type of syringe shown in the figure. Place an arrow at the appropriate level of measurement on the syringe for the volume given.

1. _____ syringe; 0.72 mL

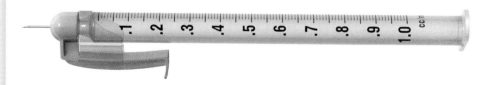

Workspace

2. _____ syringe; 6.8 mL

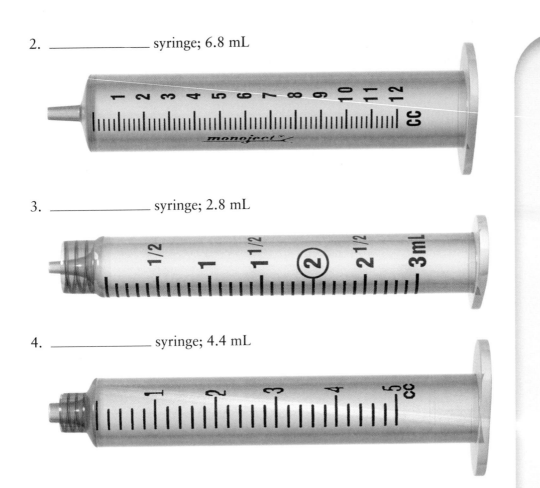

3. _____ syringe; 2.8 mL

4. _____ syringe; 4.4 mL

5. The prescriber ordered 34 units of Regular insulin and 18 units of Humulin N subcutaneously 30 minutes ac breakfast. Read the labels and do the following:

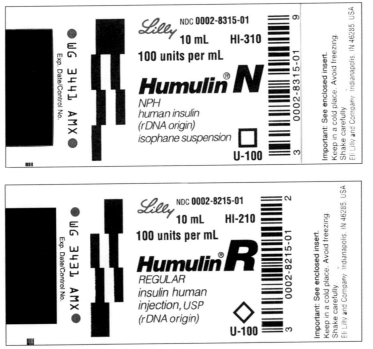

(Copyright Eli Lilly and Company. Used with permission.)

(a) Select the appropriate syringe to administer this dose in one injection.

(b) Indicate the measurement of the Regular insulin.

(c) Indicate the measurement of the Humulin N insulin.

(d) Determine how many units the patient will receive.

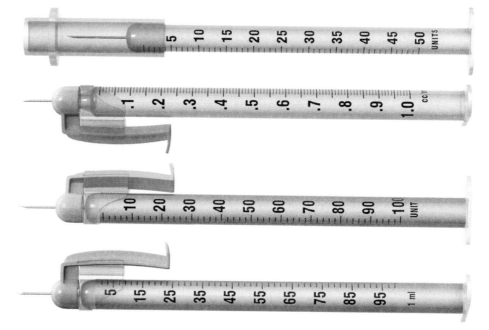

## Exercises

Reinforce your understanding in class or at home.

In problems 1 through 14, identify the type of syringe shown in the figure. Then, for each quantity, place an arrow at the appropriate level of measurement on the syringe.

1. _____ syringe; 0.62 mL

2. _____ syringe; 28 units

3. _____ syringe; 3.6 mL

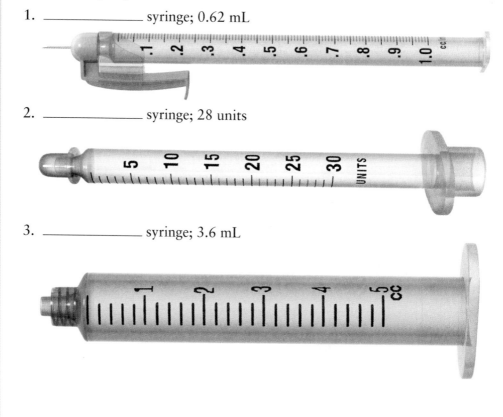

4. _____ syringe; 1.4 mL

5. _____ syringe; 13 mL

6. _____ syringe; 9.6 mL

7. _____ syringe; 32 units

8. _____ syringe; 56 units

9. _____ syringe; 0.37 mL

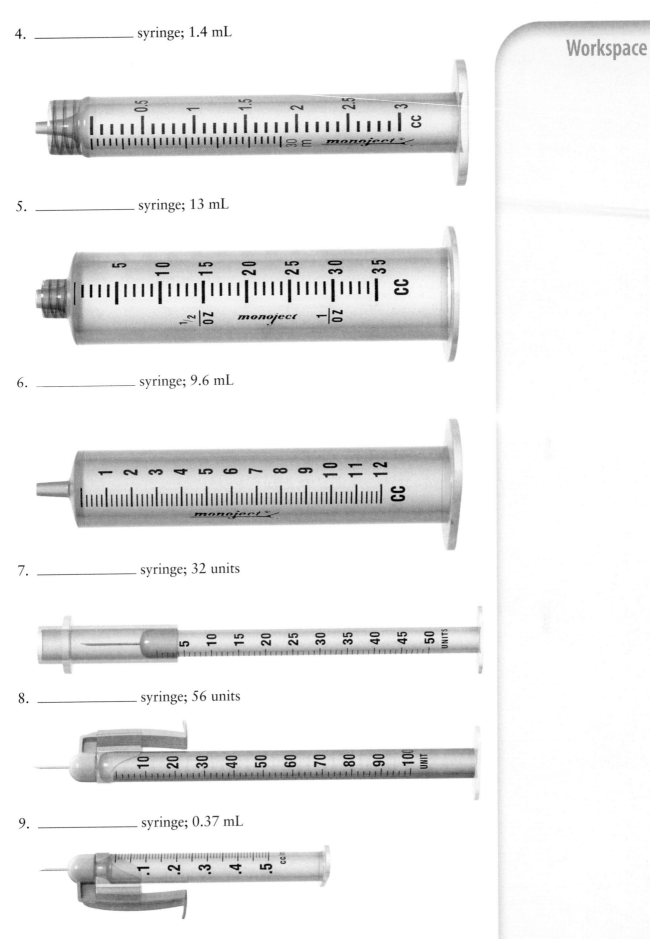

**Workspace**

10. _____ syringe; 51 units

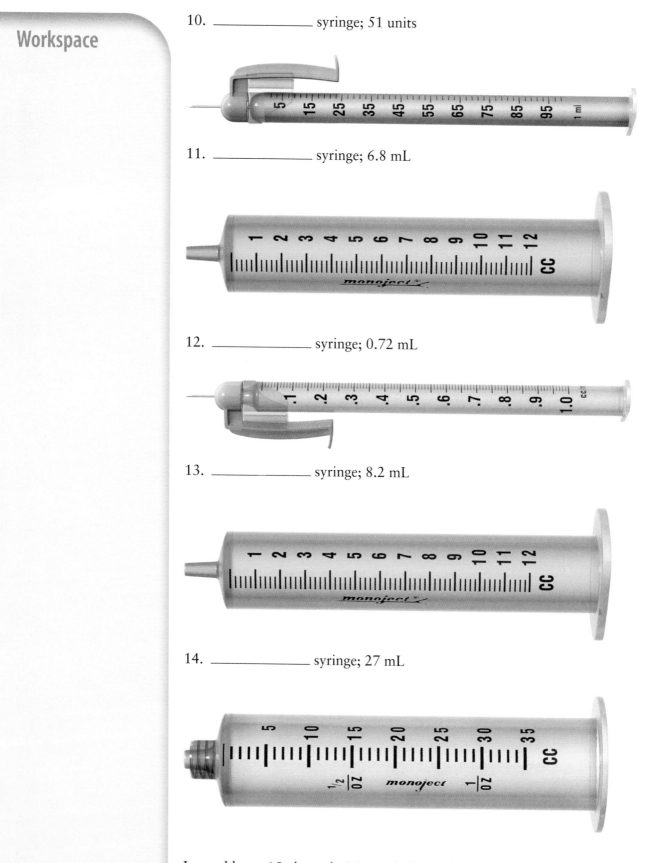

11. _____ syringe; 6.8 mL

12. _____ syringe; 0.72 mL

13. _____ syringe; 8.2 mL

14. _____ syringe; 27 mL

In problems 15 through 20, read the order, use the appropriate label in ● **Figure 7.38**, calculate the dosage if necessary, and place an arrow at the appropriate level of measurement on the syringe.

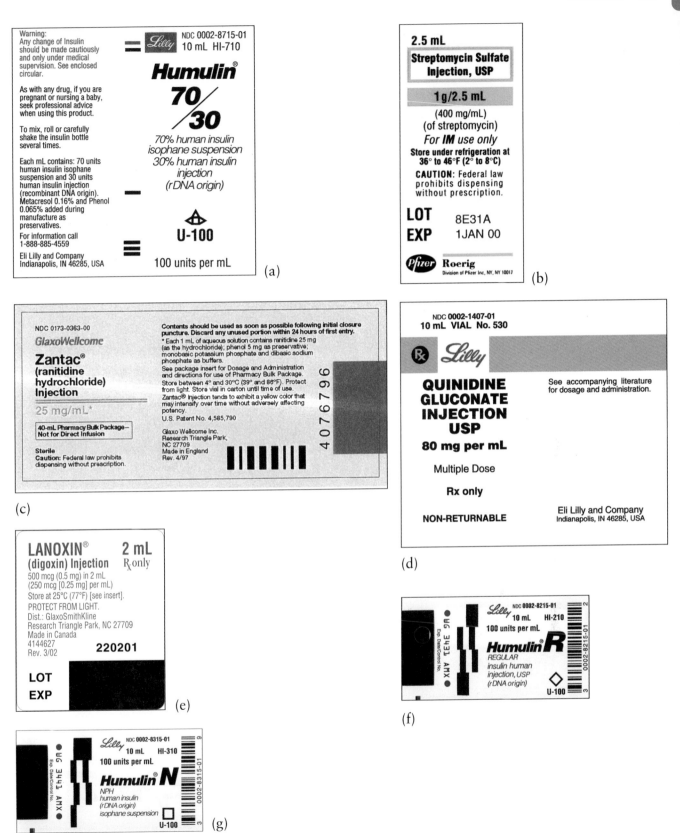

**(a)**

Warning:
Any change of Insulin should be made cautiously and only under medical supervision. See enclosed circular.

As with any drug, if you are pregnant or nursing a baby, seek professional advice when using this product.

To mix, roll or carefully shake the insulin bottle several times.

Each mL contains: 70 units human insulin isophane suspension and 30 units human insulin injection (recombinant DNA origin). Metacresol 0.16% and Phenol 0.065% added during manufacture as preservatives.

For information call 1-888-885-4559

Eli Lilly and Company Indianapolis, IN 46285, USA

*Lilly* NDC 0002-8715-01
10 mL HI-710

**Humulin®**
**70/30**

70% human insulin isophane suspension
30% human insulin injection
(rDNA origin)

**U-100**

100 units per mL

**(b)**

2.5 mL

**Streptomycin Sulfate Injection, USP**

**1 g/2.5 mL**

(400 mg/mL)
(of streptomycin)
*For IM use only*
Store under refrigeration at 36° to 46°F (2° to 8°C)
CAUTION: Federal law prohibits dispensing without prescription.

**LOT** 8E31A
**EXP** 1JAN 00

*Pfizer* **Roerig**
Division of Pfizer Inc, NY, NY 10017

**(c)**

NDC 0173-0363-00
**GlaxoWellcome**

**Zantac®**
(ranitidine hydrochloride)
Injection

25 mg/mL*

40-mL Pharmacy Bulk Package—
Not for Direct Infusion

**Sterile**
**Caution:** Federal law prohibits dispensing without prescription.

Contents should be used as soon as possible following initial closure puncture. Discard any unused portion within 24 hours of first entry.
* Each 1 mL of aqueous solution contains ranitidine 25 mg (as the hydrochloride); phenol 5 mg as preservative; monobasic potassium phosphate and dibasic sodium phosphate as buffers.
See package insert for Dosage and Administration and directions for use of Pharmacy Bulk Package.
Store between 4° and 30°C (39° and 86°F). Protect from light. Store vial in carton until time of use.
Zantac® Injection tends to exhibit a yellow color that may intensify over time without adversely affecting potency.
U.S. Patent No. 4,585,790

Glaxo Wellcome Inc.
Research Triangle Park,
NC 27709
Made in England
Rev. 4/97

4076796

**(d)**

NDC 0002-1407-01
10 mL VIAL No. 530

**R** *Lilly*

**QUINIDINE GLUCONATE INJECTION USP**

**80 mg per mL**

Multiple Dose

**Rx only**

**NON-RETURNABLE**

See accompanying literature for dosage and administration.

Eli Lilly and Company
Indianapolis, IN 46285, USA

**(e)**

**LANOXIN®** 2 mL
(digoxin) Injection  Rₓ only
500 mcg (0.5 mg) in 2 mL
(250 mcg [0.25 mg] per mL)
Store at 25°C (77°F) [see insert].
PROTECT FROM LIGHT.
Dist.: GlaxoSmithKline
Research Triangle Park, NC 27709
Made in Canada
4144627
Rev. 3/02      220201

**LOT**
**EXP**

**(f)**

*Lilly* NDC 0002-8215-01
10 mL HI-210
100 units per mL

**Humulin® R**
REGULAR
insulin human injection, USP
(rDNA origin)

**U-100**

Exp. Date/Control No.
8E31A AMX

0002-8215-01

**(g)**

*Lilly* NDC 0002-8315-01
10 mL HI-310
100 units per mL

**Humulin® N**
NPH
human insulin
(rDNA origin)
isophane suspension

**U-100**

Exp. Date/Control No.
8E31A AMX

0002-8315-01

● **Figure 7.38**
**Drug labels for Exercises 15–20.**

*(07–38a Copyright Eli Lilly and Company. Used with permission.   07–38b Reg. Trademark of Pfizer Inc. Reproduced with permission.*
*07–38c Reproduced with permission of GlaxoSmithKlin.   07–38d Copyright Eli Lilly and Company. Used with permission.*
*07–38e Reproduced with permission of GlaxoSmithKlin.   07–38f Copyright Eli Lilly and Company. Used with permission.*
*07–38g Copyright Eli Lilly and Company. Used with permission.)*

15. Order: Give 26 units of Humulin 70/30 subcutaneously, 30 minutes ac breakfast

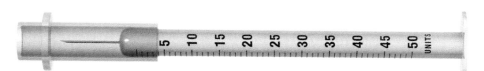

16. Order: Streptomycin 600 mg IM daily

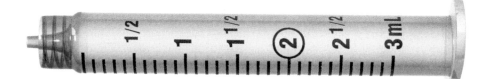

17. Order: Give 14 units of Regular insulin and 44 units of NPH insulin subcutaneously 30 minutes ac breakfast

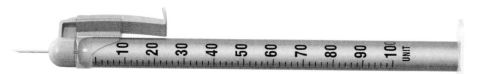

18. Order: ranitidine hydrochloride 50 mg IVPB q6h

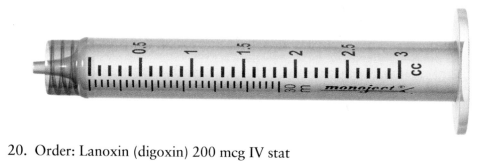

19. Order: quinidine gluconate 200 mg IV stat

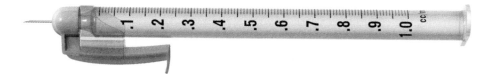

20. Order: Lanoxin (digoxin) 200 mcg IV stat

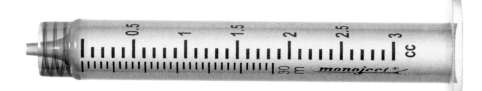

# Additional Exercises

Now, test yourself!
In problems 1–15 identify the type of syringe shown in the figure. Then, for each quantity, place an arrow at the appropriate level of measurement on the syringe.

1. _____ syringe; 42 units

2. _____ syringe; 14 units

3. _____ syringe; 3.6 mL

4. _____ syringe; 1.8 mL

5. _____ syringe; 7.2 mL

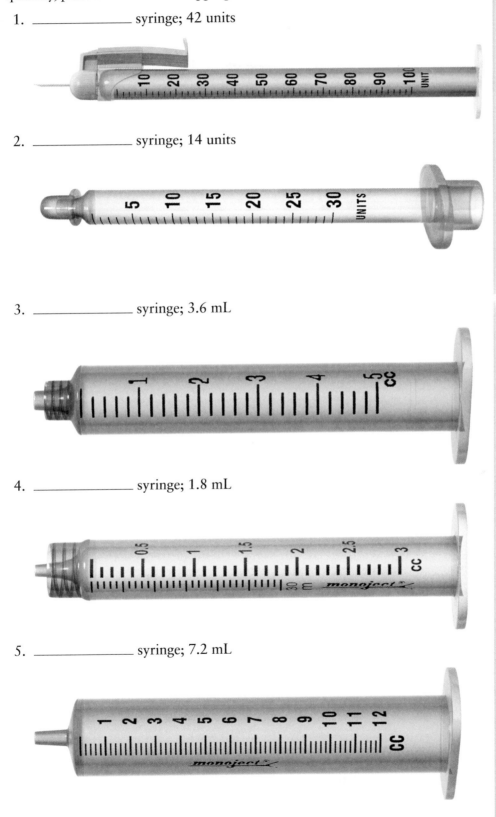

6. _____ syringe; 16 mL

7. _____ syringe; 12 units

8. _____ syringe; 54 units

9. _____ syringe; 0.35 mL

10. _____ syringe; 31 units

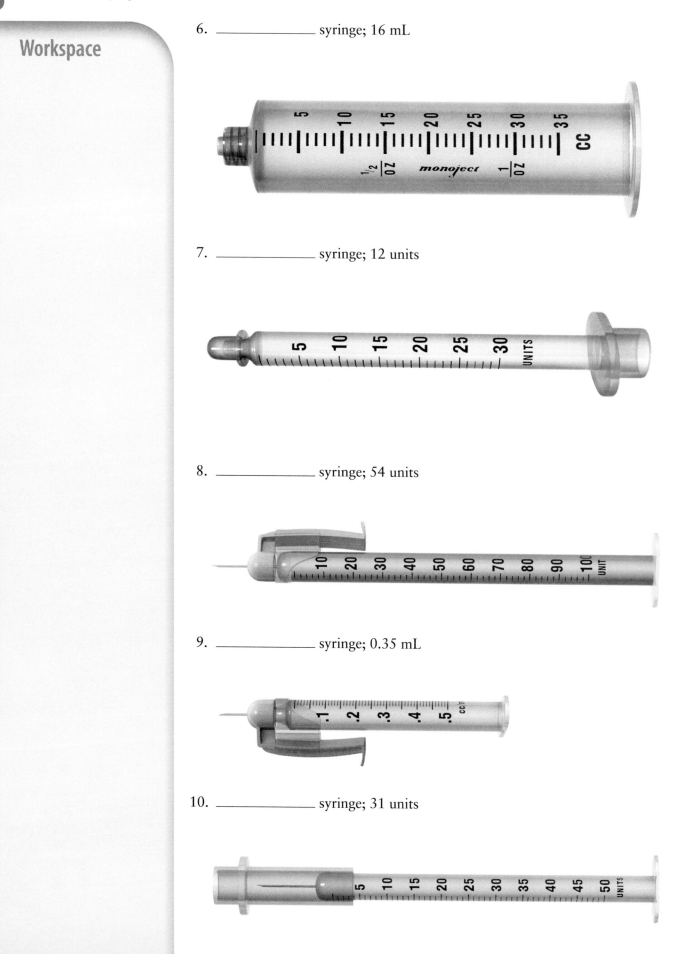

11. _____ syringe; 4.4 mL

12. _____ syringe; 16 units

13. _____ syringe; 8.8 mL

14. _____ syringe; 22 mL

15. _____ syringe; 0.38 mL

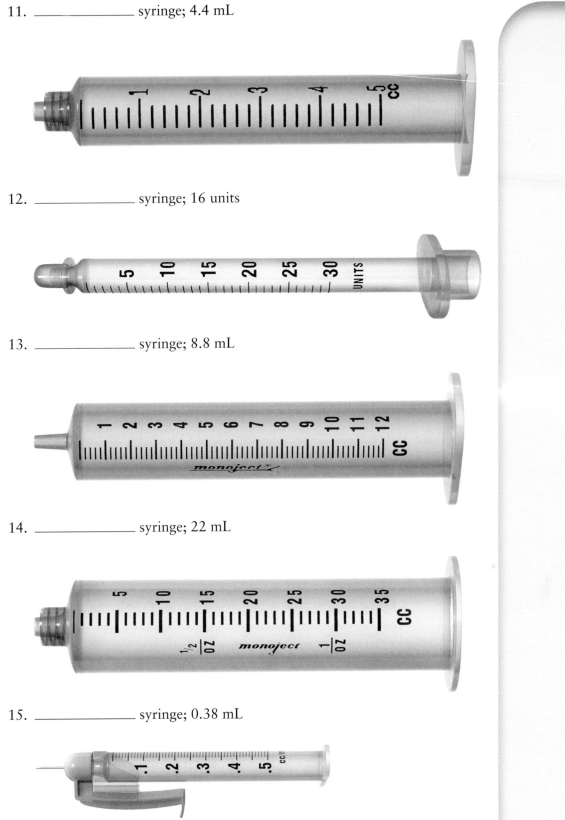

In problems 16 through 20, read the order and use the appropriate label in
● **Figure 7.39** calculate the dosage if necessary, and place an arrow at the
appropriate level of measurement on the syringe.

16. Order: Humulin R 8 units subcutaneously 15 minutes ac breakfast

17. Order: Humulin N 38 units subcut ac dinner

18. Order: fentanyl citrate 75 mcg IM 30 min before surgery

19. Order: Quinidine 400 mg IM q4h prn

20. Order: Humulin 70/30 U-100 insulin 46 units subcutaneously ac dinner

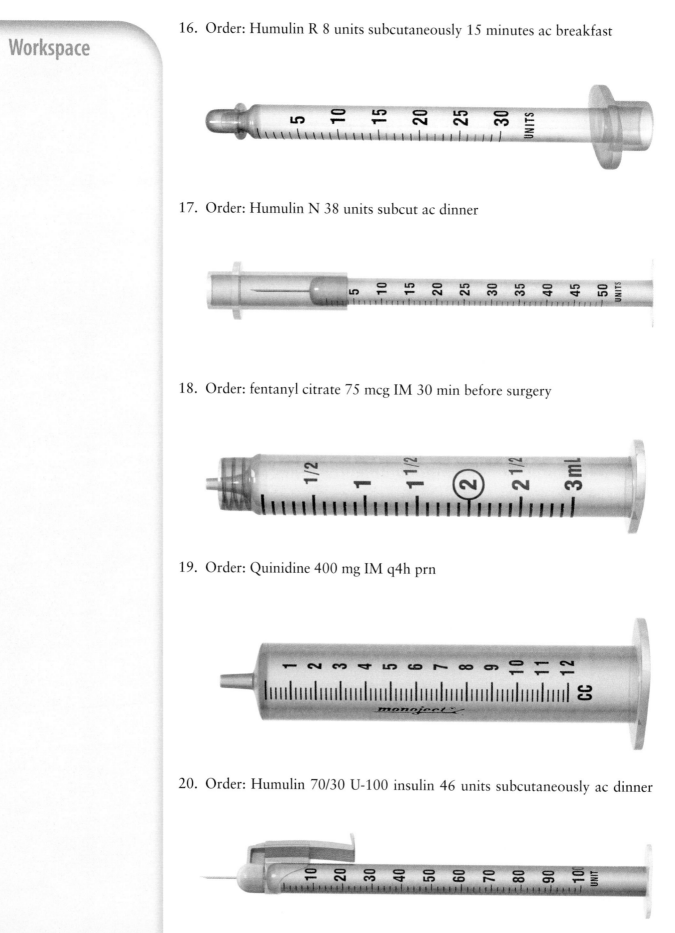

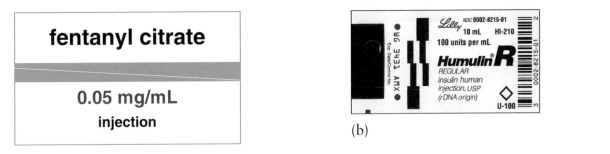

(a)

(b)

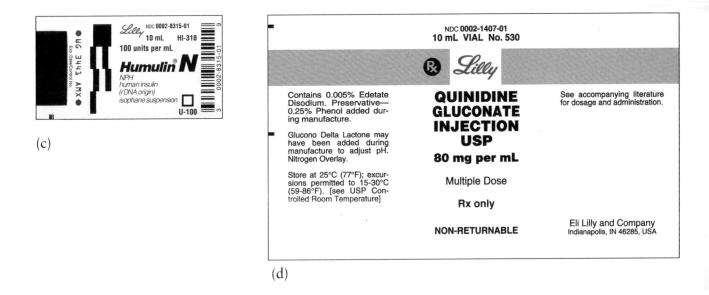

(c)

(d)

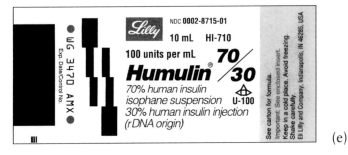

(e)

● **Figure 7.39**
**Drug labels for Additional Exercises 15–20.**

*(07-39b Copyright Eli Lilly and Company. Used with permission.    07-39c Copyright Eli Lilly and Company. Used with permission.*
*07-39d Copyright Eli Lilly and Company. Used with permission.    07-39e Copyright Eli Lilly and Company. Used with permission.)*

# Cumulative Review Exercises

Review your mastery of previous chapters.

1. Prescriber's order: *Administer Humulin R (regular insulin [rDNA origin])*
   *subcutaneously as per the following blood glucose results:*

   For glucose less than 160 mg/dL    — no insulin

   glucose 160 mg/dL–220 mg/dL    — give 2 units

Workspace

*glucose 221 mg/dL–280 mg/dL       — give 4 units*
*glucose 281 mg/dL–340 mg/dL       — give 6 units*
*glucose 341 mg/dL–400 mg/dL       — give 8 units*
*glucose greater than 400 mg/dL    — notify MD stat*

How many units will you administer if the patient's glucose level at lunchtime is

(a) *152 mg/dL*

(b) *174 mg/dL*

(c) *343 mg/dL*

2. 1,600 mL = _____ L

3. The prescriber ordered *Prilosec 40 mg PO daily.* Each capsule contains 20 mg. How many capsules will the patient receive in two weeks? _____

4. The order reads *morphine sulfate 4 mg subcutaneously q4h prn pain.* What is the maximum number of times the patient may receive this medication in one day? _____

5. The prescriber ordered *Biaxin 300 mg PO q12h.* The label reads 375 mg/mL. How many milliliters will you administer? _____

6. Prescriber's order: *Reglan (metoclopramide) 10 mg, 30 minutes ac meals and at bedtime.* The label reads 5 mg/tab. How many tablets will the patient receive per day? _____

7. The prescriber ordered 120 mL $H_2O$ PO q2h for 10h. How many ounces should the patient receive? _____

8. Convert 8 fluid oz to mL. _____

9. The prescriber ordered *Ceclor (cefaclor) oral suspension 225 mg PO B.I.D.* The label reads 375 mg/5 mL. How many milliliters will you administer? _____

10. Which of the following has the greatest weight? 0.3 mg, 0.05 mg, 0.125 mg _____

11. The prescriber ordered *Amoxicillin 750 mg PO q12h.* Each capsule contains 250 mg. How many capsules will you administer to the patient? _____

12. The prescriber ordered 0.3 mg of clonidine hydrochloride. If each tablet contains 0.1 mg, how many tablets will you administer to the patient? _____

13. Read the information on the label in ● **Figure 7.40** and calculate the number of capsules equal to 0.002 g. _____

14. The prescriber ordered *Vistaril 75 mg IM stat.* The label reads 50 mg/mL. How many milliliters will you administer? _____

15. Read the label in ● **Figure 7.41** How many milligrams equal 1 mL? _____

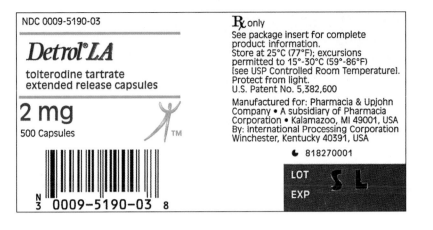

**Figure 7.40**
**Drug label for Detrol.**

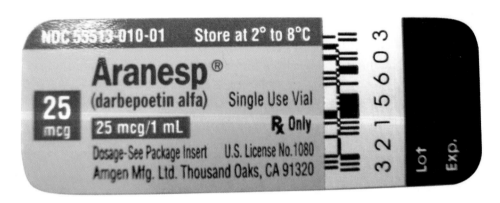

**Figure 7.41**
**Drug label for Aranesp.**

*(Published with permission of Amgen Inc.)*

**MediaLink**
www.prenhall.com/giangrasso

Animated examples, interactive practice questions with animated solutions, and challenge tests for this chapter can be found on the Pearson Dosage Calculation Tutor that accompanies this text. Additional, unique, interactive resources and activities can be found on the Companion Web site.

Workspace

# Preparation of Solutions

## Learning Outcomes

After completing this chapter, you will be able to

1. Describe the strength of a solution as a ratio, fraction, and as a percent.
2. Determine the amount of solute in a given amount of solution.
3. Determine the amount of solution that would contain a given amount of solute.
4. Do the calculations necessary to prepare solutions from pure drugs.
5. Do the calculations necessary to prepare solutions for irrigations, soaks, and nutritional feedings.

In this chapter you will learn about solutions. Although solutions are generally prepared by the pharmacist, healthcare providers should understand the concepts involved, and be able to prepare solutions.

Drugs are manufactured in both pure and diluted forms. A pure drug contains only the drug and nothing else. A pure drug can be diluted by dissolving a quantity of pure drug in a liquid to form a solution. The pure drug (either dry or liquid) is called the *solute*. The liquid added to the pure drug to form the solution is called the *solvent* or *diluent*.

# Determining the Strength of a Solution

To make a cup of coffee, you might dissolve 2 teaspoons of instant coffee granules in a cup of hot water. The instant coffee granules (*solute*), are added to the hot water (*solvent*) to form the cup of coffee (*solution*). If instead of 2 teaspoons of instant coffee granules, you add either 1 or 3 teaspoons of instant coffee granules to the cup of hot water, the coffee solution will taste quite different. The **strength or concentration** of the coffee could be described in terms of *teaspoons per cup* (*t/cup*). Thus, a coffee solution with a strength of *1 t/cup* is a "*weaker*" solution than a coffee solution with a strength of *2 t/cup*, and a strength of *3 t/cup* is "*stronger*" *than a strength of 2 t/cup.*

Important terms for the elements of a solution:

- The **solute** is the solid or liquid to be dissolved or diluted. Some solutes are: various powdered drugs, chemical salts, and liquid nutritional supplements.

- The **solvent** (**diluent**) is the liquid which dissolves the solid solute, or dilutes the liquid solute. Two commonly used solvents are sterile water and normal saline.

- The **solution** is the liquid resulting from the combination of the solute and solvent.

The strength of a drug is stated on the label. Liquid drugs are solutions. The strength of these solutions compares the *amount of drug (solute)* in the solution to the *volume of solution*. Some examples of drug strengths or concentrations are: *Lanoxin 500 mcg/2 mL, KCl 2 mEq/mL, Garamycin 80 mg/2 ml,* and *heparin 10,000 units/mL.*

Suppose a vial is labeled *furosemide 5 mg/mL.* This means that there are 5 milligrams of furosemide in each milliliter of the solution. If a second vial is labeled *furosemide 10 mg/mL,* then this second solution is "stronger" than the first because there are 10 mg of furosemide in each milliliter of the solution. If an order is *furosemide 10 mg po stat,* then, to receive 10 mg of the drug, the patient would receive either 2 mL of the "weaker" first solution, or 1 mL of the "stronger" second solution.

## Strengths of Solutions as Ratios, Fractions, and Percents

Sometimes the strength of a solution is specified without using explicit units of measurement like milligrams or milliliters, but by comparing the number of parts of *solute* to the number of parts of *solution*. This method of stating strength is generally expressed by using either *ratios, fractions,* or *percents.* Some examples of these strengths are *epinephrine 1:1,000 (ratio), Enfamil* $\frac{1}{2}$ *strength (fraction),* and *0.9% NaCl (percent).*

If a solution contains *1 part solute* in *2 parts of solution,* the strength could be expressed in the form of the *ratio 1:2* (read "1 to 2"), the *fraction* $\frac{1}{2}$ *strength* or (because $\frac{1}{2} = 50\%$) the *percentage 50%.* See ● **Figure 8.1.**

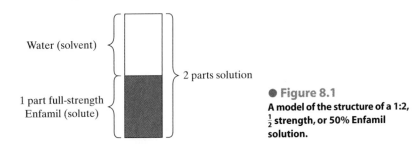

Water (solvent) }

} 2 parts solution

1 part full-strength Enfamil (solute) }

● **Figure 8.1**
**A model of the structure of a 1:2,** $\frac{1}{2}$ **strength, or 50% Enfamil solution.**

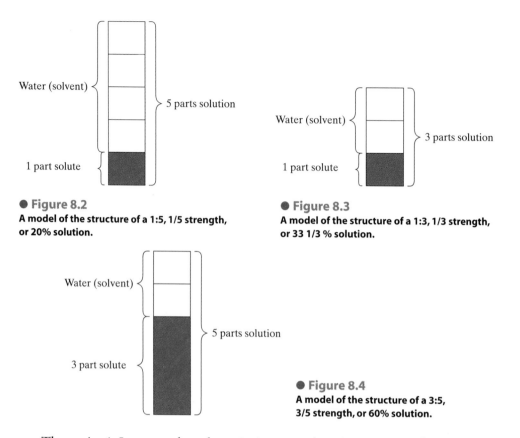

● **Figure 8.2**
A model of the structure of a 1:5, 1/5 strength, or 20% solution.

● **Figure 8.3**
A model of the structure of a 1:3, 1/3 strength, or 33 1/3 % solution.

● **Figure 8.4**
A model of the structure of a 3:5, 3/5 strength, or 60% solution.

The ratio *1:5* means that there is 1 part *solute* in 5 parts *solution*. This solution is also referred to as a *1/5* strength solution or as a *20%* solution. See ● **Figure 8.2**.

A *1/3* strength solution can be expressed as a *1:3* solution. This has 1 part *solute* for 3 parts *solution*. Since 1/3 = 33 1/3%, this is a *33 1/3%* solution. See ● **Figure 8.3**.

A *60%* solution can be referred to (in fractional form) as a 60/100 solution, and after reducing this fraction becomes *3/5*. In ratio form this strength would be *3:5*. This solution has 3 parts *solute* for 5 parts *solution*. See ● **Figure 8.4**.

### EXAMPLE 8.1

Fill in the missing items in each line by following the pattern of the first line.

| The solution contains: | The strength of the solution is | | |
|---|---|---|---|
| | ratio | fraction | percent |
| 1 part solute in 2 parts solution | | | |
| | 1:4 | | |
| | | 1/5 | |
| | | | 3% |
| | | | 5% |
| | | 2/5 | |
| 1 part solute in 1,000 parts solution | | | |

Here are the answers.

| The solution contains: | The strength of the solution is | | |
|---|---|---|---|
| | ratio | fraction | percent |
| 1 part solute in 2 parts solution | 1:2 | 1/2 | 50% |
| 1 part solute in 4 parts solution | 1:4 | 1/4 | 25% |
| 1 part solute in 5 parts solution | 1:5 | 1/5 | 20% |
| 3 parts solute in 100 parts solution | 3:100 | 3/100 | 3% |
| 1 part solute in 20 parts solution | 1:20 | 1/20 | 5% |
| 2 parts solute in 5 parts solution | 2:5 | 2/5 | 40% |
| 1 part solute in 1,000 parts solution | 1:1,000 | 1/1,000 | 0.1% |

## Liquid Solutes

For a solute that is in liquid form, the ratio 1:40 means there is 1 milliliter of solute in every 40 milliliters of solution. So 40 milliliters of a 1:40 acetic acid solution means that 1 milliliter of pure acetic acid is diluted with water to make a total of 40 milliliters of solution. You would prepare this solution by placing 1 milliliter of pure acetic acid in a graduated cylinder and adding water until the level in the graduated cylinder reaches 40 milliliters. ● **Figure 8.5.**

A 1% solution means that there is 1 part of the solute in 100 parts of solution. So you would prepare 100 mL of a 1% creosol solution by placing 1 milliliter of pure creosol in a graduated cylinder and adding water until the level in the graduated cylinder reaches 100 mL. ● **Figure 8.6.**

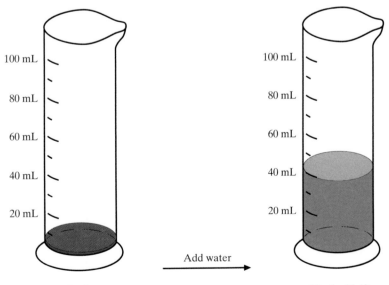

100 mL
80 mL
60 mL
40 mL
20 mL

1 mL of pure
acetic acid (solute)

Add water

100 mL
80 mL
60 mL
40 mL
20 mL

40 mL of 1:40
acetic acid (solution)

● **Figure 8.5**
**Preparing a 1:40 solution from a liquid solute.**

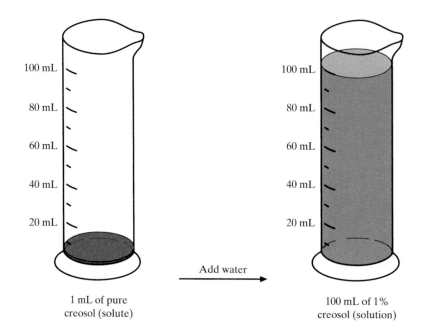

Add water

● **Figure 8.6**
**Preparing a 1% solution from a liquid solute.**

1 mL of pure
creosol (solute)

100 mL of 1%
creosol (solution)

### EXAMPLE 8.2

**40 mL of an iodine solution contain 10 mL of (solute) pure iodine. Express the strength of this solution as a ratio, a fraction, and a percentage.**

The strength of a solution may be expressed as the ratio of the *amount of pure drug in the solution to the total amount of the solution.* The amount of the solution is always expressed in milliliters, and because iodine is a liquid in pure form, the amount of iodine is also expressed in milliliters.

There are 10 mL of pure iodine in the 40 mL of the solution, so the strength of this solution, expressed as a ratio, is ten to forty. The ratio may also be written as *10:40, 10 to 40,* or in fractional form as $\frac{10}{40}$. This fraction could then be simplified to $\frac{1}{4}$, which is equal to 25%.

So, the strength of this iodine solution may be expressed as the ratio 1:4, the fraction $\frac{1}{4}$ strength, and as the percentage 25%.

## Dry Solutes

The ratio 1:20 means 1 part of the solute in 20 parts of solution, or 2 parts of the solute in 40 parts of solution, or 3 parts in 60, or 4 parts in 80, or 5 parts in 100, and so on. When a pure drug is in *dry* form, the ratio 1:20 means 1 g of pure drug in every 20 mL of solution. So 100 mL of a 1:20 potassium permanganate solution means 5 g of pure potassium permanganate dissolved in water to make a total of 100 mL of the solution. A 1:20 solution is the same as a 5% solution. If each tablet is 5 g, then you would prepare this solution by placing 1 tablet of the pure potassium permanganate in a graduated cylinder and adding some water to dissolve the tablet; then add more water until the level in the graduated cylinder reaches 100 mL.

Because a 5% potassium permanganate solution means 5 g of pure potassium permanganate in 100 mL of solution, the strength is also written as $\frac{5\,g}{100\,mL}$ or $\frac{1\,g}{20\,mL}$. ● **Figure 8.7.**

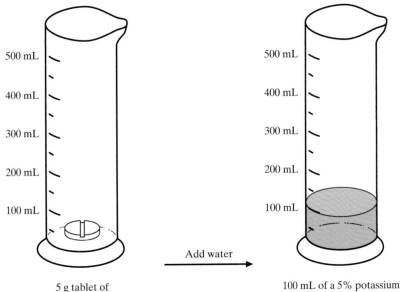

● **Figure 8.7**
**Preparing a 5% solution from a pure, dry drug.**

5 g tablet of
potassium permanganate (solute)

Add water

100 mL of a 5% potassium
permanganate (solution)

## EXAMPLE 8.3

One liter of an isotonic normal saline solution contains 9,000 mg of sodium chloride. Express the strength of this solution both as a ratio and as a percentage.

The strength of a solution may be expressed as the ratio of the *amount of solute* in the solution to the *total amount of the solution.* Since sodium chloride (NaCl) is a *solid* in pure form, the amount of NaCl (9,000 mg) must be expressed in *grams* (9 g). The *amount of the solution* (1 L) must always be expressed in *milliliters* (1,000 mL).

Since there are 9 g of pure NaCl in 1,000 mL of the solution, the strength of this solution, expressed as a ratio, is *nine to one thousand.*

This ratio may also be written as *9 to 1,000, 9:1,000,* or in fractional form as $\frac{9}{1,000}$. This fraction could be written in decimal form as 0.009, which is equal to 0.9%.

So, the strength of this isotonic normal saline solution may be expressed as the ratio *9:1,000* or the percentage *0.9%.*

## EXAMPLE 8.4

Read the label in ● Figure 8.8 and verify that the two strengths stated on the label are equivalent.

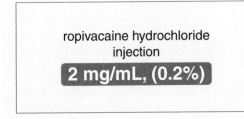

ropivacaine hydrochloride
injection
**2 mg/mL, (0.2%)**

● **Figure 8.8**
**Drug label for ropivacaine hydrochloride.**

The two strengths stated on this label are *2 mg/mL and 0.2%*. To show that they are equivalent, take either one of these strengths and show how to change it to the other. For example, if you start with 0.2%, you must change this to 2 mg/mL.

A solution whose strength is 0.2% has 0.2 g of solute (ropivacaine HCl) in 100 mL of solution. As a fraction, this is $\frac{0.2\,g}{100\,mL}$.

You need to change this fraction to mg/mL. But 0.2 g can be converted to 200 mg by moving the decimal point three places.

$$\frac{0.2\,g}{100\,mL} = \frac{200\,mg}{100\,mL} \text{ or } \frac{2\,mg}{1\,mL}$$

So, the two strengths stated on the label, 2 mg/mL and 0.2%, are equivalent.

## Determining the Amount of Solute in a Given Amount of Solution

Ratio and proportion can be used to determine the amount of solute in a given amount of a solution of known strength. This is useful in preparing solutions from pure drugs.

The units of measurement for the amount of solution (volume), strength of the solution, and amount of solute are listed as follows:

Amount of solution: Use *milliliters.*

Strength: Always write as a fraction for calculations.

For liquid solutes:
1:40 acetic acid solution is written as $\frac{1\,mL}{40\,mL}$

5% acetic acid solution is written as $\frac{5\,mL}{100\,mL}$
For dry or powder solutes:
1:20 potassium permanganate solution is written as $\frac{1\,g}{20\,mL}$

12% potassium permanganate solution is written as $\frac{12\,g}{100\,mL}$

Amount of solute: Use *milliliters* for liquids.
Use *grams* for tablets or powders.

In order to prepare a given amount of a solution of a given strength, you must first determine the amount of pure drug that will be in that solution. The following examples illustrate how this is done.

---

**EXAMPLE 8.5**

**How would you prepare 500 mL of a 0.45% sodium chloride solution using 2.25 g sodium chloride tablets?**

The 0.45% strength means that there is 0.45 g of sodium chloride in every 100 mL of this solution *(0.45 g = 100 mL)*. You need to determine the number of grams of sodium chloride which are in 500 mL of this strength solution *(? g = 500 mL).*

Think of the problem as:

$$0.45\,g = 100\,mL$$
$$x\,g = 500\,mL$$

Because the number of grams of solute is proportional to the number of milliliters of solution, a proportion could be used to solve the problem. The proportion could be set up as

$$\frac{g}{mL} = \frac{g'}{mL'}$$

Substituting, you get

$$\frac{0.45\,g}{100\,mL} = \frac{x\,g}{500\,mL}$$

Eliminate the units of measurement and cross multiply

$$\frac{0.45}{100} = \frac{x}{500}$$

$$(x)(100) = (0.45)(500)$$
$$100x = 225$$
$$x = 2.25$$

So, 500 mL of the solution must contain 2.25 g of sodium choride.

Since each tablet contains 2.25 g, you would need 1 tablet.

So, you would place 1 tablet into a graduated cylinder, add some water to dissolve the tablet, and then add water until the 500 mL level is reached.

## EXAMPLE 8.6

Read the label in ● Figure 8.9. How many grams of dextrose are contained in 30 mL of this solution?

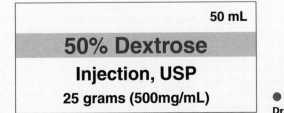

● **Figure 8.9**
**Drug label for 50% dextrose.**

The 50% strength means that there are 50 g of dextrose in every 100 mL of this solution *(50 g = 100 mL)*. You need to determine the number of grams of dextrose which are in 30 mL of this strength solution *(? g = 30 mL)*.

Think of the problem as:

$$50\,g = 100\,mL$$
$$x\,g = 30\,mL$$

The proportion could be set up as

$$\frac{g}{mL} = \frac{g'}{mL'}$$

Substituting, you get

$$\frac{50\,g}{100\,mL} = \frac{x\,g}{30\,mL}$$

Eliminate the units of measurement and cross multiply

$$\frac{50}{100} = \frac{x}{30}$$
$$100x = 1,500$$
$$x = 15$$

So, 15 g of dextrose are contained in 30 mL of a 50% dextrose solution.

## EXAMPLE 8.7

**How would you prepare 2,000 mL of a 1:10 Clorox solution?**

Because Clorox is a liquid in its pure form, it is measured in milliliters. So, 1:10 strength means 1 mL of Clorox in each 10 mL of the solution *(1 mL of Clorox = 10 mL of solution)*. You need to determine the number of mL of Clorox that are in 2,000 mL of this solution *(? mL of Clorox = 2,000 mL of solution)*.

Think of the problem as:

$$1\,mL\,(Clorox) = 10\,mL\,(solution)$$
$$x\,mL\,(Clorox) = 2,000\,mL\,(solution)$$

Because the number of milliliters of solute is proportional to the number of milliliters of solution, a proportion could be used to solve the problem. The proportion could be set up as

$$\frac{mL(Clorox)}{mL(solution)} = \frac{mL(Clorox)'}{mL(solution)'}$$

Substituting, you get

$$\frac{1\,mL(Clorox)}{10\,mL(solution)} = \frac{x\,mL(Clorox)}{2,000\,mL(solution)}$$

Eliminate the units of measurement and cross multiply

$$\frac{1}{10} = \frac{x}{2{,}000}$$

$$10x = 2{,}000$$

$$x = 200$$

So, you need 200 mL of Clorox to prepare 2,000 mL of a 1:10 solution. This means that 200 mL of Clorox is diluted with water to 2,000 mL of solution.

## EXAMPLE 8.8

**How would you prepare 250 mL of a $\frac{1}{2}$% Lysol solution?**

Because Lysol is a liquid in its pure form, it is measured in milliliters. So, $\frac{1}{2}$% (0.5%) strength means 0.5 mL of Lysol is contained in each 100 mL of the solution *(0.5 mL of Lysol = 100 mL of solution)*. You need to determine the number of mL of Lysol which are contained in 250 mL of this solution *(? mL of Lysol = 250 mL of solution)*.

Think of the problem as:

$$0.5\,mL\,(\text{Lysol}) = 100\,mL\,(\text{solution})$$

$$x\,mL\,(\text{Lysol}) = 250\,mL\,(\text{solution})$$

The proportion could be set up as

$$\frac{mL(Lysol)}{mL(solution)} = \frac{mL(Lysol)'}{mL(solution)'}$$

Substituting, you get

$$\frac{0.5\,mL(Lysol)}{100\,mL(solution)} = \frac{x\,mL(Lysol)}{250\,mL(solution)}$$

Eliminate the units of measurement and cross multiply

$$\frac{0.5}{100} = \frac{x}{250}$$

$$100x = 125$$

$$x = 1.25$$

So, you need 1.25 mL of Lysol to prepare 250 mL of a $\frac{1}{2}$% Lysol solution. This means that 1.25 mL of Lysol is diluted with water to 250 mL of solution.

## EXAMPLE 8.9

Read the label in ● Figure 8.10 and determine the number of milligrams of lidocaine that are contained in 5 mL of this lidocaine solution.

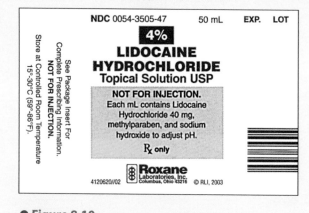

● **Figure 8.10**
**Drug label for lidocaine.**
*(Courtesy of Roxane Laboratories Inc.)*

Because lidocaine is a solid in its pure form, it is measured in grams. So, 4% strength means 4 g of lidocaine in each 100 mL of the solution *(4 g of lidocaine = 100 mL of solution)*. You need to determine the number of mg of lidocaine which are in 5 mL of this solution *(? mg of lidocaine = 5 mL of solution)*.

This problem expresses quantities of lidocaine in two different units of measure: grams *(4 g)* and milligrams *(? mg)*. In order to set up a proportion, you need to use a single unit of measurement for the lidocaine. To do this, change 4 g to 4,000 mg (by moving the decimal point three places). Now you can think of the problem as:

$$4,000 \, \text{mg (lidocaine)} = 100 \, \text{mL (solution)}$$

$$x \, \text{mg (lidocaine)} = 5 \, \text{mL (solution)}$$

The proportion could be set up as

$$\frac{mg}{mL} = \frac{mg'}{mL'}$$

Substituting, you get

$$\frac{4,000 \, mg}{100 \, mL} = \frac{x \, mg}{5 \, mL}$$

Eliminate the units of measurement and cross multiply

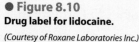

$$100x = 20,000$$

$$x = 200$$

So, 200 mg of lidocaine are contained in 5 mL of a 4% lidocaine solution.

# Determining the Amount of Solution That Contains a Given Amount of Solute

In the previous examples, you were given a volume of solution of known strength and had to find the amount of solute in that solution. Now, the process will be reversed. In the following examples, you will be given an amount of the solute in a solution of known strength and have to find the volume of that solution.

## EXAMPLE 8.10

**How many milliliters of a 20% magnesium sulfate solution will contain 40 g of the pure drug magnesium sulfate?**

The 20% strength means that there is 20 g of magnesium sulfate in every 100 mL of this solution *(20 g = 100 mL)*. You need to determine the number of milliliters of this solution that contain 40 g of the pure drug magnesium sulfate *(40 g = ? mL)*.

Think of the problem as:

$$20\,g = 100 \text{ mL}$$
$$40\,g = x \text{ mL}$$

The proportion could be set up as

$$\frac{g}{mL} = \frac{g'}{mL'}$$

Substituting, you get

$$\frac{20\ g}{100\ mL} = \frac{40\ g}{x\ mL}$$

Eliminate the units of measurement and cross multiply

$$\frac{20}{100} \diagdown \frac{40}{x}$$

$$4{,}000 = 20x$$
$$200 = x$$

So, 200 mL of a 20% magnesium sulfate solution contain 40 g of magnesium sulfate.

## EXAMPLE 8.11

**How many milliliters of a 1:40 acetic acid solution will contain 25 mL of acetic acid?**

The 1:40 strength means that there is 1 mL of acetic acid in every 40 mL of this solution *(1 mL of acetic acid = 40 mL of solution)*. You need to determine the number of milliliters of this solution that contain 25 mL of the pure acetic acid *(25 mL of acetic acid = x mL of solution)*.

Think of the problem as:

$$1 \, \text{mL (acetic acid)} = 40 \, \text{mL (solution)}$$
$$25 \, \text{mL (acetic acid)} = x \, \text{mL (solution)}$$

The proportion could be set up as

$$\frac{mL \, (acetic \, acid)}{mL \, (solution)} = \frac{mL \, (acetic \, acid)'}{mL \, (solution)'}$$

Substituting you get

$$\frac{1 \, mL}{40 \, mL} = \frac{25 \, mL}{x \, mL}$$

Eliminate the units of measurement and cross multiply

$$\frac{1}{40} = \frac{25}{x}$$

$$1,000 = 1x$$

$$1,000 = x$$

So, 1,000 mL of a *1:40* acetic acid solution contain 25 mL of acetic acid.

## NOTE

Because the strength (4 *mg*/5 *mL*) stated on the zoledronic acid label in Figure 8.11 uses mg/mL instead of g/mL, it is not a *4:5* solution. A 4:5 solution would have a strength of $\frac{4 \, g}{5 \, mL}$.

## EXAMPLE 8.12

How many milliliters of the zoledronic acid solution (● Figure 8.11) contain 10 mg of the pure drug?

### zoledronic acid
#### Injection
#### 4 mg/5 mL

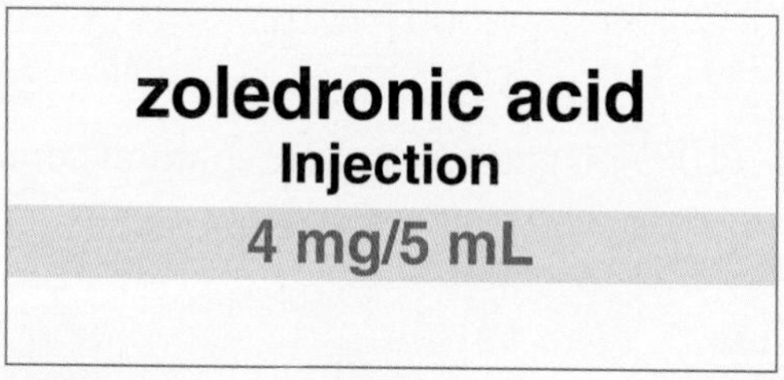

● **Figure 8.11**
**Drug label for zoledronic acid.**

The *4 mg/5 mL* strength means that there is 4 mg of the pure drug (zoledronic acid) in every 5 mL of this solution. You need to determine the number of milliliters of this solution that contain 10 mg of the pure drug.

Think of the problem as:

$$4\,mg\,(drug) = 5\ mL\ (solution)$$

$$10\,mg\,(drug) = x\ mL\,(solution)$$

The proportion could be set up as

$$\frac{mg}{mL} = \frac{mg'}{mL'}$$

Substituting, you get

$$\frac{4\ mg}{5\ mL} = \frac{10\ mg}{x\ mL}$$

Eliminate the units of measurement and cross multiply

$$\frac{4}{5} = \frac{10}{x}$$

$$50 = 4x$$

$$\frac{50}{4} = x$$

$$12.5 = x$$

So, 12.5 mL of the solution contain 10 mg of the pure drug.

## Irrigating Solutions, Soaks, and Oral Feedings

Sometimes healthcare professionals are required to prepare irrigating solutions, soaks, and nutritional feedings. These may be supplied in ready-to-use form, or they can be prepared from dry powders or from liquid concentrates.

**Irrigating solutions and soaks** are used for sterile irrigation of body cavities, wounds, indwelling catheters; washing and rinsing purposes; or for soaking of surgical dressings, instruments, and laboratory specimens.

**Enteral feedings** are nutritional solutions which can be supplied in ready-to-use form, or they may be reconstituted from powders or from liquid concentrates. The nutritional solutions may be administered either orally or parenterally.

### EXAMPLE 8.13

**Using a full-strength hydrogen peroxide solution, how would you prepare 300 mL of 2/3 strength hydrogen peroxide solution for a wound irrigation, using normal saline as the diluent?**

The 2/3 strength means that there is 2 mL of full-strength hydrogen peroxide in every 3 mL of the 2/3 strength solution *(2 mL of full-strength hydrogen peroxide = 3 mL of 2/3 strength solution)*. You need to determine the number of milliliters of full-strength hydrogen

**ALERT**

Full-strength (ready-to-use) hydrogen peroxide is generally supplied as a 3% solution. This stock solution may be diluted to form weaker solutions depending on the application. These dilutions must be performed using aseptic techniques.

peroxide which are contained in 300 mL of the 2/3 strength solution (*? mL of full-strength hydrogen peroxide = 300 mL of 2/3 strength solution*).

Think of the problem as:

2 mL (full-strength hydrogen peroxide) = 3 mL (2/3 strength solution)

$x$ mL (full-strength hydrogen peroxide) = 300 mL (2/3 strength solution)

The proportion could be set up as

$$\frac{mL\,(full\text{-}strength)}{mL\,(2/3\,strength\,solution)} = \frac{mL\,(full\text{-}strength)'}{mL\,(2/3\,strength\,solution)'}$$

Substituting, you get

$$\frac{2\,mL\,(full\text{-}strength)}{3\,mL\,(2/3\,strength\,solution)} = \frac{x\,mL\,(full\text{-}strength)}{300\,mL\,(2/3\,strength\,solution)}$$

Eliminate the units of measurement and cross multiply

$$\frac{2}{3} = \frac{x}{300}$$

$$3x = 600$$

$$x = 200$$

So, 200 mL of full-strength hydrogen peroxide would be diluted with 100 mL of normal saline to make 300 mL of a 2/3 strength solution.

### EXAMPLE 8.14

**How many ounces of $\frac{1}{4}$ strength Sustacal can be made from a 12-ounce can of full-strength Sustacal?**

The $\frac{1}{4}$ strength means that there is 1 ounce of full-strength Sustacal in every 4 ounces of this solution (*1 oz of full-strength Sustacal = 4 oz of $\frac{1}{4}$ strength solution*). You need to determine the number of ounces of $\frac{1}{4}$ strength Sustacal that can be made from 12 oz of full-strength Sustacal (*12 oz of full-strength Sustacal= ? oz of $\frac{1}{4}$ strength solution*).

Think of the problem as:

1 oz (full-strength Sustacal) = 4 oz ($\frac{1}{4}$ strength solution)

12 oz (full-strength Sustacal) = $x$ oz ($\frac{1}{4}$ strength solution)

The proportion could be set up as

$$\frac{oz\,(full\text{-}strength)}{oz\,(1/4\,strength\,solution)} = \frac{oz\,(full\text{-}strength)'}{oz\,(1/4\,strength\,solution)'}$$

Substituting, you get

$$\frac{1\,oz\,(\textit{full-strength})}{4\,oz\,(1/4\,strength\,solution)} = \frac{12\,oz\,(\textit{full-strength})}{x\,oz\,(1/4\,strength\,solution)}$$

Eliminate the units of measurement and cross multiply

$$\frac{1}{4} = \frac{12}{x}$$

$$48 = 1x$$

$$x = 48\,ounces$$

So, 48 ounces of $\frac{1}{4}$ strength Sustacal can be made from a 12-ounce can of full-strength Sustacal.

## EXAMPLE 8.15

How would you prepare 240 mL of $\frac{1}{2}$ strength Ensure from full-strength Ensure? Which size can(s) of Ensure would you use in order to minimize the amount of discarded Ensure if the supply consists of 8- and 12-oz cans?

The $\frac{1}{2}$ strength means that there is 1 ounce of full-strength Ensure in every 2 ounces of this solution. You need to determine the number of ounces of full-strength Ensure that are contained in 240 mL of the $\frac{1}{2}$ strength solution.

Think of the problem as:

1 oz (full-strength Ensure) = $2\,oz$ ($\frac{1}{2}$ strength solution)

$x$ oz (full-strength Ensure) = $240\,mL$ ($\frac{1}{2}$ strength solution)

This problem expresses the quantities of $\frac{1}{2}$ strength Ensure in two different units of measure: ounces *(2 oz)* and milliliters *(240 mL)*. In order to set up a proportion, you need to use a single unit of measurement for the $\frac{1}{2}$ strength Ensure; either ounces or milliliters. One way to do this is to use the equivalence 30 mL = 1 oz to change 240 milliliters to 8 ounces.

Now think of the problem as:

1 oz (full-strength Ensure) = $2\,oz$ ($\frac{1}{2}$ strength solution)

$x$ oz (full-strength Ensure) = $8\,oz$ ($\frac{1}{2}$ strength solution)

Now, a proportion could be set up as

$$\frac{1\,oz\,(\textit{full-strength})}{2\,oz\,(1/2\,strength\,solution)} = \frac{x\,oz\,(\textit{full-strength})}{8\,oz\,(1/2\,strength\,solution)}$$

Eliminate the units of measurement and cross multiply

$$\frac{1}{2} = \frac{x}{8}$$

$$2x = 8$$

$$x = 4 \text{ ounces}$$

So, 4 oz of full-strength Ensure are contained in 240 mL of $\frac{1}{2}$ strength Ensure. To prepare the solution, add 4 ounces of water to 4 ounces of full-strength Ensure to make 8 ounces of the $\frac{1}{2}$-strength solution. Because 4 ounces of full-strength Ensure are needed, using a 8-oz can would result in discarding 4 oz of Ensure, while using a 12-oz can would result in discarding 8 oz of Ensure. Therefore, use one 8-oz can to minimize waste.

# Summary

In this chapter, you learned that there are three important quantities associated with a solution: the *strength* of the solution, the *amount of solute* dissolved in the solution, and the total *volume of the solution*. If any two of these three quantities are known, the remaining quantity can be found.

- The *strength* of a solution is the ratio of the *amount of solute* dissolved in the solution to the total *volume of the solution*.
- The strength of a solution may be expressed in the form of a *ratio*, *fraction*, or *percentage*.
- A $\frac{1}{2}$ *strength* solution is a *1:2* or a *50%* solution, and should not be confused with a $\frac{1}{2}$ % solution.
- The amount of solute dissolved in the solution should be expressed in *milliliters* if the solute is a *liquid*.
- The amount of solute dissolved in the solution should be expressed in *grams* if the solute is a *solid* or *powder*.
- The *volume of a solution* should be expressed in *milliliters*.
- To determine the amount of solute contained in a given amount of a solution of known strength, use the strength as the known equivalence.
- To determine amount of a solution of known strength containing a given amount of solute, use the strength as the known equivalence.

- Use aseptic technique when diluting stock solutions for irrigations, soak, and nutritional liquids.
- The strength of a particular solution may be written in many different forms. The following strengths are all equivalent:

*Using* stated Units of Measurement

Rates $\begin{cases} 500 \text{ mg/mL} \\ 500 \text{ mg per mL} \\ \dfrac{500\ mg}{1\ mL} \end{cases}$

Equivalence    500 mg = 1 mL

*Without* stated Units of Measurement

| | |
|---|---|
| Fraction | $\frac{1}{2}$ strength |
| Ratio | 1:2 |
| Precentage | 50% |

# Case Study 8.1

Read the Case Study and answer the questions. The answers are found in Appendix A.

A 75-year-old female is admitted to a long-term care facility status post-mitral valve replacement. She has a past medical history of osteoarthritis; hypertension; atrial fibrillation; and insulin-dependent diabetes mellitus. Skin assessment reveals a 3 cm wound on the right heel. She is alert and oriented to person, place, time, and recent memory and she rates her pain level as 6 on a scale of 0–10. Vital signs are: T 98.7 °F; P 68; R 18; B/P 124/76.

Her orders are as follows:

- Persantine (dipyridamole) 75 mg PO, q.i.d.
- Cordarone (amiodarone hydrochloride) 400 mg PO daily; notify MD if P less than 60
- Cardizem SR(diltiazem) 180 mg PO daily
- Relafen (nabumetone) 1,000 mg PO daily
- KCl oral solution 20 mEq PO b.i.d.
- Multi-vitamin 1 tab PO daily
- Tylenol 650 mg PO q4h prn T above 101
- Humulin R insulin 10 units and Humulin N insulin 38 units subcutaneous 30 minutes ac breakfast
- Humulin R insulin 10 units and Humulin N insulin 30 units 30 minutes ac dinner
- Pneumovax 0.5 mL IM stat × 1 dose

- Cleanse right heel with NS solution (0.9% NaCl) and apply a DSD daily
- 1,800 calorie ADA 2 g sodium diet

Refer to the labels in ● Figure 8.12 when necessary to answer the following questions:

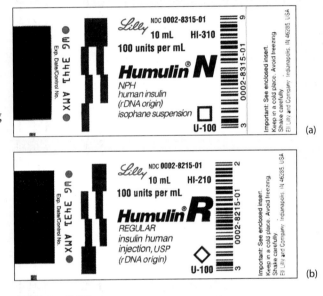

● Figure 8.12

**Drug labels for Case Study 8.1.**

(08–12a Copyright Eli Lilly and Company. Used with permission. 08–12b Copyright Eli Lilly and Company. Used with permission.)

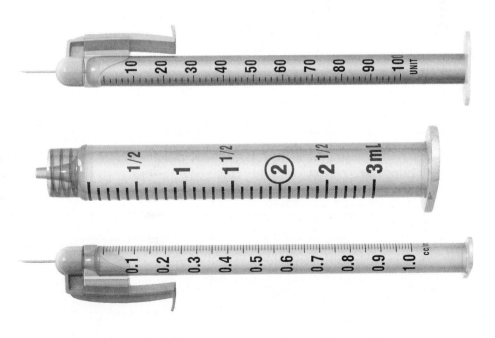

1. The Pneumovax vial contains 2.5 mL. Choose the appropriate syringe from those above and place an arrow at the dose.

2. Cardizem SR is available in 60 mg and 120 mg tablets. Which strength will you use and how many tablets for the daily dose?

3. The KCl solution label reads 40 mEq/15 mL. How many milliliters will you administer?

4. The dipyridamole is available in 25, 50, and 75 mg tablets. Which strength tablets will you administer and how many?

5. The strength of the nabumetone tablets is 500 mg. How many tablets will you administer?

6. Describe how you will measure the morning insulin. Select the appropriate syringe from those below and mark the dose of Humulin R and Humulin N.

7. How many grams of sodium chloride (NaCl) are in 1 liter of the saline solution?

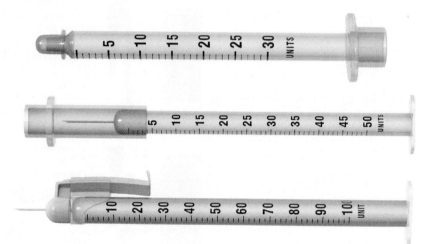

## Practice Sets

Workspace

The answers to *Try These for Practice*, *Exercises*, and *Cumulative Review Exercises* are found in Appendix A. Ask your instructor for the answers to the *Additional Exercises*.

### Try These for Practice

Test your comprehension after reading the chapter.

1. 320 mL of a solution contain 80 mg of a pure drug. Express the strength of this solution as a percent. _____

2. How would 1 liter of a 10% solution be prepared from tablets each containing 5 grams of the pure drug? _____

3. How many milliliters of a 25% potassium permanganate solution contains 20 grams of potassium permanganate? _____

4. The nutritional formula Sustacal is available in 4- and 12-ounce cans. How would you prepare 720 mL of 1/3 strength Sustacal? What size can(s) would you use in order to minimize the amount of discarded Sustacal? _____

5. Read the label in ● **Figure 8.13** and show how you would determine that two of the strengths mentioned on the label are equivalent (use 500 mcg/2 mL and 0.25 mg/mL). _____

**LANOXIN®       2 mL**
**(digoxin) Injection     R̖only**
500 mcg (0.5 mg) in 2 mL
(250 mcg [0.25 mg] per mL)
Store at 25°C (77°F) [see insert].
PROTECT FROM LIGHT.
Dist.: GlaxoSmithKline
Research Triangle Park, NC 27709
Made in Canada
4144627          **220201**
Rev. 3/02

**LOT**
**EXP**

● **Figure 8.13**
**Drug label for Lanoxin.**
*(Reproduced with permission of GlaxoSmithKline.)*

## Exercises

Reinforce your understanding in class or at home.

1. 750 mL of a solution contain 15 mL of a pure drug. Express the strength of this solution both as a ratio and as a percentage.

2. Two liters of a solution contain 60 g of a pure drug. Express the strength of this solution both as a ratio and as a percentage.

3. How would 300 mL of a 0.9% sodium chloride solution be prepared using sodium chloride crystals?

4. Read the label in ● **Figure 8.14** and determine the number of milligrams of hydroxyzine pamoate that are contained in the vial of Vistaril.

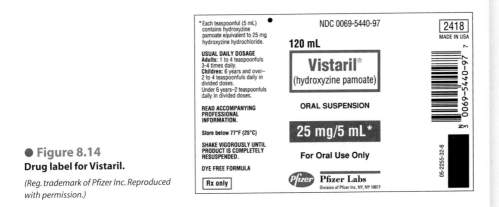

● **Figure 8.14**
**Drug label for Vistaril.**
*(Reg. trademark of Pfizer Inc. Reproduced with permission.)*

5. How many milliliters of Vistaril (see Figure 8.14) contain 20 mg of hydroxyzine pamoate?

6. How would 400 mL of a 50% solution be prepared from a drug that in its pure form is a liquid?

7. How many milliliters of a 6% solution contain 18 g of the pure drug?

8. Read the label in ● **Figure 8.15**. How many milliliters of the lidocaine hydrochloride solution contain 300 mg of lidocaine hydrochloride?

Workspace

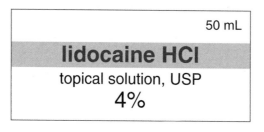

● **Figure 8.15**
**Drug label for 4% lidocaine HCl.**

9. Read the label in ● **Figure 8.16** and verify that the two strengths stated on the lidocaine label are equivalent.

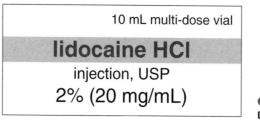

● **Figure 8.16**
**Drug label for 2% lidocaine HCl.**

10. A drug has a strength of 125 mg/mL. Write this strength in the form of a ratio, a fraction, and a percentage.

11. The nutritional formula Sustacal is supplied in 10 ounce cans. How would you prepare 1,600 mL of a 3/4 strength Sustacal solution?

12. If 600 mL of a solution contain 120 mL of a pure drug, express the strength of this solution both as a ratio and as a percentage.

13. If 1 L of a solution contains 2,000 mg of a pure drug, express the strength of this solution both as a ratio and as a percentage.

14. How would 800 mL of a 10% solution be prepared using tablets each containing 20 g?

15. Read the label in ● **Figure 8.17** and determine how many milligrams of metoprolol tartrate are contained in 12 mL of the solution.

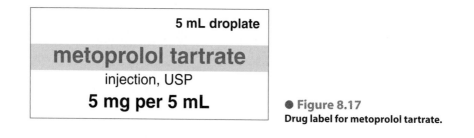

● **Figure 8.17**
**Drug label for metoprolol tartrate.**

16. Read the label in Figure 8.17 and determine the number of milliliters of the solution that would contain 35 mg of pure metoprolol tartrate.

17. How would you prepare 1,200 mL of a 25% solution from a pure drug in solid form?

18. A drug label states the strength of the solution is 10 mg/mL or 1%. Verify that the two stated strengths are equivalent.

19. A drug has a strength of 25 mg/mL. Write this strength in the form of a ratio, a fraction, and a percentage.

20. The nutritional formula Isomil is supplied in 4-, 8-, and 12-ounce cans. How would you prepare 6 oz of a 2/3 strength Isomil solution. What size can(s) would you use in order to minimize the amount of discarded Isomil?

## Additional Exercises

Now, test yourself!

1. Prepare 2 L of a 1:50 solution of Lysol from a 100% solution.

2. A drug has a strength of 200 mg/mL. Write this strength in the form of a ratio, a fraction, and a percentage.

3. From full-strength hydrogen peroxide, how would you prepare 480 mL of 1/3 strength hydrogen peroxide for skin cleansing? Use normal saline as the diluent.

4. Describe how you would prepare 240 mL of a $\frac{1}{2}$ strength solution of Ensure from full-strength Ensure.

5. How many grams of amino acids are contained in 500 mL of an 8.5% amino acid solution?

6. A patient is receiving 250 mL of a 10% Intralipid solution. How many grams of lipids will this patient receive?

7. How many milliliters of a 20% glucose solution will contain 50 g of glucose?

8. Physician's order:

    *magnesium sulfate 2 g in 10 mL D$_5$W IV push in 10 minutes*

    The label on the vial reads 50% magnesium sulfate. How many milliliters will you prepare?

**Workspace**

9. A patient has an order for 200 mL of a 2% lidocaine solution. How many milligrams of lidocaine are contained in this order?

_____

10. A patient receives 4 mL of 1% lidocaine as a nerve block. How many grams of lidocaine did the patient receive?

_____

11. Describe how 100 mL of 0.9% NaCl would be prepared from sodium chloride crystals.

_____

12. How many grams of dextrose are contained in 4,000 mL of a 25% dextrose solution?

_____

13. Prepare 240 mL of a $\frac{1}{3}$ strength solution of Ensure from an 8-oz can of Ensure.

_____

14. The nutritional formula Isomil is supplied in 4-, 8-, and 12-ounce cans. How would you prepare 8 oz of 1/3 strength Isomil? What size can(s) would you use in order to minimize the amount of discarded Isomil?

_____

15. Use the information on the label in ● **Figure 8.18** to determine the number of grams of calcium chloride contained in 2 mL of the solution.

_____

| 1 gram |
| **calcium chloride** |
| injection, USP |
| 10%             100 mg/mL |

● **Figure 8.18**
**Drug label for calcium chloride.**

16. Read the label in ● **Figure 8.19** and determine the number of milliliters of the solution that will contain 0.001 g of epinephrine.

_____

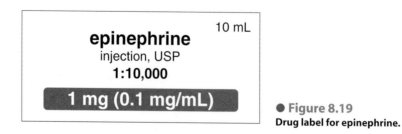

● **Figure 8.19**
**Drug label for epinephrine.**

17. Read the label in ● Figure 8.20. How many grams of Mannitol are contained in 25 mL of this solution?

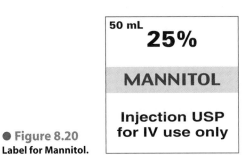

**● Figure 8.20**
**Label for Mannitol.**

18. How many milliliters of a 1:30 acetic acid solution will contain 20 g of acetic acid?

_____

19. A client must have a foot soak. Prepare 4,000 mL of a 4% solution of potassium permanganate solution from 5 g tablets.

_____

20. Describe how to prepare 3,500 mL of a 1:1,000 aluminum acetate solution, an antiseptic, from 0.5 g tablets.

_____

# Cumulative Review Exercises

Review your mastery of previous chapters.

1. Read the information on the label in ● Figure 8.21 and calculate the amount of dextrose in 25 mL of this solution.

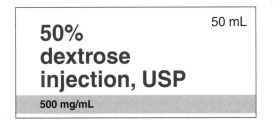

**● Figure 8.21**
**Drug label for dextrose.**

2. From a supply of full-strength hydrogen peroxide, how would you prepare 6 ounces of $\frac{1}{4}$ strength hydrogen peroxide for wound irrigation? Use normal saline as the solvent.

3. Your patient has an order for a tube feeding of 200 mL of $\frac{3}{4}$ strength Isocal, a nutritional supplement. Each can contains 200 mL of Isocal. How many milliliters of $H_2O$ and how many milliliters of Isocal will you need to make a $\frac{3}{4}$ strength solution? (Hint: $\frac{3}{4}$ strength means 75% solution.)

4. 2 glasses =_____ ounces

5. 0.0006 g =_____ mg

6. 5 ft 6 in =_____ in

7. The label on a vial containing a drug indicates a strength of 25 mg/mL. How many milliliters of this solution will contain 62.5 mg of the drug?

8. A patient is 6 feet tall. What is the patient's height in centimeters?

9. A patient must receive 9 mg of a drug subcut daily in 3 divided doses. If the drug is supplied in a vial labeled 5 mg/mL, how many milliliters would you administer, and which syringe would you use?

10. The order reads *atropine sulfate 0.4 mg sc stat*. Express this dose in grams.

11. The order is *digoxin 0.25 mg PO q.i.d.* Convert this dose to micrograms.

12. You have 2 mL of epinephrine 1:10,000. How many milligrams of epinephrine are contained in this solution?

13. A physician orders 0.6 g of a drug PO b.i.d. for three days. How many grams of the drug will the patient receive in three days?

14. The antianxiety drug *Tranxene (clorazepate) 15 mg PO at bedtime* has been prescribed for a patient. The label reads 7.5 mg per tablet. How many tablets will you give your patient?

15. The order is 600 mg of a drug PO b.i.d. The label reads 0.2 g in 5 mL. How many milliliters will you give your patient?

**MediaLink**
www.prenhall.com/giangrasso

Animated examples, interactive practice questions with animated solutions, and challenge tests for this chapter can be found on the Pearson Dosage Calculation Tutor that accompanies this text. Additional, unique, interactive resources and activities can be found on the Companion Web site.

# Chapter

# Parenteral Medications

## Learning Outcomes

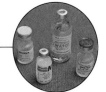

After completing this chapter, you will be able to

1. Calculate doses for parenteral medications in liquid form.
2. Interpret the directions on drug labels and package inserts for reconstituting medications supplied in powdered form.
3. Label reconstituted multi-dose medication containers with the necessary information.
4. Choose the most appropriate diluent volume when reconstituting a multiple-strength medication.
5. Calculate doses of parenteral medications measured in units.

This chapter introduces the calculations you will use to prepare and administer parenteral medications safely. Chapter 2 discussed the most common parenteral sites: intramuscular (IM), subcutaneous (subcut), intravenous (IV), intradermal (ID), intracardiac (IC), intrathecal, and epidural. This chapter will focus on calculations for administering medications via the subcutaneous and intramuscular routes.

# Parenteral Medications

Parenteral medications are those that are injected into the body by various routes. Drugs for parenteral medications may be packaged in a variety of forms, including ampules, vials, and prefilled cartridges or syringes. Prefilled cartridges and syringes were discussed in Chapter 7.

An *ampule* is a glass container that holds a single dose of medication. It has a narrowed neck that is designed to snap open. The medication is aspirated into a syringe by gently pulling back on the plunger, which creates a negative pressure and allows the liquid to be pulled into the syringe (● **Figure 9.1**).

A *vial* is a glass or plastic container that has a rubber membrane on the top. This membrane is covered with a lid that maintains the sterility of the membrane until the vial is used for the first time. Multidose vials contain more than one dose of a medication. Single-dose vials contain one dose of medication, and many drugs are now prepared in single-dose format to reduce the chance of error. The medication in a vial may be supplied in liquid or powdered form (● **Figure 9.2**).

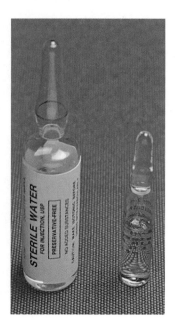

● **Figure 9.1**
**Ampules.**

**NOTE**

Single-dose ampules and vials may contain a little more drug than indicated on the label. Therefore, if the order is for the exact amount of medication stated on the label, it is very important to carefully measure the amount of medication to be withdrawn. Before a fluid can be extracted from a vial, that same volume of air must be injected into the vial.

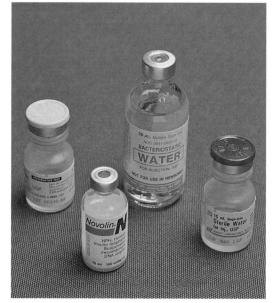

● **Figure 9.2**
**Vials.**

## Parenteral Medications Supplied as Liquids

When parenteral medications are in liquid form, you must calculate the volume of the solution that contains the prescribed amount of the medication. To perform this calculation you also need to know the strength of the solution. You will use ratio and proportion to calculate the volume that will be administered.

The following rough guidelines for the volumes generally administered subcutaneously or intramuscularly can be used to test the reasonableness of your calculated dosages.

| | | |
|---|---|---|
| Subcut: | Infant: | less than 0.1 mL |
| | Child: | less than 0.5 mL |
| | Adult: | from 0.5 mL to 1 mL |
| IM: | Infant: | less than 1 mL |
| | Child: | less than 2 mL |
| | Adult: | less than 3 mL (in the deltoid less than 2 mL) |

**NOTE**

An IM dose which is larger than 3 mL should be divided into two syringes and administered at two different injection sites.

## EXAMPLE 9.1

The prescriber ordered *hydromorphone hydrochloride 4 mg IM q4h prn*. Read the label in ● Figure 9.3 and calculate how many milliliters of this narcotic analgesic you will administer and indicate this dose on the 0.5 mL syringe.

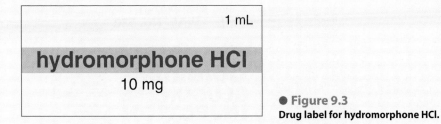

1 mL

# hydromorphone HCl
## 10 mg

● **Figure 9.3**
**Drug label for hydromorphone HCl.**

Begin by determining how many milliliters of the solution in the vial contain the prescribed quantity of the medication prescribed. That is, you want to convert 4 mg to an equivalent in milliliters. The label indicates a strength of 10 mg in 1 mL.

Think of the problem as:

$$4 \text{ mg (hydromorphone)} = x \text{ mL (solution)} \quad \text{(dose)}$$
$$10 \text{ mg (hydromorphone)} = 1 \text{ mL (solution)} \quad \text{(strength)}$$

The proportion could be set up as

$$\frac{mg}{mL} = \frac{mg'}{mL'}$$

Substituting, you get

$$\frac{4\ mg}{x\ mL} = \frac{10\ mg}{1\ mL}$$

Eliminate the units of measurement and cross multiply

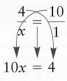

$$10x = 4$$

Divide both sides by the coefficient of $x$

$$x = \frac{4}{10}$$
$$x = 0.4$$

So, you would administer 0.4 mL to the patient.

0.4 mL

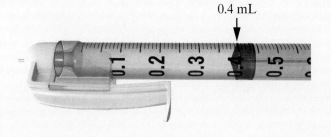

**NOTE**

Whenever you have any doubt about the accuracy of your calculations, ask another professional (nurse, pharmacist, or prescriber) for help.

## EXAMPLE 9.2

The prescriber ordered *quinidine gluconate 600 mg IM stat and 400 mg IM q4h prn*. Read the label in ● Figure 9.4 and calculate the number of milliliters of this antiarrhythmic drug you will administer to the patient as needed.

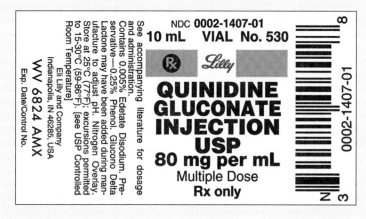

● **Figure 9.4**

**Drug label for quinidine gluconate.**

*(Copyright Eli Lilly and Company. Used with permission.)*

Begin by determining how many milliliters of the liquid in the vial contain the prescribed quantity of the medication (400 mg of quinidine gluconate—the question asks for the prn dose!). That is, you want to convert 400 mg to an equivalent in milliliters. The strength on the label is 80 mg per mL.

Think of the problem as:

400 mg (quinidine) = x mL (solution)    (dose)

80 mg (quinidine) = 1 mL (solution)    (strength)

The proportion could be set up as

$$\frac{mg}{mL} = \frac{mg'}{mL'}$$

Substituting, you get

$$\frac{400\ mg}{x\ mL} = \frac{80\ mg}{1\ mL}$$

Eliminate the units of measurement and cross multiply

$$\frac{400}{x} \diagup \frac{80}{1}$$

$$80x = 400$$

Divide both sides by the coefficient of x

$$x = \frac{400}{80}$$

$$x = 5$$

So, you would administer 5 mL to the patient. Because of the large volume, the dosage would be divided in two syringes.

## EXAMPLE 9.3

The prescriber ordered *prochlorperazine 7 mg IM q4h prn.* Read the label in ● Figure 9.5 and calculate the number of milliliters of this antiemetic you would administer to the patient, and indicate which size syringe should be used.

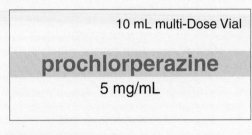

10 mL multi-Dose Vial

**prochlorperazine**

5 mg/mL

● **Figure 9.5**
**Drug label for prochlorperazine.**

Begin by determining how many milliliters of the liquid in the vial contain the prescribed quantity of the medication. That is, you want to convert 7 mg to an equivalent in milliliters. The strength on the label is 5 mg/mL.

Think of the problem as:

7 mg (prochlorperazine) = *x* mL (solution)    (dose)
5 mg (prochlorperazine) = 1 mL (solution)    (strength)

The proportion could be set up as

$$\frac{mg}{mL} = \frac{mg'}{mL'}$$

Substituting, you get

$$\frac{7\ mg}{x\ mL} = \frac{5\ mg}{1\ mL}$$

Eliminate the units of measurement and cross multiply

$$\frac{7}{x} = \frac{5}{1}$$

$$5x = 7$$

Divide both sides by the coefficient of *x*

$$x = \frac{7}{5}$$

$$x = 1.4$$

So, you would administer 1.4 mL using a 3 mL syringe.

**ALERT**

Always check to see whether the amount of drug prescribed is larger (or smaller) than the amount of drug mentioned in the strength available. In Example 9.3, the amount of drug in the order (7 mg) is *larger* than the amount of drug (5 mg) in the strength (5 mg/1 mL), therefore the amount to be administered must be *larger* than 1 mL.

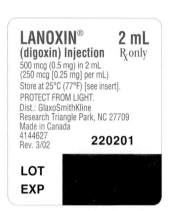

LANOXIN® **2 mL**
(digoxin) Injection    R only
500 mcg (0.5 mg) in 2 mL
(250 mcg [0.25 mg] per mL)
Store at 25°C (77°F) [see insert].
PROTECT FROM LIGHT.
Dist.: GlaxoSmithKline
Research Triangle Park, NC 27709
Made in Canada
4144627
Rev. 3/02    **220201**

LOT
EXP

● **Figure 9.6**
**Drug label for Lanoxin.**

*(Reproduced with permission of GlaxoSmithKline.)*

## EXAMPLE 9.4

The prescriber ordered *Lanoxin (digoxin) 600 mcg IV push stat.* Read the label in ● Figure 9.6 and determine how many milliliters of this anti-arrythmic cardiac glycoside you will prepare, and indicate the dose on the 3 mL syringe.

Begin by determining how many milliliters of the solution in the vial contain the prescribed quantity of the medication. That is, you want to convert 600 mcg to an equivalent in milliliters. Because the order includes mcg, use the first strength on the label, 500 mcg in 2 mL.

$$600 \text{ mcg} = x \text{ mL} \quad \text{(dose)}$$
$$500 \text{ mcg} = 2 \text{ mL} \quad \text{(strength)}$$

$$\frac{600 \text{ mcg}}{x \text{ mL}} = \frac{500 \text{ mcg}}{2 \text{ mL}}$$

$$500x = 1200$$
$$x = \frac{1200}{500}$$
$$x = 2.4$$

So, you would give the patient 2.4 mL.

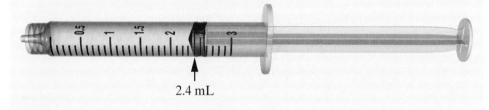

2.4 mL

## EXAMPLE 9.5

The prescriber ordered *Tigan (trimethobenzamide hydrochloride) 200 mg IM stat.* You have a 20 mL multidose vial, and the label indicates that the strength is 100 mg/mL. How many milliliters of this antiemetic drug will you prepare?

Begin by determining how many milliliters of the solution in the vial contain the prescribed quantity of the medication. That is, you want to convert 200 mg to an equivalent in milliliters.

$$200 \text{ mg} = x \text{ mL} \quad \text{(dose)}$$
$$100 \text{ mg} = 1 \text{ mL} \quad \text{(strength)}$$

$$\frac{200 \text{ mg}}{x \text{ mL}} = \frac{100 \text{ mg}}{1 \text{ mL}}$$

$$100x = 200$$
$$x = \frac{200}{100}$$
$$x = 2$$

So, you would give the patient 2 mL.

## EXAMPLE 9.6

The order for an adult with adrenal insufficiency is *dexamethasone sodium phosphate 5 mg IM q12h*. The patient weighs 100 kg, and the strength in the vial is 4 mg/mL.

(a)  If the recommended daily dosage is 0.03–0.15 mg/kg, is the prescribed dosage safe?

(b)  How many milliliters will you administer?

(a)  Using the recommended daily dosage, calculate the minimum and maximum number of milligrams the patient should receive each day.

*Minimum Daily Dosage*

Because the *minimum* recommended daily dosage (0.03 mg/kg) is based on the size of the patient (100 kg), multiply these as follows:

$$100 \, kg \times \frac{0.03 \, mg}{kg} = 3 \, mg$$

*Maximum Daily Dosage*

Because the *maximum* recommended daily dosage (0.15 mg/kg) is based on the size of the patient (100 kg), multiply these as follows:

$$100 \, kg \times \frac{0.15 \, mg}{kg} = 15 \, mg$$

So, the safe dose range for this patient is 3–15 mg daily.

The prescribed dosage is safe because the prescribed dosage of 5 mg q12h means the patient would receive 10 mg per day, which is in the safe dose range of 3–15 mg per day.

(b)

$$4 \text{ mg} = 1 \text{ mL} \quad \text{(strength)}$$
$$5 \text{ mg} = x \text{ mL} \quad \text{(dose)}$$

$$\frac{4 \, mg}{1 \, mL} = \frac{5 \, mg}{x \, mL}$$

$$5 = 4x$$

$$\frac{5}{4} = x$$

$$1.25 = x$$

So, you would administer 1.3 mL.

# Parenteral Medications Supplied in Powdered Form

Some parenteral medications are unstable when stored in liquid form, so they are packaged in powdered form. Before they can be administered, the powder in the vial must be diluted with a liquid (*diluent* or *solvent*). This process is referred to as *reconstitution*.

Sterile water and 0.9% sodium chloride (normal saline) are the most commonly used *diluents*. Both the type and amount of diluent to be used must be determined when reconstituting parenteral medications. This information is found on the medication label or package insert. Because many reconstituted parenteral medications can be administered intramuscularly or intravenously, it is essential to verify the route ordered **before** reconstituting the medication, because different routes may require different strengths.

Drugs dissolve completely in the diluent. Some drugs do not add any volume to the amount of diluent added, while other drugs increase the amount of total volume. This increase in volume is called the *displacement factor*. For example, directions for a 1 g powdered medication may state to add 2 mL of diluent to provide an approximate volume of 2.5 mL. When the 2 mL of diluent is added, the 1 g of powdered drug displaces an additional 0.5 mL for a total volume of 2.5 mL. The available strength after reconstitution is 1 g in 2.5 mL or 400 mg/mL. If there are no directions for reconstitution on the label or package insert, consult appropriate resources such as the PDR or the pharmacist before reconstituting.

To reconstitute a powdered medication:

- Follow the directions on the label or package insert exactly as specified.
- Check the expiration dates of the drug and the diluent.
- Add the diluent to the vial.
- Shake, roll, or invert the vial as directed.
- Make sure that the powder is fully dissolved.

When you reconstitute a multiple-dose vial of powdered medication, it is important that you clearly label the vial with the following:

1. date and time of preparation
2. strength of the solution
3. date and time that the reconstituted solution will expire
4. storage directions
5. your initials

**ALERT**

Proper labeling of reconstituted medication is critical for safe administration.

Suppose that at 6 P.M. on January 23, 2008, Marie Colon, R.N., reconstitutes a drug to a strength of 50 mg/mL, which will retain its potency for one week if kept refrigerated. Nurse Colon would write the following information on the label:

> *1/23/2008, 1800h, 50 mg/mL,*
> *Expires 1/30/2008, 1800h,*
> *Keep refrigerated, MC*

Some medications are manufactured in a vial that contains a single dose of medication in which the vial has two compartments, separated by a rubber stopper. The top portion contains a sterile liquid (diluent), and the bottom portion contains the medication in powder form. When pressure is applied to the top of the vial, the rubber stopper that separates the medication from the diluent is released. This allows the diluent and powder to mix. ●**Figure 9.7.**

## How to use a Mix-O Vial

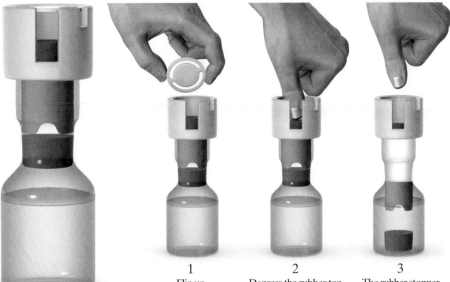

| 1 | 2 | 3 |
|---|---|---|
| Flip up and remove the protective cover. | Depress the rubber top so the diluent can mix into the chamber. | The rubber stopper will drop and help mix the drug. |

● **Figure 9.7**
**How to prepare a Mix-O Vial.**

### EXAMPLE 9.7

The prescriber ordered *Kefzol 265 mg IM q8h*. The directions on the label state: "For IM use, add 2.5 mL of sterile water for injection and shake well. The resulting solution has an approximate volume of 3 mL yielding a strength of 330 mg/mL." Describe how you would prepare this cephalosporin antibiotic. How many milliliters will you administer to the patient?

To prepare the solution, inject 2.5 mL of air into a vial of sterile water for injection and withdraw 2.5 mL of sterile water. Then add the 2.5 mL of sterile water to the Kefzol 1 g vial and shake well. ● **Figure 9.8**.

Now the vial contains a reconstituted solution in which 1 mL = 330 mg.

To calculate the number of milliliters containing the prescribed dose, you need to convert 265 mg to milliliters.

$$265 \text{ mg} = x \text{ mL} \quad \text{(dose)}$$

$$330 \text{ mg} = 1 \text{ mL} \quad \text{(strength)}$$

$$\frac{265 \text{ mg}}{x \text{ mL}} = \frac{330 \text{ mg}}{1 \text{ mL}}$$

$$330x = 265$$

$$x = \frac{265}{330}$$

$$x \approx 0.803$$

So, you would withdraw 0.8 mL (265 mg) from the vial and administer it to the patient.

### NOTE

The label in Example 9.7 states that when 2.5 mL of diluent is added, the resulting solution has an approximate volume of 3 mL. This is due to the displacement factor of 0.5 mL, which adds 0.5 mL to the 2.5 mL of added diluent, to yield a total solution of 3 mL.

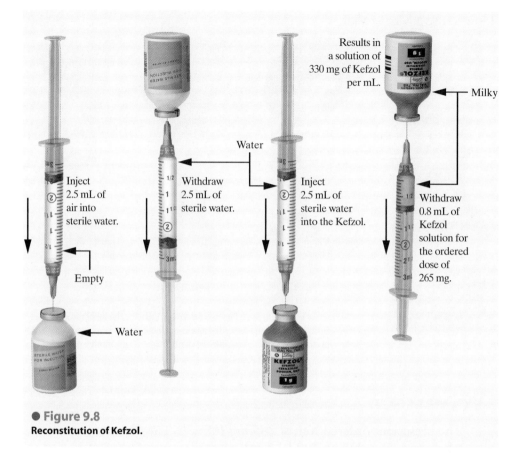

● **Figure 9.8**
**Reconstitution of Kefzol.**

**NOTE**

If the vial label does not contain reconstitution directions, refer to the drug package insert or contact the pharmacist. If directions are given for both IM and IV reconstitution, be careful to use the directions appropriate for the route prescribed.

## EXAMPLE 9.8

Order: *cefotetan disodium 1 g IM q12h*. Read the drug label and the reconstitution portion of the package insert in ● Figure 9.9. The package insert indicates that the reconstituted medication must be refrigerated, and it will expire in 2 days.

2 grams

**cefotetan disodium**
for injection

| Vial Size | Diluent Added (mL) | Volume Obtained (mL) | Concentration (mg/mL) |
|-----------|--------------------|--------------------|----------------------|
| 1 g | 2 | 2.5 | 400 |
| 2 g | 3 | 4 | 500 |

● **Figure 9.9**
**Drug label and reconstitution portion of the package insert for cefotetan disodium.**

(a)  How much diluent must be added to the vial?

(b)  If nurse Susan Green reconstitutes the cefotetan disodium at 0600 h on February 1, 2009, complete the label she will put on the vial.

(c)  Determine how many milliliters of this cephalosporin antibiotic you would give the patient.

(a)  First, prepare the solution. Since the vial contains 2 g, inject 3 mL of air into a vial of sterile water for injection and withdraw 3 mL of sterile water. Add the 3 mL of sterile water to the Cefotan 2 g vial and shake well.

(b)  Nurse Green would write the following on the label:

> 2/1/2009, 0600h, Reconstituted strength 500 mg/mL, Expires
> 2/3/2009, 0600h, Keep refrigerated, SG

(c)  The strength is 500 mg/mL, and the order is for 1 g (1,000 mg).

Think:

$$500 \text{ mg} = 1 \text{ mL} \quad \text{(strength)}$$
$$1,000 \text{ mg} = x \text{ mL} \quad \text{(dose)}$$

$$\frac{500 \text{ mg}}{1 \text{ mL}} = \frac{1,000 \text{ mg}}{x \text{ mL}}$$

$$1,000 = 500x$$
$$\frac{1,000}{500} = x$$
$$2 = x$$

So, you would administer 2 mL to the patient.

## EXAMPLE 9.9

An order requires 80 mg of a drug to be administered IM stat. The vial has the following three choices of strength after reconstitution:

> 10 mg/mL
> 20 mg/mL
> 40 mg/mL

For each of the three strengths:

(a)  Determine the required volume of the solution to be administered

(b)  Choose the most appropriate strength

(a)  Using 10 mg/mL (weakest strength)

Think:

$$10 \text{ mg} = 1 \text{ mL} \quad \text{(strength)}$$
$$80 \text{ mg} = x \text{ mL} \quad \text{(dose)}$$

One way to set up the proportion is

$$\frac{10 \ mg}{1 \ mL} = \frac{80 \ mg}{x \ mL}$$

$$80 = 10x$$

$$8 \ \text{mL} = x$$

Using 20 mg/mL (relatively moderate strength)

Think:

$$20 \ \text{mg} = 1 \ \text{mL} \quad \text{(strength)}$$
$$80 \ \text{mg} = x \ \text{mL} \quad \text{(dose)}$$

One way to set up the proportion is

$$\frac{20 \ mg}{1 \ mL} = \frac{80 \ mg}{x \ mL}$$

$$80 = 20x$$

$$4 \ \text{mL} = x$$

Using 40 mg/mL (strongest strength)

Think:

$$40 \ \text{mg} = 1 \ \text{mL} \quad \text{(strength)}$$
$$80 \ \text{mg} = x \ \text{mL} \quad \text{(dose)}$$

One way to set up the proportion is

$$\frac{40 \ mg}{1 \ mL} = \frac{80 \ mg}{x \ mL}$$

$$80 = 40x$$

$$2 \ \text{mL} = x$$

In summary:

(Weakest)     10 mg/mL requires 8 mL
(Moderate)   20 mg/mL requires 4 mL
(Strongest)  40 mg/mL requires 2 mL

(b) **Weakest: 10 mg/mL** requires 8 mL to be administered. However, IM volumes are generally less that 3 mL. Therefore, this strength *should not be selected.*

**Moderate: 20 mg/mL** requires 4 mL to be administered. However, IM volumes are generally less that 3 mL. Therefore, this strength is a *poor choice.* However, the 4 mL could be divided into two syringes and administered at two different sites.

**Strongest: 40 mg/mL** requires 2 mL to be administered. This is less than 3 mL and is the *best choice.*

**NOTE**

In Example 9.9, the *stronger* the strength (concentration) of the reconstituted drug, the *smaller* the volume to be administered.

NOTE

When reconstituting a multiple-strength parenteral medication, select a solution strength that results in a volume appropriate for the route of administration, for example, a volume of no more than 3 mL per IM dose. Also, consider the patient's age and size.

## EXAMPLE 9.10

A prescriber ordered *Pfizerpen (penicillin potassium) 200,000 units IM stat and q6h.* Read the label in ● Figure 9.10 and calculate how many milliliters of this penicillin antibiotic you will administer to the patient.

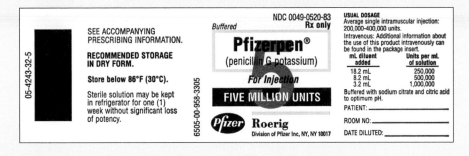

● **Figure 9.10**
**Drug label for Pfizerpen.**

*(Reg. trademark of Pfizer Inc. Reproduced with permission.)*

First, reconstitute the solution. The label lists three options: 250,000 units/mL, 500,000 units/mL, and 1,000,000 units/mL. If you choose the first option, 18.2 mL of diluent must be added to obtain a dosage strength of 250,000 units/mL.

Now, inject 18.2 mL of air into a vial of sterile water for injection and then withdraw 18.2 mL of sterile water. Add the sterile water to the Pfizerpen vial and shake well. Now the vial contains a solution in which 1 mL = 250,000 units

$$250{,}000 \text{ units} = 1 \text{ mL} \quad \text{(strength)}$$
$$200{,}000 \text{ units} = x \text{ mL} \quad \text{(dose)}$$

$$\frac{250{,}000 \text{ units}}{1 \text{ mL}} = \frac{200{,}000 \text{ units}}{x \text{ mL}}$$

$$200{,}000 = 250{,}000x$$
$$\frac{200{,}000}{250{,}000} = x$$
$$0.8 = x$$

So, you would withdraw 0.8 mL from the vial and administer it to the patient.

NOTE

Some medications must be reconstituted immediately before administering them because they lose potency rapidly. Ampicillin, for example, must be used within one hour of being reconstituted.

In Example 9.10, if a *stronger concentration* had been chosen for the reconstitution, then a *smaller volume* of the solution would be administered. The calculations would be similar to those just completed. The last two lines of the following table show the volumes for the other two options.

| Concentration | Amount of diluent | Strength of the solution | Volume to administer |
|---|---|---|---|
| Weakest | 18.2 mL | 250,000 units/mL | 0.8 mL |
| Moderate | 8.2 mL | 500,000 units/mL | 0.4 mL |
| Strongest | 3.2 mL | 1,000,000 units/mL | 0.2 mL |

## EXAMPLE 9.11

The prescriber ordered *Solu-Medrol (methylprednisolone sodium succinate) 200 mg IM q6h.* You have a mix-o-vial of Solu-Medrol 500 mg. The directions on the label state: "Each 4 mL when mixed contains methylprednisolone sodium succinate equivalent to 500 mg methylprednisolone (125 mg per mL)." How many milliliters will you administer?

First, reconstitute the solution. Depress the rubber stopper and allow the diluent into the bottom chamber of the vial and be sure that the powder is dissolved. See Figure 9.7.

Now the vial contains a solution in which 1 mL = 125 mg

$$125 \text{ mg} = 1 \text{ mL} \quad \text{(strength)}$$

$$200 \text{ mg} = x \text{ mL} \quad \text{(dose)}$$

$$\frac{125 \text{ mg}}{1 \text{ mL}} = \frac{200 \text{ mg}}{x \text{ mL}}$$

$$200 = 125x$$

$$\frac{200}{125} = x$$

$$1.6 = x$$

So, you would administer 1.6 mL of Solu-Medrol.

**ALERT**

Heparin flush solutions (for example, Hep-Lock or Hep-Flush) are used for maintaining the patency of indwelling intravenous catheters. They are available in 10 units/mL and 100 units/mL. Heparin for injection and heparin flush solutions are different drugs and can never be used interchangeably.

# Heparin

Heparin sodium is a high-alert medication. It is a potent anticoagulant that inhibits clot formation and blood coagulation. Heparin can be administered subcutaneously or intravenously.

Like insulin, penicillin, and some other medications, heparin is supplied and ordered in units. Heparin is available in single and multidose vials, as well as in commercially prepared IV solutions. Heparin is *never given intramuscularly because of the danger of hematomas.* Heparin is available in a variety of strengths, ranging from 10 units/mL for a flush to 40,000 units/mL for injection. The wide range of available strengths can lead to dire consequences for the patient if the wrong strength is administered. Heparin is also available in prepackaged syringes. Lovenox (enoxaprin) and Fragmin (dalteparin sodium) are examples of low molecular weight heparin, which are used to prevent and treat deep vein thrombosis (DVT), unstable angina, or acute coronary syndromes.

Heparin requires close monitoring of the patient's blood work because of the bleeding potential associated with anticoagulant drugs. In order to assure the accuracy of dose measurement, a 0.5 mL or a 1 mL (tuberculin) syringe should be used to administer heparin. Healthcare providers should know and follow agency policies when administering heparin.

## EXAMPLE 9.12

The prescriber ordered *heparin 2,000 units subcutaneously q12h.* The label on the multidose vial reads 5,000 units/mL. How many milliliters will you administer to the patient?

The strength is 5,000 units/mL. You need to convert the order, 2,000 units, to milliliters.

$$5{,}000 \text{ units} = 1 \text{ mL} \quad \text{(strength)}$$
$$2{,}000 \text{ units} = x \text{ mL} \quad \text{(dose)}$$

One way to set up the proportion is

$$\frac{5{,}000 \; units}{1 \; mL} = \frac{2{,}000 \; units}{x \; mL}$$

$$2{,}000 = 5{,}000x$$
$$\frac{2{,}000}{5{,}000} = x$$
$$0.4 = x$$

So, you would administer 0.4 mL of heparin to the patient.

### EXAMPLE 9.13

The prescriber ordered *heparin 2,000 units subcutaneously q12h.* The label on the multidose vial reads 10,000 units/mL. How many milliliters will you administer to the patient?

The strength is 10,000 units/mL. You need to convert the order, 2,000 units, to milliliters.

$$10{,}000 \text{ units} = 1 \text{ mL} \quad \text{(strength)}$$
$$2{,}000 \text{ units} = x \text{ mL} \quad \text{(dose)}$$

One way to set up the proportion is

$$\frac{10{,}000 \; units}{1 \; mL} = \frac{2{,}000 \; units}{x \; mL}$$

$$2{,}000 = 10{,}000x$$
$$\frac{2{,}000}{10{,}000} = x$$
$$0.2 = x$$

So, you would administer 0.2 mL of heparin to the patient.

**NOTE**

Observe that in Examples 9.12 and 9.13 the orders for heparin are exactly the same (2,000 units subcutaneously q12h). However, the available dosage strengths are different. In Example 9.13 the strength is twice the strength of that in Example 9.12. Therefore, in Example 9.13, only half the amount of solution (0.2 mL instead of 0.4 mL) is needed. It is of the utmost importance to carefully read the label in determining the correct dose.

### EXAMPLE 9.14

Order: *heparin 150 units/kg subcut q12h* for a patient who weighs 92 pounds. See ● Figure 9.11 and determine the number of milliliters of heparin you will need to administer this dose.

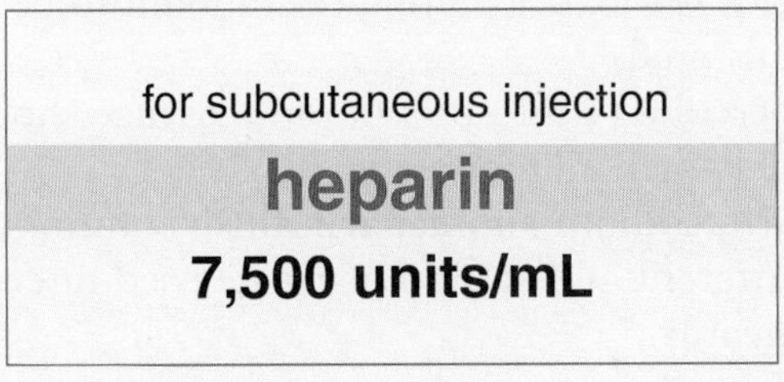

for subcutaneous injection

### heparin

**7,500 units/mL**

● **Figure 9.11**
**Drug label for heparin.**

Because this example contains a lot of information, you may find it useful to summarize it as follows:

| | |
|---|---|
| Size of the patient: | 92 lb |
| Order: | 150 units/kg |
| Strength of the drug: | 7,500 units/mL |
| Find: | ? mL to be administered |

First, change the weight of 92 pounds to kilograms by dividing by 2.2.

$$\frac{92}{2.2} \approx 41.82$$

So, the patient weighs 41.82 kg.

Because the order is based on the size of the patient, *multiply the size of the patient by the order to obtain the dose:*

$$41.82 \; kg \times \frac{150 \; units}{kg} \approx 6{,}273 \; units$$

Now, you need to convert 6,273 units to milliliters. Use the strength of 7,500 units/mL to form a proportion. Think:

$$6{,}273 \; units = x \; mL \quad (dose)$$
$$7{,}500 \; units = 1 \; mL \quad (strength)$$

$$\frac{7{,}500 \; units}{1 \; mL} = \frac{6{,}273 \; units}{x \; mL}$$

$$6{,}273 = 7{,}500x$$
$$\frac{6{,}273}{7{,}500} = x$$
$$0.8364 = x$$

Therefore, you would need 0.84 mL.

# Summary

In this chapter, you learned how to calculate doses for administering parenteral medications in liquid form, the procedure for reconstituting medications in powdered form, and how to calculate dosages for medications supplied in units.

- Medications supplied in powdered form must be reconstituted following the manufacturer's directions.
- You must determine the best dosage strength when there are several options for reconstituting the medication.
- After reconstituting a multiple-dose vial, label the medication vial with the dates and times of both preparation and expiration, storage directions, your initials, and strength.

- When directions on the label are provided for both IM and IV reconstitution, be sure to read the order and the label carefully to determine the necessary amount of diluent to use.
- Heparin is measured in USP units.
- It is especially important that heparin orders be carefully checked with the available dosage strength before calculating the amount to be administered.
- A tuberculin (1 mL) or a 0.5 mL syringe should be used when administering heparin.
- Heparin sodium and heparin flush solutions are different and should never be used interchangeably.

## Case Study 9.1

Read the Case Study and answer the questions. The answers are found in Appendix A.

A 64-year-old man is referred by his physician to the hospital for an emergency appendectomy following a CAT scan. The patient reports a past medical history of hypertension, hypercholesterolemia, and BPH (benign prostatic hypertrophy). He is 6 feet tall and weighs 150 lb, has no known drug or food allergies, and is to be transported to the operating room following his admission lab work and physical exam. His vital signs are: T 98.4°F; B/P 130/86; P 96; R 18.

**Pre-op orders:**

- NPO
- CBC, serum electrolytes, type and screen
- IV RL @ 125 mL/h
- morphine 2 mg IVP stat
- Transfer to OR

**Post-op orders:**

- NPO, progress to clear liquids as tolerated

- IV D5/NS @ 125 mL/h
- V/S q4h
- Flagyl (metronidazole) 7.5 mg/kg IVPB q6h
- Avelox (moxifloxacin) 400 mg IV daily for 5 days
- metoprolol 5 mg IVP q4h, hold for SBP below 110 or HR below 60
- heparin 5,000 units subcutaneously q12h
- Toradol (ketorolac tromethamine) 30 mg IM q6h prn moderate pain
- Percocet 1 tab PO q4h prn pain
- Ambien (zolpidem) 5 mg PO before bedtime
- Avodart (dutasteride) 0.5 mg PO every other day
- Norvasc (amlodipine) 10 mg PO daily
- Vasotec (enalapril maleate) 5 mg PO daily
- Lipitor (atorvastatin calcium) 20 mg PO every day

Refer to the labels in ● **Figure 9.12** when necessary to answer the following questions.

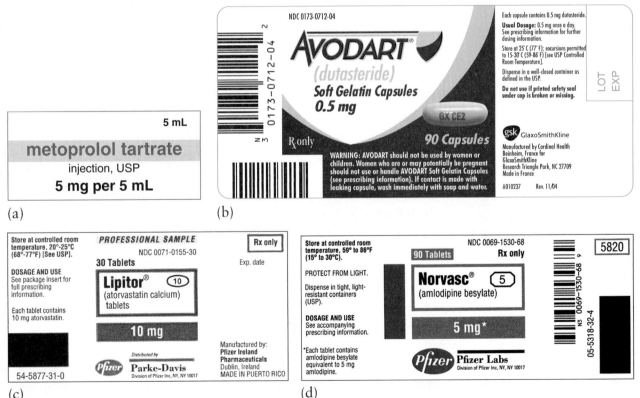

● **Figure 9.12**

**Drug labels for Case Study 9.1.**

(09-12b Reproduced with permission of GlaxoSmithKline.    09-12c Reg. Trademark of Pfizer Inc. Reproduced with permission.    09-12d Reg. Trademark of Pfizer Inc. Reproduced with permission.)

1. The morphine is supplied in vials labeled 5 mg/mL.
   (a) How many milliliters are needed for the prescribed dose?
   (b) What type of syringe will you use to administer the dose?
2. The heparin vial is labeled 20,000 units/mL.
   (a) How many milliliters will you prepare?
   (b) What type of syringe will you use to administer the dose?
3. How many milliliters are needed to prepare the dose of the metoprolol?
4. What is the number of milligrams of Flagyl to be administered?
5. The Toradol vial is labeled 30 mg/mL. What is the maximum number of milliliters of Toradol that the patient may receive in 24 hours?

6. How many grams of Norvasc will be administered in one week?
7. How many capsules of dutasteride will you administer for each dose?
8. How many tablets of amlodipine will you administer each day?
9. The Vasotec is supplied in 2.5 mg, 5 mg, 10 mg, and 20 mg tablets.
   (a) Which dosage strength will you use?
   (b) How many tablets will you administer?
10. How many tablets of atorvastatin will you administer?

**Workspace**

## Practice Sets

The answers to *Try These for Practice, Exercises,* and *Cumulative Review Exercises* are found in Appendix A. Ask your instructor for the answers to the *Additional Exercises*.

### Try These for Practice

Test your comprehension after reading the chapter.

1. Order:
   *penicillin G 150,000 units IM q12h*

   The label on a 5,000,000 unit vial of penicillin G reads: "Preparation for solution: Add 23 mL, 18 mL, 8 mL, or 3 mL diluent to provide 200,000 units, 250,000 units, 500,000 units, or 1,000,000 units per mL. Keep in the refrigerator 1 week without significant loss of potency."

   (a) If Nurse Mary Jones chooses to reconstitute to a strength of 250,000 units/mL, how much diluent would she add to the vial?
   (b) How many milliliters would she administer?
   (c) How many full doses would be available in the vial?
   (d) If she reconstituted the drug at 0900h on May 5, 2010, write the reconstitution label that she would put on the vial.

2. Order:
   *Claforan (cefotaxime) 500 mg IM q6h.* See portion of the package insert in ● **Figure 9.13.**

   (a) Which vial would you choose for reconstitution?
   (b) How much diluent must be added to the vial?
   (c) What is the reconstituted volume in the vial?

| CLAFORAN for IM or IV administration should be reconstituted as follows: | | | |
|---|---|---|---|
| Strength | Diluent (mL) | Withdrawable volume (mL) | Approximate concentration (mg/mL) |
| 2g vial* (IM) | 5 | 6.0 | 330 |
| 1g vial* (IV) | 10 | 10.4 | 95 |

● **Figure 9.13**
**Portion of package insert for Claforan.**

(d) What is the strength of the reconstituted solution?
(e) How many milliliters would you administer?
(f) How many full doses are in the vial?

3. Order:
*Ativan (lorazepam) 0.05 mg/kg IM two hours before surgery.*

The patient weighs 135 pounds, and the label on the 10 mL multidose vial reads: "2 mg per 2 mL."

(a) How many milligrams will you prepare?
(b) How many milliliters will you administer?

4. Order:
*Heparin 8,000 units subcutaneously q12h.*

The vial is labeled 10,000 units/mL.

(a) How many milliliters will you administer?
(b) What size syringe will you use?

5. Order:
*Pipracil (piperacillin sodium) 2 g IM stat with probenecid 1 g PO 30 minutes before giving the Pipracil.*

The package insert for the 2 g Pipracil vial states: "Add 4 mL of diluent to yield 1 g/2.5 mL." The label on the probenecid bottle reads: "0.5 g tablet."

(a) How many tablets of probenecid will you administer?
(b) How many milliliters of Pipracil contain the prescribed dose?

## Exercises

Reinforce your understanding in class or at home.

1. The prescriber ordered *ampicillin 750 mg IM q6h*.

   The directions for the 1 g ampicillin vial state, "reconstitute with 3.5 mL of diluent to yield 250 mg/mL." How many milliliters will contain the prescribed dose?

2. The prescriber ordered *Unasyn 1.5 g IM q6h*.

   The package insert states: Add 3.2 mL of sterile water for injection to yield 375 mg/mL (250 mg ampicillin and 125 mg sulbactam/mL). Calculate how many milliliters you will administer.

3. The prescriber ordered *Aranesp 0.49 mcg/kg subcutaneously once per week* for a patient who weighs 155 pounds.

   (a) How many mcg will you administer?
   (b) Read the label in ● **Figure 9.14** and calculate how many milliliters you will administer.

NDC 55513-011-01    Store at 2° to 8°C

**Aranesp®**

**40 mcg** (darbepoetin alfa)    Single Use Vial

40 mcg/1 mL    R Only

Dosage–See Package Insert    U.S. License No.1080
Amgen Mfg. Ltd. Thousand Oaks, CA 91320

3210003    LOT    EXP.

● **Figure 9.14**
**Drug label for Aranesp.**
*(Published with permission of Amgen Inc.)*

4. The prescriber ordered *Claforan (cefotaxime) 1,200 mg IM q12h*. The directions for the 1 g vial state: "Add 3.2 mL of diluent to yield an approximate concentration of 300 mg/mL. The directions for the 2 g vial state: Add 5 mL of diluent to yield an approximate concentration of 330 mg/mL."

   (a) Which vial will you use?
   (b) How many milliliters will you administer?

5. The prescriber ordered *streptomycin 500 mg IM q12h for 7 days*. Read the label in ● **Figure 9.15** and calculate how many milliliters of this antibiotic you will administer.

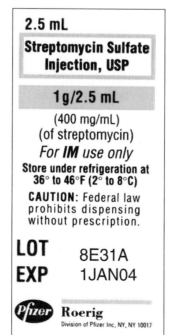

**2.5 mL**

**Streptomycin Sulfate Injection, USP**

**1 g/2.5 mL**

(400 mg/mL)
(of streptomycin)
*For IM use only*
Store under refrigeration at
36° to 46°F (2° to 8°C)

**CAUTION:** Federal law prohibits dispensing without prescription.

**LOT**    8E31A
**EXP**    1JAN04

*Pfizer* **Roerig**
Division of Pfizer Inc, NY, NY 10017

● **Figure 9.15**
**Drug label for streptomycin.**
*(Reg. Trademark of Pfizer Inc. Reproduced with permission.)*

6. The prescriber ordered *Stelazine (trifluoperazine hydrochloride) 1.4 mg IM (give deep IM) q6h prn.* The label on the 10 mL multidose vial reads 2 mg/mL injection.

 (a) Calculate the number of milliliters that contain this dose.
 (b) How many full doses are in the vial?

7. The prescriber ordered *Enbrel (etanercept) 50 mg subcutaneously once a week.* Read the label in ● Figure 9.16 and calculate how many vials you will use.

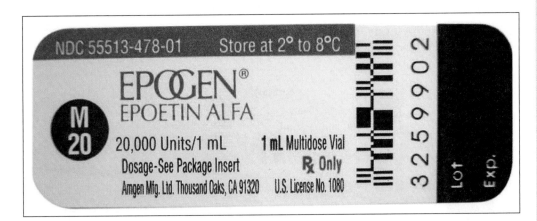

● **Figure 9.16**
**Drug label for Enbrel.**

*(Published with permission of Amgen Inc.)*

8. The prescriber ordered *Epogen (epoetin alfa) 6,000 units subcutaneously three times a week.* Use the label in ● Figure 9.17 and do the following:

 (a) Calculate how many milliliters contain this dose.
 (b) Determine what size syringe you will use to administer this medication.

● **Figure 9.17**
**Drug label for Epogen.**

*(Published with permission of Amgen Inc.)*

9. The prescriber ordered *gentamicin 60 mg IM q12h*. The drug is supplied in a 20 mL multidose vial. The label reads 40 mg/mL. How many milliliters will you administer?

10. The prescriber ordered *morphine sulfate 5 mg subcutaneously q4h prn*. The drug is supplied in a 1 mL vial that is labeled 15 mg/mL.

    (a) How many milliliters will you administer?
    (b) What size syringe will you use?

11. The prescriber ordered *Lasix (furosemide) 30 mg IM stat*. The drug is supplied in a vial labeled 40 mg/mL. How many milliliters will you administer?

12. A patient is to receive *Ativan (lorazepam) 3 mg IM, 2 hours before surgery*. The drug is supplied in a vial labeled 4 mg/mL. How many milliliters will you administer?

13. Use the insulin "sliding scale" below to determine how much insulin you will give to a patient whose blood glucose is 320.

    Order: *Give Humulin R Unit-100 insulin subcutaneously for blood glucose levels as follows:*

    | | |
    |---|---|
    | *glucose less than 160* | *—no insulin* |
    | *glucose 160–220* | *—2 units* |
    | *glucose 221–280* | *—4 units* |
    | *glucose 281–340* | *—6 units* |
    | *glucose 341–400* | *—8 units* |
    | *glucose more than 400* | *—hold insulin and call MD stat* |

14. The prescriber ordered *heparin 3,500 units subcutaneously q12h*. The label on the vial states 5,000 units/mL.

    (a) How many milliliters will you administer?
    (b) What size syringe will you use?

15. The prescriber ordered *Humulin N 25 units subcutaneously ac breakfast*.

    Use the label in ● **Figure 9.18** to determine the following:

    (a) How many units will you administer?
    (b) What size syringe will you use?

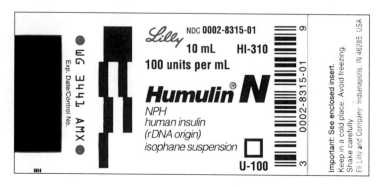

● **Figure 9.18**
**Drug label for Humulin N insulin.**

*(Copyright Eli Lilly and Company. Used with permission.)*

16. Read the information in ● Figure **9.19** and use the highest concentration to determine how many milliliters contain 650,000 units.

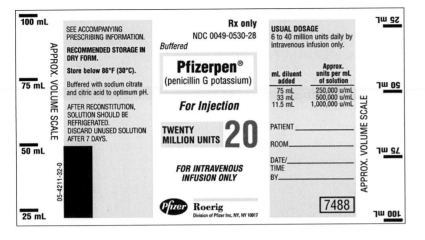

● Figure 9.19

**Drug label for Pfizerpen.**    *(Reg. trademark of Pfizer Inc. Reproduced with permission.)*

17. A patient is to receive *atropine sulfate 0.2 mg IM 30 minutes before surgery*. The vial is labeled 0.4 mg/mL.

    (a) How many milliliters will you administer?
    (b) What size syringe will you use?

18. A patient weighs 110 pounds. The daily recommended safe dose range for a certain drug is 0.03–0.04 mg/kg.

    (a) What is the minimum number of mg of this drug that this patient should receive each day?
    (b) What is the maximum number of mg of this drug that this patient should receive each day?

19. The order is *Thorazine (chlorpromazine hydrochloride) 40 mg IM q6h prn for agitation*. The vial is labeled 25 mg/mL.

    (a) How many milliliters will you administer?
    (b) What size syringe will you use?

20. Use the information in ● Figure **9.20** and answer the following:

    (a) How much diluent must be added to the vial to prepare a 250,000 units/mL strength?
    (b) How much diluent must be added to the vial to prepare a 500,000 units/mL strength?
    (c) What is the total dose of this vial?
    (d) The order is *penicillin G 2,000,000 units IM stat*. How will you prepare this dose?

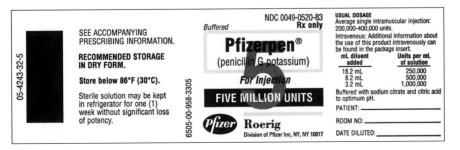

● Figure 9.20

**Drug label for Pfizerpen.**    *(Reg. trademark of Pfizer Inc. Reproduced with permission.)*

# Additional Exercises

Now, test yourself!

1.  The prescriber ordered *Brethine (terbutaline sulfate) 0.25 mg subcutaneous stat.* The vial is labeled 1 mg/mL.

    (a)  How many milliliters will you administer? _____
    (b)  What size syringe will you use? _____

2.  Order: *streptomycin 500 mg IM daily for 8 days.* Read the label in
    ● **Figure 9.21** and calculate how many vials of this antibiotic you would
    need for your patient over the eight days. _____

    | |
    |---|
    | **2.5 mL** |
    | **Streptomycin Sulfate Injection, USP** |
    | **1 g/2.5 mL** |
    | (400 mg/mL) (of streptomycin) *For **IM** use only* |
    | **Store under refrigeration at 36° to 46°F (2° to 8°C)** |
    | **CAUTION:** Federal law prohibits dispensing without prescription. |
    | **LOT**  8E31A  **EXP**  1JAN04 |
    | Pfizer **Roerig** Division of Pfizer Inc, NY, NY 10017 |

    ● **Figure 9.21**
    **Drug label for streptomycin.**
    *(Reg. trademark of Pfizer Inc. Reproduced with permission.)*

3.  Order: *ampicillin 500 mg IM q6h*

    The directions on the 2 g vial read, add 7 mL of diluent and each mL =
    250 mg.

    (a)  How many milliliters of diluent will be added to the vial?
    (b)  What is the strength of the reconstituted solution?
    (c)  How many milliliters should be administered?
    (d)  How many full doses are available in the vial?

4.  A patient is to receive *Inapsine (droperidol) 2.5 mg IM 30 minutes before
    surgery.* The label reads 5 mg/2 mL.

    (a)  How many milliliters will you need? _____
    (b)  What size syringe will you use? _____

5.  The prescriber ordered *Bactocill (oxacillin sodium) 400 mg IM q4h.*

    The package insert for the 1 g vial states: "Add 5.7 mL of sterile water for
    injection. Each 1.5 mL contains 250 mg oxacillin."

    (a)  How many milliliters will you need? _____
    (b)  What size syringe will you use? _____

6. Order: *Tigan 200 mg IM stat, then 100 mg q6h prn nausea.* The Tigan strength is 100 mg/mL.

   (a) How many milliliters would you administer immediately?
   (b) How many milliliters would you administer in case of nausea?

7. Order: *Lovenox (enoxaprin sodium) 30 mg subcutaneous q12h.*

   The label on the 0.4 mL prefilled syringe reads 40 mg/0.4 mL. How much solution should be discarded to administer the prescribed dose?

   _____

8. Order: *Dilaudid-HP (hydromorphone HCl) 3 mg subcutaneous q4 h prn pain.* Read the label in ● **Figure 9.22** and calculate how many milliliters you will administer.

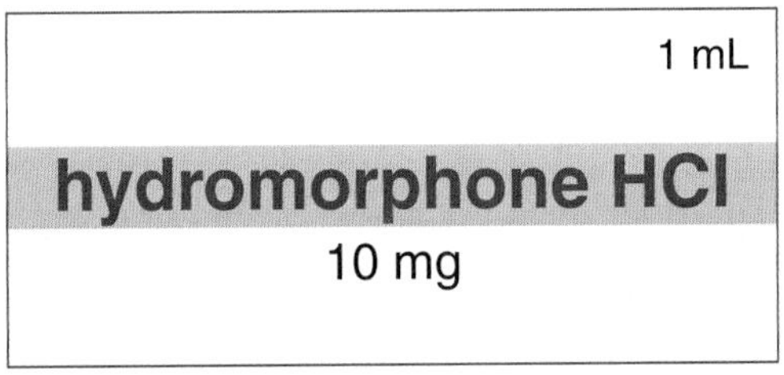

   _____

   | 1 mL |
   | **hydromorphone HCl** |
   | 10 mg |

   ● **Figure 9.22**
   **Drug label for hydromorphone HCl.**

9. The prescriber ordered *Rocephine (ceftriaxone) 250 mg IM stat.*

   The package insert states that when "1.8 mL of diluent is added to a 500 mg vial, 1 mL of solution contains approximately 250 mg of ceftriaxone." How many milliliters will contain the prescribed dose?

   _____

10. The prescriber ordered *Energix-B (hepatitis B vaccine) 20 mcg IM stat.*

    The multidose vial label reads "25 adult doses 20 mcg/mL." How many milliliters will you administer?

    _____

11. A patient is to receive *Loxitane (loxapine HCl) 30 mg IM q6h.*

    The label reads 50 mg/mL. How many milliliters should the patient receive?

    _____

12. The prescriber ordered *Vitamin B (thiamine HCl) 50 mg IM t.i.d.*

    The label reads 100 mg/mL. How many milliliters will you administer?

    _____

13. Read the cefazolin sodium label in ● **Figure 9.23**. If you add 45 mL of diluent to the 10 g vial, how many milliliters will contain 500 mg?

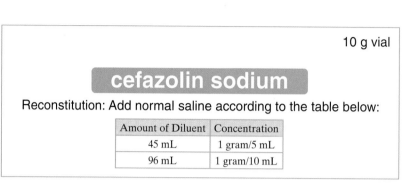

● **Figure 9.23**
**Drug label for cefazolin sodium.**

14. The prescriber ordered *Demerol (meperidine HCl) 75 mg IM q4h prn pain.*

    The vial is labeled 100 mg/mL. How many milliliters will you administer?

15. A patient who has rheumatoid arthritis weighs 150 pounds. The maximum recommended safe dose of cyclosporine is 2.5–4 mg/kg/d. Would a daily dose of 1 g of cyclosporine be safe for this patient?

16. Order: *Cogentin (benztropine mesylate) 1 mg IM now.*

    The label on the 2 mL ampule reads 1 mg/mL. How many milliliters is the patient receiving?

17. The prescriber ordered *cyanocobalamin 30 mcg IM daily for 5 days, then 200 mcg per month.*

    The label on the vial states 100 mcg/mL. How many milliliters contain the daily dose?

18. Order: *Pentam (pentamidine isethionate) 3 mg/kg IM q.i.d.*

    The label reads: Add 3 mL of sterile water to each 300 mg vial. Calculate how many milliliters you will administer to the patient who weighs 90 pounds.

19. Order: *Bicillin L-A (penicillin G benzathine) 1.2 million units IM q4 weeks.*

    The label vial reads 2,400,000 units/4 mL. Calculate the number of milliliters you will administer.

    _____

20. Order: *Methergine (methylergonovine maleate) 0.2 mg IM q4h for three doses.*

    The drug label reads 0.2 mg/mL.

    (a) How many milliliters will you administer per dose? _____
    (b) What is the total number of milligrams the patient will receive for the three doses?

    _____

## Cumulative Review Exercises

Review your mastery of previous chapters.

Read the label in ● **Figure 9.24** to answer questions 1 through 4.

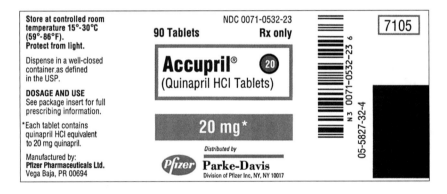

● **Figure 9.24**
**Drug label for Accupril.**

*(Reg. trademark of Pfizer Inc. Reproduced with permission.)*

1. What is the generic name of this drug? _____

2. What is the route of administration? _____

3. What is the name of the manufacturer? _____

4. A patient is to receive 80 mg q12h. How many tablets will he receive every 24 hours? _____

5. The prescriber ordered *Antivert (meclazine HCl) 25 mg PO daily prn vertigo.*

   Read the label in ● **Figure 9.25** and calculate how many tablets you will administer.

**Workspace**

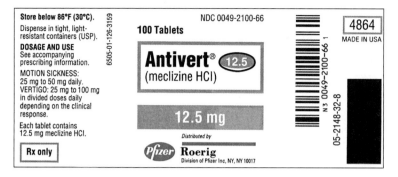

● **Figure 9.25**
**Drug label for Antivert.**

*(Reg. trademark of Pfizer Inc. Reproduced with permission.)*

Read the label in ● **Figure 9.26** to answer questions 6 through 9.

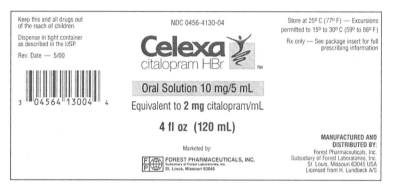

● **Figure 9.26**
**Drug label for Celexa.**

*(Courtesy of Forest Pharmaceuticals, Inc.)*

6. What is the trade name of the drug? _____

7. What is the strength of the drug? _____

8. A patient is to receive 20 mg PO daily. How many milliliters will you administer? _____

9. A patient is to receive 20 mg PO daily. How many doses of medication will this container supply? _____

10. The prescriber ordered *Mycobutin (rifabutin) 300 mg PO b.i.d.*

    Read the label in ● **Figure 9.27** and calculate the number of capsules the patient will receive.

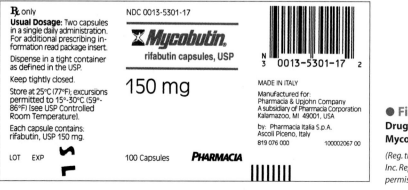

● **Figure 9.27**
**Drug label for Mycobutin.**

*(Reg. trademark of Pfizer Inc. Reproduced with permission.)*

11. The label on a reconstituted medication states that the strength is 500,000 units/mL. How many milliliters equal 200,000 units? _____

12. Order: *Solu-Medrol 125 mg IM once daily.* The label on the 500 mg vial reads: Reconstitute with 8 mL of bacteriostatic water for injection with benzyl alcohol and 62.5 mg per mL.

   (a) How much diluent should be added to the vial?
   (b) How many milliliters should be administered?
   (c) How many full doses are available in the vial?

13. A patient had a clear liquid dinner consisting of 4 oz of apple juice, 8 oz of chicken broth, and 6 oz of hot tea. Calculate the total intake in mL.

14. The order is *ampicillin sodium 500 mg IM q6h.* The label on the 500 mg vial indicates for reconstitution to add 1.8 mL of diluent, and 250 mg = 1 mL.

   (a) How much diluent should be added to the vial?
   (b) What is the concentration after reconstitution?
   (c) How many milliliters should be administered?
   (d) How many full doses are available in the vial?

15. Order: *Nubain (nalbuphine HCl) 5 mg subcut q4h prn pain.* The label on the 10 mL multiple dose vial reads 20 mg/mL.

   (a) How many milliliters should be administered?
   (b) How many full doses are available in the vial?

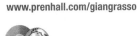

**MediaLink**
www.prenhall.com/giangrasso

Animated examples, interactive practice questions with animated solutions, and challenge tests for this chapter can be found on the Pearson Dosage Calculation Tutor that accompanies this text. Additional, unique, interactive resources and activities can be found on the Companion Web site.

# Infusions and Pediatric Dosages

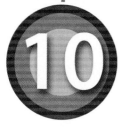

**Chapter**

# 10 Flow Rates and Durations of Enteral and Intravenous Infusions

## Learning Outcomes

After completing this chapter, you will be able to

1. Describe the basic concepts and standard equipment used in administering enteral and intravenous (IV) infusions.
2. Quickly convert flow rates between gtt/min and mL/h.
3. Calculate the flow rates of enteral and IV infusions.
4. Calculate the durations of enteral and IV infusions.
5. Determine fluid replacement volumes.

This chapter introduces the basic concepts and standard equipment used in intravenous and enteral therapy. You will also learn how to calculate flow rates for these infusions and to determine how long it will take for a given amount of solution to infuse (its duration).

280

# Introduction to Intravenous and Enteral Solutions

Fluids can be given to a patient slowly over a period of time through a vein (*intravenous*) or through a tube inserted into the alimentary tract (*enteral*). The rate at which these fluids flow into the patient is very important and must be controlled precisely.

## Enteral Feedings

When a patient cannot ingest food or if the upper gastrointestinal tract is not functioning properly, the prescriber may write an order for an *enteral* feeding (*"tube feeding"*). Enteral feedings provide nutrients and other fluids by way of a tube inserted directly into the gastrointestinal system (alimentary tract).

There are various types of tube feedings. A gastric tube may be inserted into the stomach through the nares (**nasogastric**, as shown in ● **Figure 10.1**) or through the mouth (**orogastric**). A longer tube may be similarly inserted, but would extend beyond the stomach into the upper small intestine, jejunum (**nasojejunum** or **orojejunum**).

For long-term feedings, tubes can be inserted surgically or laproscopically through the wall of the abdomen and directly into either the stomach (gastrostomy) or through the stomach and on to the jejunum (jejunostomy). These tubes are sutured in place and are referred to as *percutaneous endoscopic gastrostomy (PEG) tubes* and *percutaneous endoscopic jejunostomy (PEJ) tubes*, respectively (● **Figure 10.2**).

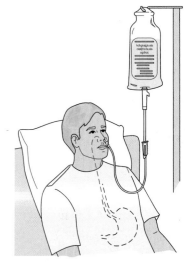

● **Figure 10.1**
**A patient with a nasogastric tube.**

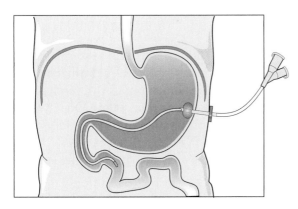

● **Figure 10.2**
*A percutaneous endoscopic jejunostomy (PEJ) tube.*

Enteral feedings may be given *continuously* (over a 24-hour period) or *intermittently* (over shorter periods, perhaps several times a day). There are many enteral feeding solutions, including Boost, Compleat, Ensure, Isocal, Resource, and Sustacal. Enteral feedings are generally administered via pump. ● **Figure 10.3**.

Orders for enteral solutions always indicate a volume of fluid to be infused over a period of time; that is, a flow rate. For example, a tube feeding order might read *Isocal 50 mL/h via nasogastric tube for 6 hours beginning 6 A.M.* This order is for an intermittent feeding in which the name of the solution is Isocal, the rate of flow is 50 mL/h, the route of administration is via nasogastric tube, and the duration is 6 hours.

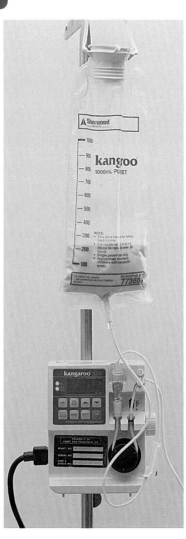

● **Figure 10.3**
**Enteral feeding via pump.**

*(Photographer; Elena Dorfman)*

# Intravenous Infusions

*Intravenous* (IV) means *through the vein*. Fluids are administered intravenously to provide a variety of fluids, including blood, water containing nutrients, electrolytes, minerals, and specific medications to the patient. IV fluids can replace lost fluids, maintain fluid and electrolyte balance, or serve as a medium to introduce medications directly into the bloodstream.

*Replacement fluids* are ordered for a patient who has lost fluids through hemorrhage, vomiting, or diarrhea. *Maintenance fluids* help sustain normal levels of fluids and electrolytes. They are ordered for patients who are at risk of becoming depleted; for example, patients who are NPO (nothing by mouth).

Intravenous infusions may be *continuous* or *intermittent*. Continuous IV infusions are used to replace or maintain fluids or electrolytes. Intermittent IV infusions—for example, IV piggyback (IVPB) and IV push (IVP)—are used to administer drugs and supplemental fluids. *Intermittent peripheral infusion devices* (saline locks or heparin locks) are used to maintain venous access without continuous fluid infusion. Intermittent IV infusions are discussed in Chapter 11.

A healthcare professional must be able to perform the calculations to determine the correct rate at which an enteral or intravenous solution will enter the body (*flow rate*). Infusion flow rates are usually measured in drops per minute (gtt/min) or milliliters per hour (mL/h). It is important to be able to convert each of these rates to the other and to determine how long a given amount of solution will take to infuse.

For example, a continuous IV order might read *IV fluids: D5W 125 mL/h for 8h*. In this case, the order is for an IV infusion in which the name of the solution is 5% dextrose in water, the rate of flow is 125 mL/h, the route of administration is intravenous, and the duration is 8 hours.

## Intravenous Solutions

A **saline solution,** which is a solution of *sodium chloride (NaCl)* in sterile water, is commonly used for intravenous infusion. Sodium chloride is ordinary table salt. Saline solutions are available in various concentrations for different purposes. A 0.9% NaCl solution is also referred to as **normal saline (NS)**. Other saline solutions commonly used include **half-normal saline** (0.45% NaCl), written as $\frac{1}{2}$ NS; and **quarter-normal saline** (0.225% NaCl), written as $\frac{1}{4}$ NS.

Intravenous fluids generally contain dextrose, sodium chloride, and/or electrolytes:

- D5W, D5/W, or 5% D/W is a 5% dextrose solution, which means that 5 g of dextrose are dissolved in water to make each 100 mL of this solution. ● **Figures 10.4a** and **10.4b**.

- NS or 0.9% NaCl is a solution in which each 100 mL contain 0.9 g of sodium chloride. ● **Figures 10.4c** and **10.4d**.

- 5% D/0.45% NaCl is a solution containing 5 g of dextrose and 0.45 g of NaCl in each 100 mL of solution ● **Figure 10.5b**.

- Ringer's lactate (RL), also called lactated Ringer's solution (LRS), is a solution containing electrolytes, including potassium chloride and calcium chloride. ● **Figure 10.5c**.

Additional information on the many other IV fluids can be found in nursing and pharmacology textbooks.

**NOTE**

Pay close attention to the abbreviations of the names of the IV solutions. *Letters* indicate the solution compounds, whereas *numbers* indicate the solution strength e.g., D5W.

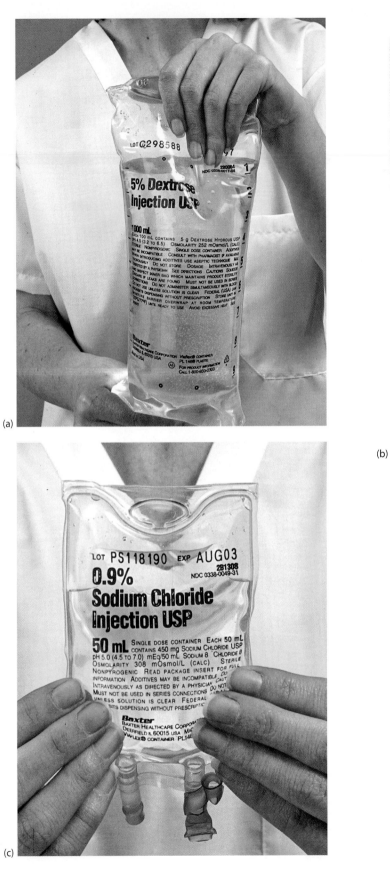

LOT          EXP

290064
NDC 0338-0017-04          **1**

**2**

**3**

## 5% Dextrose
## Injection USP

**4**

**1000 mL**
EACH 100 mL CONTAINS    5 g DEXTROSE HYDROUS USP
pH 4.0 (3.2 TO 6.5)    OSMOLARITY 252 mOsmol/L (CALC)
STERILE   NONPYROGENIC   SINGLE DOSE CONTAINER   ADDITIVES
MAY BE INCOMPATIBLE   CONSULT WITH PHARMACIST IF AVAILABLE
WHEN INTRODUCING ADDITIVES USE ASEPTIC TECHNIQUE   MIX
THOROUGHLY    DO NOT STORE    DOSAGE    INTRAVENOUSLY AS
DIRECTED BY A PHYSICIAN   SEE DIRECTIONS  CAUTIONS  SQUEEZE
AND INSPECT INNER BAG WHICH MAINTAINS PRODUCT STERILITY
DISCARD IF LEAKS ARE FOUND    MUST NOT BE USED IN SERIES
CONNECTIONS   DO NOT ADMINISTER SIMULTANEOUSLY WITH BLOOD
DO NOT USE UNLESS SOLUTION IS CLEAR   FEDERAL (USA) LAW
PROHIBITS DISPENSING WITHOUT PRESCRIPTION   STORE UNIT IN
MOISTURE BARRIER OVERWRAP AT ROOM TEMPERATURE
(25°C/77°F) UNTIL READY TO USE   AVOID EXCESSIVE HEAT   SEE
INSERT

**5**

**6**

**7**

**8**

*Baxter*
BAXTER HEALTHCARE CORPORATION   VIAFLEX® CONTAINER
DEERFIELD IL 60015 USA          PL 146® PLASTIC
MADE IN USA                     FOR PRODUCT INFORMATION
                                CALL 1-800-933-0303

**9**

(b)

⊡ 1000 mL  NDC 0074-7983-09

0—                              —0

1—                              —1

2—  **0.9%**                    —2
    **Sodium Chloride**
    Injection, USP

3—                              —3

    EACH 100 ML CONTAINS SODIUM CHLORIDE
4—  900 mg IN WATER FOR INJECTION.       —4
    ELECTROLYTES PER 1000 mL: SODIUM 154 mEq;
    CHLORIDE 154 mEq.
    308 mOsm/LITER (CALC).   pH 5.6 (4.5–7.0)
5—  ADDITIVES MAY BE INCOMPATIBLE. CONSULT   —5
    WITH PHARMACIST, IF AVAILABLE. WHEN
    INTRODUCING ADDITIVES, USE ASEPTIC
6—  TECHNIQUE, MIX THOROUGHLY AND DO NOT     —6
    STORE. SINGLE-DOSE CONTAINER. FOR
    INTRAVENOUS USE. USUAL DOSE: SEE INSERT.
    STERILE, NONPYROGENIC. CAUTION: FEDERAL
7—  (USA) LAW PROHIBITS DISPENSING WITHOUT   —7
    PRESCRIPTION. USE ONLY IF SOLUTION IS CLEAR
    AND CONTAINER IS UNDAMAGED. MUST NOT
8—  BE USED IN SERIES CONNECTIONS.           —8
                              PATENT PENDING
    ©ABBOTT 1988                PRINTED IN USA
9—  ABBOTT LABORATORIES, NORTH CHICAGO, IL60064, USA   9

(d)

● **Figure 10.4**
**Examples of IV bags and labels.**

*(10-04a Al Dodge/Al Dodge.   10-04b Courtesy of Baxter Healthcare Corporation. All
rights reserved.   10-04c Al Dodge/Al Dodge.   10-04d Reproduced with permission of
Abbott Laboratories)*

● **Figure 10.5**
**Examples of intravenous fluids.**

*(Reproduced with permission of Abbott Laboratories.)*

## ALERT

In Figure 10.5, solutions (a) and (b) both contain 5% dextrose and $\frac{1}{2}$ NS. However, solution (a) also contains 20 mEq of potassium chloride, which is a high-alert medication. Do not confuse these two solutions.

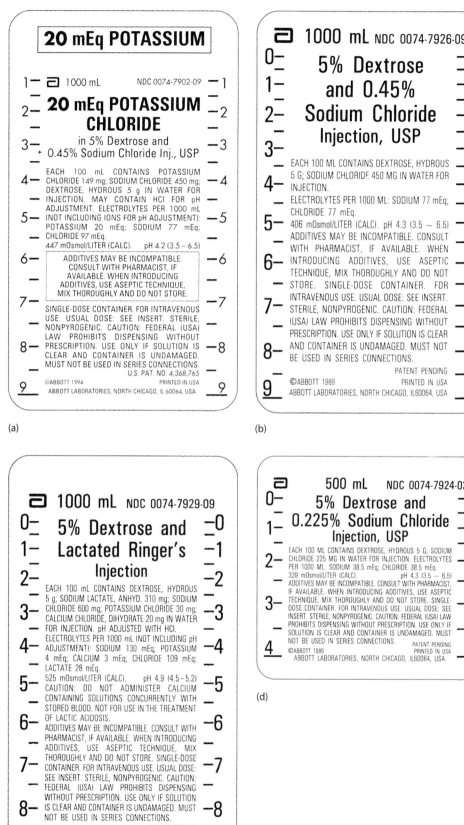

**20 mEq POTASSIUM**

1 — ⌐ 1000 mL          NDC 0074-7902-09 — 1

2 — **20 mEq POTASSIUM** — 2
**CHLORIDE**

3 — in 5% Dextrose and — 3
0.45% Sodium Chloride Inj., USP

4 — EACH 100 mL CONTAINS POTASSIUM — 4
CHLORIDE 149 mg; SODIUM CHLORIDE 450 mg;
DEXTROSE, HYDROUS 5 g IN WATER FOR
INJECTION. MAY CONTAIN HCI FOR pH
ADJUSTMENT. ELECTROLYTES PER 1000 mL
5 — (NOT INCLUDING IONS FOR pH ADJUSTMENT): — 5
POTASSIUM 20 mEq; SODIUM 77 mEq;
CHLORIDE 97 mEq.
447 mOsmol/LITER (CALC).          pH 4.2 (3.5 – 6.5)

6 — ADDITIVES MAY BE INCOMPATIBLE. — 6
CONSULT WITH PHARMACIST, IF
AVAILABLE. WHEN INTRODUCING
ADDITIVES, USE ASEPTIC TECHNIQUE,
MIX THOROUGHLY AND DO NOT STORE.

7 — SINGLE-DOSE CONTAINER. FOR INTRAVENOUS — 7
USE. USUAL DOSE: SEE INSERT. STERILE,
NONPYROGENIC. CAUTION: FEDERAL (USA)
LAW PROHIBITS DISPENSING WITHOUT
8 — PRESCRIPTION. USE ONLY IF SOLUTION IS — 8
CLEAR AND CONTAINER IS UNDAMAGED.
MUST NOT BE USED IN SERIES CONNECTIONS.
U.S. PAT. NO. 4,368,765
9 — ©ABBOTT 1994          PRINTED IN USA — 9
ABBOTT LABORATORIES, NORTH CHICAGO, IL 60064, USA

(a)

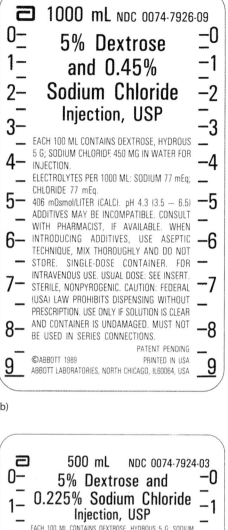

ⓐ 1000 mL  NDC 0074-7926-09

0 — **5% Dextrose** — 0
1 — **and 0.45%** — 1
2 — **Sodium Chloride** — 2
**Injection, USP**
3 — — 3
EACH 100 ML CONTAINS DEXTROSE, HYDROUS
5 G; SODIUM CHLORIDE 450 MG IN WATER FOR
4 — INJECTION. — 4
ELECTROLYTES PER 1000 ML: SODIUM 77 mEq;
CHLORIDE 77 mEq.
5 — 406 mOsmol/LITER (CALC). pH 4.3 (3.5 – 6.5) — 5
ADDITIVES MAY BE INCOMPATIBLE. CONSULT
WITH PHARMACIST, IF AVAILABLE. WHEN
6 — INTRODUCING ADDITIVES, USE ASEPTIC — 6
TECHNIQUE, MIX THOROUGHLY AND DO NOT
STORE. SINGLE-DOSE CONTAINER. FOR
INTRAVENOUS USE. USUAL DOSE: SEE INSERT.
7 — STERILE, NONPYROGENIC. CAUTION: FEDERAL — 7
(USA) LAW PROHIBITS DISPENSING WITHOUT
PRESCRIPTION. USE ONLY IF SOLUTION IS CLEAR
AND CONTAINER IS UNDAMAGED. MUST NOT
8 — BE USED IN SERIES CONNECTIONS. — 8
PATENT PENDING
9 — ©ABBOTT 1989          PRINTED IN USA — 9
ABBOTT LABORATORIES, NORTH CHICAGO, IL60064, USA

(b)

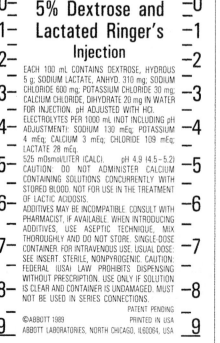

ⓐ 1000 mL  NDC 0074-7929-09

0 — **5% Dextrose and** — 0
1 — **Lactated Ringer's** — 1
**Injection**
2 — — 2
EACH 100 mL CONTAINS DEXTROSE, HYDROUS
5 g; SODIUM LACTATE, ANHYD. 310 mg; SODIUM
3 — CHLORIDE 600 mg; POTASSIUM CHLORIDE 30 mg; — 3
CALCIUM CHLORIDE, DIHYDRATE 20 mg IN WATER
FOR INJECTION. pH ADJUSTED WITH HCI.
ELECTROLYTES PER 1000 mL (NOT INCLUDING pH
4 — ADJUSTMENT): SODIUM 130 mEq; POTASSIUM — 4
4 mEq; CALCIUM 3 mEq; CHLORIDE 109 mEq;
LACTATE 28 mEq.
5 — 525 mOsmol/LITER (CALC).      pH 4.9 (4.5 – 5.2) — 5
CAUTION: DO NOT ADMINISTER CALCIUM
CONTAINING SOLUTIONS CONCURRENTLY WITH
STORED BLOOD. NOT FOR USE IN THE TREATMENT
6 — OF LACTIC ACIDOSIS. — 6
ADDITIVES MAY BE INCOMPATIBLE. CONSULT WITH
PHARMACIST, IF AVAILABLE. WHEN INTRODUCING
ADDITIVES, USE ASEPTIC TECHNIQUE, MIX
7 — THOROUGHLY AND DO NOT STORE. SINGLE-DOSE — 7
CONTAINER. FOR INTRAVENOUS USE. USUAL DOSE:
SEE INSERT. STERILE, NONPYROGENIC. CAUTION:
FEDERAL (USA) LAW PROHIBITS DISPENSING
WITHOUT PRESCRIPTION. USE ONLY IF SOLUTION
8 — IS CLEAR AND CONTAINER IS UNDAMAGED. MUST — 8
NOT BE USED IN SERIES CONNECTIONS.
PATENT PENDING
9 — ©ABBOTT 1989          PRINTED IN USA — 9
ABBOTT LABORATORIES, NORTH CHICAGO, IL60064, USA

(c)

ⓐ  500 mL   NDC 0074-7924-03

0 — **5% Dextrose and** — 0
1 — **0.225% Sodium Chloride** — 1
**Injection, USP**
2 — EACH 100 mL CONTAINS DEXTROSE, HYDROUS 5 G; SODIUM — 2
CHLORIDE 225 MG IN WATER FOR INJECTION. ELECTROLYTES
PER 1000 ML: SODIUM 38.5 mEq; CHLORIDE 38.5 mEq.
329 mOsmol/LITER (CALC).          pH 4.3 (3.5 – 6.5)
ADDITIVES MAY BE INCOMPATIBLE. CONSULT WITH PHARMACIST,
IF AVAILABLE. WHEN INTRODUCING ADDITIVES, USE ASEPTIC
TECHNIQUE, MIX THOROUGHLY AND DO NOT STORE. SINGLE-
3 — DOSE CONTAINER. FOR INTRAVENOUS USE. USUAL DOSE: SEE — 3
INSERT. STERILE, NONPYROGENIC. CAUTION: FEDERAL (USA) LAW
PROHIBITS DISPENSING WITHOUT PRESCRIPTION. USE ONLY IF
SOLUTION IS CLEAR AND CONTAINER IS UNDAMAGED. MUST
NOT BE USED IN SERIES CONNECTIONS.      PATENT PENDING
4 — ©ABBOTT 1989          PRINTED IN USA — 4
ABBOTT LABORATORIES, NORTH CHICAGO, IL60064, USA

(d)

# Equipment for IV Infusions

Equipment used for the administration of continuous IV infusions includes the IV solution and IV tubing, a drip chamber, at least one injection port, and a roller clamp. The tubing connects the IV solution to the hub of an IV catheter at the infusion site. The rate of flow of the infusion is regulated by an electronic infusion device (pump or controller) or by gravity. ● **Figures 10.6** and **10.9**.

**ALERT**

No intravenous solution should infuse for more than 24 hours.

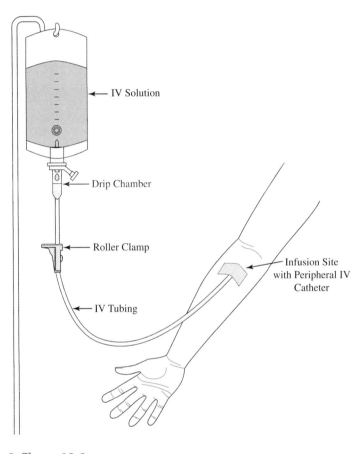

● **Figure 10.6**
**Primary intravenous line (gravity flow).**

Labels: IV Solution, Drip Chamber, Roller Clamp, IV Tubing, Infusion Site with Peripheral IV Catheter

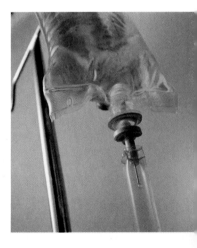

● **Figure 10.7**
**Tubing with drip chamber.**

*(Photodisc/Getty Images)*

The drip chamber (Figure 10.6) is located at the site of the entrance of the tubing into the container of intravenous solution. It allows you to count the number of drops per minute that the client is receiving (flow rate).

A roll valve clamp or clip is connected to the tubing and can be manipulated to increase or decrease the flow rate.

The size of the drop that IV tubing delivers is not standard; it depends on the way the tubing is designed. ● **Figure 10.7**. Manufacturers specify the number of drops that equal 1 mL for their particular tubing. This equivalent is called the tubing's drop factor (● **Figure 10.8** and Table 10.1). You must know the tubing's **drop factor** when calculating the flow rate of solutions in drops per minute (gtt/min) or microdrops per minute (mcgtt/min).

It is difficult to visually make an accurate count of the drops falling per minute when setting the flow rate on a gravity system infusion. In addition, the flow rate

**ALERT**

Be sure to follow the procedures for eliminating all air in the tubing.

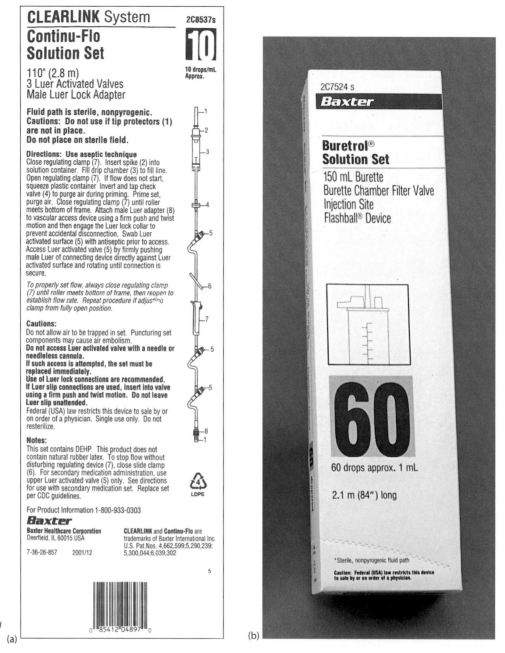

● **Figure 10.8**

**Samples of IV tubing containers with drop factors of 10 and 60.**

*(10-8a Courtesy of Baxter Healthcare Corporation. All rights reserved.    10-8b Al Dodge/Al Dodge)*

of a gravity system infusion depends on the *relative heights* of the IV bag and the infusion site; changes in the relative position of either may cause flow rate changes. For these two reasons, the use of IV pumps is becoming more common.

---

### NOTE

60 microdrops = 1 mL is a universal equivalent for IV tubing calibrated in microdrops.

### Table 10.1 **Common Drop Factors**

| | |
|---|---|
| 10 gtt = 1mL | |
| 15 gtt = 1 mL | macrodrops |
| 20 gtt = 1 mL | |
| 60 mcgtt = 1 mL | microdrops |

# Infusion Pumps

An intravenous infusion can flow solely by the force of gravity or by an electronic infusion pump. There are many different types of electronic infusion pumps. ● **Figure 10.9**.

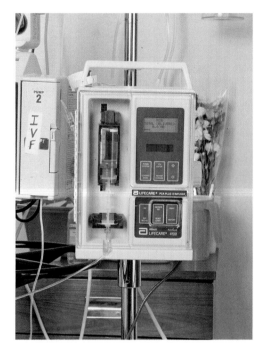

● **Figure 10.9**
**Volumetric infusion pump.**

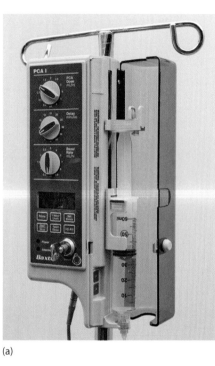

(a)

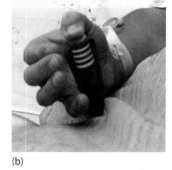

(b)

● **Figure 10.10**
**Patient-Controlled Analgesia (PCA) (a) pump (b) control button.**

These electrically operated devices allow the rate of flow (usually specified in mL/h) to be simply keyed into the device by the user. The pumps can more precisely regulate the flow rate than can the gravity systems. For example, pumps detect an interruption in the flow (constriction) and sound an alarm to alert the nursing staff and the patient, sound an alarm when the infusion finishes, indicate the volume of fluid already infused, and indicate the time remaining for the infusion to finish. "Smart" pumps may contain libraries of safe dosage ranges that will help prevent the user from keying in an unsafe dosage.

A *Patient Controlled Analgesia (PCA) pump* (see ● **Figure 10.10**) allows a patient to self-administer pain-relieving drugs. The dose is predetermined by the physician, and the pump is programmed accordingly. To receive the drug when pain relief is needed, the patient presses the button on the handset, which is connected to the PCA pump. A lockout device in the pump prevents patient overdose.

**ALERT**

A facility might use many different types of infusion pumps. The healthcare provider must learn how to program all of them. Be sure to use the specific tubing supplied by the manufacturer for each pump.

# Calculating the Flow Rate of Infusions

The next three examples will employ techniques that were presented in Chapter 3 for the conversion of flow rates.

### EXAMPLE 10.1

Set the pump in mL/h if the infusion contains 400 mL to be infused in 8 hours.

The flow rate as a fraction is

$$\frac{400 \; mL}{8 \; h}$$

The units of the fraction are already in mL/h, therefore, you need only work with the numbers. Break up the fraction as follows:

$$\frac{400 \; mL}{8 \; h} = \frac{400}{8} \; \frac{mL}{h}$$

Because

$$\frac{400}{8} = 50$$

$$\frac{400 \; mL}{8 \; h} = 50 \; \frac{mL}{h}$$

So, set the pump to 50 mL/h.

### EXAMPLE 10.2

(a)  Change 3 mL/min to an equivalent rate in mL/h.
(b)  Change 120 mL/h to an equivalent rate in mL/min.

(a)  The problem is

$$\frac{3 \; mL}{min} = \frac{? \; mL}{h}$$

The units in the denominators do not match; you must change minutes to hours. Because 60 minutes = 1 h, multiply the given rate by $\frac{60}{60}$ as follows:

$$\frac{3 \; mL}{1 \; min} = \frac{3 \; mL}{1 \; min} \times \frac{60}{60} = \frac{180 \; mL}{60 \; min}$$

Replace 60 min with 1 h.

$$\frac{180 \; mL}{60 \; min} = \frac{180 \; mL}{1 \; h}$$

Therefore, 3 mL/min is equivalent to the rate of 180 mL/h.

(b) The problem is

$$\frac{120\ mL}{1\ h} = \frac{?\ mL}{min}$$

The units in the denominators do not match; you must change h to min. Because 1 h = 60 minutes, *replace 1 h by 60 minutes* in the given rate as follows:

$$\frac{120\ mL}{1\ h} = \frac{120\ mL}{60\ min} = \frac{120}{60}\ \frac{mL}{min}$$

Because

$$\frac{120}{60} = 2$$

$$\frac{120}{60}\ \frac{mL}{min} = 2\ \frac{mL}{min}$$

Therefore, 120 mL/h is equivalent to the rate of 2 mL/min.

## EXAMPLE 10.3

A patient must receive a tube feeding of *Ensure 240 mL in 90 minutes*. The calibration of the tubing is 20 drops per milliliter. Because enteral feedings are generally placed on an infusion pump and are measured in mL/h, calculate the flow rate in milliliters per hour.

The problem is

$$\frac{240\ mL}{90\ min} = ?\ \frac{mL}{h}$$

The units in the denominators do not match; you must change 90 minutes to hours.

Use the proportion

$$\frac{x\ h}{90\ min} = \frac{1\ h}{60\ min}$$

$$90 = 60x$$

$$1.5 = x$$

The problem becomes

$$\frac{240\ mL}{1.5\ h} = ?\ \frac{mL}{h}$$

Because

$$\frac{240}{1.5} = 160$$

$$\frac{240\ mL}{1.5\ h} = 160\ \frac{mL}{h}$$

Therefore, the flow rate is 160 mL/h.

# Changing between Milliliters per Hour and Drops per Minute

The next example illustrates how the ratio and proportion method can be used to perform a flow rate conversion from mL/h to gtt/min.

### EXAMPLE 10.4

**Change 150 mL/h to an equivalent rate in gtt/min if the drop factor is 10 gtt/mL.**

The problem is

$$\frac{150 \; mL}{h} = \frac{? \; gtt}{min}$$

To make the units in the denominators match, substitute 60 minutes for 1 hour in the given rate

$$\frac{150 \; mL}{1 \; h} = \frac{150 \; mL}{60 \; min} = \frac{150}{60} \; \frac{mL}{min}$$

because

$$\frac{150}{60} = 2.5$$

$$\frac{150}{60} \; \frac{mL}{min} = 2.5 \; \frac{mL}{min}$$

Now, the units in the denominator match, and the problem becomes

$$\frac{2.5 \; mL}{min} = \frac{x \; gtt}{min}$$

The units in the numerators do not match. To change the numerator from 2.5 mL to $x$ gtt, use the fact that the number of milliliters and the number of drops are proportional.

Think:

$$2.5 \; mL = x \; gtt$$

$$1 \; mL = 10 \; gtt \; (\text{drop factor})$$

Set up a proportion and cross multiply

$$\frac{2.5 \; mL}{x \; gtt} = \frac{1 \; mL}{10 \; gtt}$$

$$x = 25$$

Therefore,

$$150 \; \frac{mL}{h} = 25 \; \frac{gtt}{min}$$

There is a much simpler way to do Example 10.4; it uses the *flow rate conversion number*.

# Flow Rate Conversion Number (FC)

The **flow rate conversion number**, abbreviated as **FC** (think: Flow Converter), is equal to the quotient of 60 and the drop factor (DF). That is,

$$FC = \frac{60}{DF}$$

For example, if the drop factor (DF) is $15$ gtt/mL, then the flow rate conversion number is obtained as follows:

$$FC = \frac{60}{15} = 4$$

Table 10.2 shows the common drop factors and their corresponding flow rate conversion numbers.

| Table 10.2 Common Drop Factors and Corresponding Flow Rate Conversion Numbers | |
| --- | --- |
| Drop Factor (DF) | Flow Rate Conversion Number (FC) |
| 10 | $\frac{60}{10} = 6$ |
| 15 | $\frac{60}{15} = 4$ |
| 20 | $\frac{60}{20} = 3$ |
| 60 | $\frac{60}{60} = 1$ |

To change flow rates between mL/h and gtt/min involves simply multiplying or dividing the given flow rate by the flow rate conversion number as follows:

*To change from mL/h to gtt/min, divide the given rate by FC.*
*To change from gtt/min to mL/h, multiply the given rate by FC.*

An easy way to remember the FC method is:

When you want <u>D</u>rops, <u>D</u>ivide.
When you want <u>M</u>illiliters, <u>M</u>ultiply.

The following example contains the same problem that was solved in Example 10.4. However, this time it is solved using the much simpler FC technique. The FC technique will be the method used throughout the book for conversions between gtt/min and mL/h.

### EXAMPLE 10.5

Change 150 mL/h to an equivalent rate in gtt/min if the drop factor is 10 gtt/mL.

The problem is

$$150 \, \frac{mL}{h} = ? \, \frac{gtt}{min}$$

**Step 1**  Because this is a conversion from mL/h to gtt/min, use the FC technique.

Use DF = 10 to calculate FC

$$FC = \frac{60}{DF}$$

$$FC = \frac{60}{10} = 6$$

**Step 2**  Because you want <u>D</u>rops per minute, <u>D</u>ivide the given flow rate by FC

$$\frac{150}{6} = 25$$

Therefore,

$$150\,\frac{mL}{h} = 25\,\frac{gtt}{min}$$

## EXAMPLE 10.6

The order is *D₅W 1,250 mL IV q12h*. The tubing is calibrated at 10 drops per milliliter. Calculate the number of drops per minute that you would administer.

The problem is

$$\frac{1,250\,mL}{12\,h} = ?\,\frac{gtt}{min}$$

Because

$$\frac{1,250}{12} \approx 104.2$$

The problem becomes

$$104.2\,\frac{mL}{h} = ?\,\frac{gtt}{min}$$

**Step 1**  Because this is a conversion from mL/h to gtt/min, use the FC technique.

Use DF = 10 to calculate FC

$$FC = \frac{60}{DF}$$

$$FC = \frac{60}{10} = 6$$

**Step 2**   Because you want <u>D</u>rops per minute, <u>D</u>ivide the given flow rate by FC

$$\frac{104.2}{6} \approx 17.4$$

Therefore,

$$150 \, \frac{mL}{h} \approx 17.4 \, \frac{gtt}{min}$$

But *drops are always rounded to the nearest whole drop.*

So, the flow rate is 17 gtt/min.

## EXAMPLE 10.7

**The order reads 125 mL 5%D/W IV in 1 hour. What is the flow rate in microdrops per minute?**

The problem is

$$\frac{125 \, mL}{1 \, h} = ? \, \frac{mcgtt}{min}$$

**Step 1**   Because this is a conversion from *mL/h* to *mcgtt/min*, use the FC technique.

It is standard that 60 mcgtt = 1 mL, therefore, use DF = 60 to calculate FC

$$FC = \frac{60}{DF}$$

$$FC = \frac{60}{60} = 1$$

**Step 2**   Because you want <u>D</u>rops per minute, <u>D</u>ivide the given flow rate by FC

$$\frac{125}{1} = 125$$

Therefore,

$$125 \, \frac{mL}{h} = 125 \, \frac{mcgtt}{min}$$

So, the flow rate is 125 *mcgtt/min.*

In Example 10.7, the drop factor is 60 because microdrops were used. Therefore, the Flow Rate Conversion Number (FC) is $\frac{60}{60}$, *which equals* 1. Whenever you multiply or divide a flow rate by 1, the flow rate does not change. That is why *125 mL/h = 125 mcgtt/min.* Therefore, *no calculations are necessary to change between mL/h and mcgtt/min.*

## EXAMPLE 10.8

The order reads: *IV fluids: 0.9% NaCl 250 mL in 4 hours.* How many microdrops per minute would you administer?

The problem is

$$\frac{250 \; mL}{4 \; h} = ? \; \frac{mcgtt}{min}$$

Because

$$\frac{250}{4} = 62.5$$

The problem becomes

$$62.5 \; \frac{mL}{h} = ? \; \frac{mcgtt}{min}$$

Because you are converting between mL/h and mcgtt/min, no calculations are necessary.

$$62.5 \; \frac{mL}{h} = 62.5 \; \frac{mcgtt}{min}$$

So, the flow rate is 63 *mcgtt/min.*

## EXAMPLE 10.9

The prescriber ordered $\frac{1}{4}$ NS *850 mL IV in 8 hours.* The label on the box containing the intravenous set to be used for this infusion is shown in ● Figure 10.11. Calculate the flow rate in drops per minute.

The problem is

$$\frac{850 \; mL}{8 \; h} = ? \; \frac{gtt}{min}$$

Because

$$\frac{850}{8} = 106.25$$

The problem becomes

$$106.25 \; \frac{mL}{h} = ? \; \frac{gtt}{min}$$

**Step 1**   Because this is a conversion from mL/h to gtt/min, use the FC technique.

Use DF = 10 to calculate FC

$$FC = \frac{60}{DF}$$

$$FC = \frac{60}{10} = 6$$

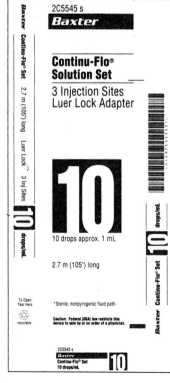

● **Figure 10.11**

**Continu-Flo Solution Set box label.**

*(Courtesy of Baxter Healthcare Corporation. All rights reserved.)*

**Step 2**   Because you want <u>D</u>rops per minute, <u>D</u>ivide the given flow rate by FC.

$$\frac{106.25}{6} \approx 17.7$$

Therefore,

$$106.25\ \frac{mL}{h} \approx 17.7\ \frac{gtt}{min}$$

But *drops are always rounded to the nearest whole drop.*

So, the flow rate is 18 gtt/min.

## EXAMPLE 10.10

(a) The order is *500 mL of 5% D/W to infuse IV in 5 hours.* Calculate the flow rate in drops per minute if the drop factor is 15 drops per milliliter.
(b) When the nurse checks the infusion 2 hours after it started, 400 mL remain to be absorbed in the remaining 3 hours. Recalculate the flow rate in drops per minute for the remaining 400 mL.

(a) The problem is

$$\frac{500\ mL}{5\ h} = ?\ \frac{gtt}{min}$$

Because

$$\frac{500}{5} = 100$$

The problem becomes

$$100\ \frac{mL}{h} = ?\ \frac{gtt}{min}$$

DF = 15, therefore

$$FC = \frac{60}{15} = 4$$

Because you want <u>D</u>rops per minute, <u>D</u>ivide the given flow rate by 4

$$\frac{100}{4} = 25$$

So, the flow rate is 25 gtt/min.

**NOTE**

Sometimes, for a variety of reasons, the infusion flow rate can change. A change may affect the prescribed duration of time in which the solution will be administered. For example, with a gravity system, raising or lowering the infusion site or moving the patient's body or bed relative to the height of the bag may change the flow rate of the IV infusion. Therefore, the flow rate must be periodically assessed, and adjustments made if necessary. Examples 10.10 and 10.11 illustrate the computations involved in this process. Be sure to check the facility policy regarding allowable flow rate adjustments.

(b) When the nurse checks the infusion, 400 mL need to be infused in 3 hours. So the problem is

$$\frac{400 \; mL}{3 \; h} = ? \; \frac{gtt}{min}$$

Because

$$\frac{400}{3} \approx 133.3$$

The problem becomes

$$133.3 \; \frac{mL}{h} = ? \; \frac{gtt}{min}$$

Because you want <u>D</u>rops per minute, <u>D</u>ivide the given flow rate by FC, which is 4.

$$\frac{133.3}{4} = 33.3$$

So, in order for the infusion to be completed within the 5-hour time period as ordered, the flow rate must be increased to 33 gtt/min.

## EXAMPLE 10.11

The order is *D5W 900 mL IV in 6 hours*. The drop factor is 10 gtt/mL. You would expect that after 3 hours, about 450 mL (half the total infusion of 900 mL) would be left in the bag. However, only 240 mL remain. Recalculate the flow rate in gtt/min so that the infusion will finish on time.

The remainder of the bag (240 mL) must infuse in the remaining time (3 hours).

The problem is

$$\frac{240 \; mL}{3 \; h} = ? \; \frac{gtt}{min}$$

Because

$$\frac{240}{3} = 80$$

The problem becomes

$$80 \; \frac{mL}{h} = ? \; \frac{gtt}{min}$$

DF = 10, therefore

$$FC = \frac{60}{10} = 6$$

Because you want <u>D</u>rops per minute, <u>D</u>ivide the given flow rate by 6

$$\frac{80}{6} = 13.3$$

So, the new flow rate is 13 *gtt/min*.

## EXAMPLE 10.12

A patient has an order for *Sustacal 240 mL in 2 hours via a feeding tube.*

Calculate the rate of flow in

(a) milliliters per hour
(b) milliliters per minute.

(a) The flow rate is 240 mL in 2 hours. No conversion of units of measurement is necessary.

$$\frac{240 \text{ mL}}{2 \text{ h}} \text{ can be simplified as follows:}$$

$$\frac{\overset{120}{\cancel{240}} \text{ mL}}{\underset{1}{\cancel{2}} \text{ h}} = \frac{120 \text{ mL}}{\text{h}}$$

So, the flow rate is 120 mL per hour.

(b) Now, change

$$\frac{120 \; mL}{1 \; h} \text{ to } ? \; \frac{mL}{min}$$

Replace 1 h by 60 min

$$\frac{120 \; mL}{1 \; h} = \frac{120 \; mL}{60 \; min}$$

$$\frac{\overset{2}{\cancel{120}} \; mL}{\underset{1}{\cancel{60}} \; min} = \frac{2 \; mL}{min}$$

So, the flow rate is 2 *mL/min*.

## EXAMPLE 10.13

An IV flow rate is 25 drops per minute. The drop factor is 10 drops per mL. What is the flow rate in milliliters per hour?

The problem is

$$25 \; \frac{gtt}{min} = ? \; \frac{mL}{h}$$

DF = 10, therefore

$$FC = \frac{60}{10} = 6$$

Because you want <u>M</u>illiliters per hour, <u>M</u>ultiply the given flow rate by 6

$$25 \times 6 = 150$$

So, the flow rate is 150 mL/h.

**EXAMPLE 10.14**

The prescriber orders *D5/0.45% NaCl IV to infuse at 21 drops per minute*. If the drop factor is 20 drops per milliliter, how many milliliters per hour will the patient receive?

The problem is

$$21 \frac{gtt}{min} = ? \frac{mL}{h}$$

DF = 20, therefore

$$FC = \frac{60}{20} = 3$$

Because you want <u>Milliliters</u> per hour, <u>Multiply</u> the given flow rate by 6

$$21 \times 3 = 63$$

So, the flow rate is 63 mL/h.

# Calculating the Duration of Flow for IV and Enteral Solutions

In the following three examples, you must determine the length of time it will take to complete an infusion.

**EXAMPLE 10.15**

The order is *NS 1,000 mL IV infuse at 125 mL/h*. How many hours will it take for this infusion to complete?

This problem involves milliliters and hours. If you double the hours (time), you double the milliliters (volume) infused. Milliliters and hours in this problem are in proportion.

Think of the problem as:

$$125 \text{ mL} = 1 \text{ h}$$
$$1,000 \text{ mL} = x \text{ h}$$

The proportion could be set up as

$$\frac{125 \text{ mL}}{1 \text{ h}} = \frac{1,000 \text{ mL}}{x \text{ h}}$$

$$1,000 = 125 x$$
$$8 = x$$

So, it will take 8 hours for this infusion to complete.

## EXAMPLE 10.16

An infusion of 5% D/W is infusing at a rate of 20 drops per minute. If the drop factor is 12 drops per milliliter, how many hours will it take for the remaining solution in the bag (● Figure 10.12) to infuse?

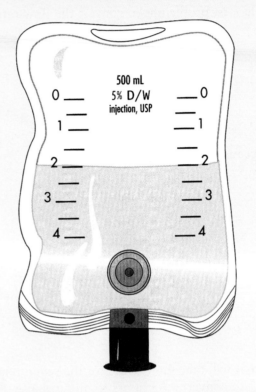

● **Figure 10.12**
**5% D/W intravenous solution.**

In Figure 10.12, you can see that 500 mL of solution were originally in the bag, and that the patient has received 200 mL. Therefore, 300 mL remain to be infused.

The first problem is to convert the flow rate to mL/h.

$$20 \, \frac{gtt}{min} = ? \, \frac{mL}{h}$$

DF = 12, therefore

$$FC = \frac{60}{12} = 5$$

Because you want <u>M</u>illiliters per hour, <u>M</u>ultiply the given flow rate by 5

$$20 \times 5 = 100$$

So, the flow rate is 100 mL/h.

Now use the proportion

$$\frac{100 \, mL}{1 \, h} = \frac{300 \, mL}{x \, h}$$

$$300 = 100 \, x$$
$$3 = x$$

So, it will take 3 hours for the remaining solution to infuse.

## EXAMPLE 10.17

A patient is to receive an IV infusion of 500 mL of 5% D/W. The flow rate is 27 drops per minute. If the drop factor is 15 drops per milliliter, how many hours will it take for this infusion to finish?

The first problem is to convert the flow rate to mL/h.

$$27 \frac{gtt}{min} = ? \frac{mL}{h}$$

DF = 15, therefore

$$FC = \frac{60}{15} = 4$$

Because you want <u>M</u>illiliters per hour, <u>M</u>ultiply the given flow rate by 5

$$27 \times 4 = 108$$

So, the flow rate is 108 mL/h.
   Now use the proportion

$$\frac{108 \ mL}{1 \ h} = \frac{500 \ mL}{x \ h}$$

$$500 = 108 \ x$$
$$4.63 \approx x$$

So, it will take 4.63 hours for the remaining solution to infuse.
   To convert 0.63 hours to minutes, use the proportion

$$\frac{1 \ h}{60 \ min} = \frac{0.63 \ h}{x \ min}$$

$$37.8 = x$$

Therefore, *0.63 hours equals about 38 minutes.*
*So, the infusion will take about 4 hours and 38 minutes.*

## EXAMPLE 10.18

An IV of 1,000 mL of 5% D/0.9% NaCl is started at 8 P.M. The flow rate is 38 drops per minute, and the drop factor is 10 drops per milliliter. At what time will this infusion finish?

For duration problems, first convert the flow rate to mL/h.

$$38 \frac{gtt}{min} = ? \frac{mL}{h}$$

DF = 10, therefore

$$FC = \frac{60}{10} = 6$$

Because you want <u>Milliliters</u> per hour, <u>Multiply</u> the given flow rate by 6

$$38 \times 6 = 228$$

So, the flow rate is 228 mL/h.

Now use the proportion

$$\frac{228 \ mL}{1 \ h} = \frac{1{,}000 \ mL}{x \ h}$$

$$1{,}000 = 228 \ x$$

$$4.39 \approx x$$

So, it will take 4.39 hours for the remaining solution to infuse.

To convert 0.39 hours to minutes, use the proportion

$$\frac{1 \ h}{60 \ min} = \frac{0.39 \ h}{x \ min}$$

$$23.4 = x$$

Therefore, 0.39 hours equals about 23 minutes.

So, the infusion will take about 4 hours and 23 minutes. Because it started at 8 P.M., it will finish at 12:23 A.M. on the following day.

## EXAMPLE 10.19

The order reads: *1,000 mL D5W IV over 8 hours.* The drop factor is 10 gtt/mL.

(a) Calculate the flow rate in gtt/min for this infusion.
(b) After 5 hours 700 mL remain to be infused. How must the flow rate be adjusted so that the infusion will finish on time?
(c) If the facility has a policy that flow rate adjustments must not exceed 25% of the original rate, was the adjustment required within the guidelines?

(a) The problem is

$$\frac{1{,}000 \ mL}{8 \ h} = ? \ \frac{gtt}{min}$$

Because

$$\frac{1{,}000}{8} = 125$$

The problem becomes

$$125 \ \frac{mL}{h} = ? \ \frac{gtt}{min}$$

DF = 10, therefore

$$FC = \frac{60}{10} = 6$$

Because you want <u>D</u>rops per minute, <u>D</u>ivide the given flow rate by 6

$$\frac{125}{6} \approx 20.8$$

So, the flow rate is 21 *gtt/min.*

(b) After 5 hours, 700 mL are left to be infused in the remaining 3 hours.

The problem is

$$\frac{700 \; mL}{3 \; h} = ? \; \frac{gtt}{min}$$

Because

$$\frac{700}{3} \approx 233.3$$

The problem becomes

$$233.3 \; \frac{mL}{h} = ? \; \frac{gtt}{min}$$

As in part (a), FC = 6

Because you want <u>D</u>rops per minute, <u>D</u>ivide the given flow rate by 6

$$\frac{233.3}{6} \approx 38.9$$

So, the new flow rate is 39 *gtt/min.*

(c) Since the facility has a policy that flow rate adjustments must not exceed 25% of the original rate, you must now calculate 25% of the original rate; that is, 25% of 21 gtt/min.

25% of 21 gtt/min = (.25 × 21) gtt/min = 5.25 gtt/min

So, the flow rate may not be changed by more than about 5 gtt/min. Therefore, the original flow rate of 21 gtt/min can be changed to no less than 16 (21 minus 5) gtt/min and no more than 26 (21 plus 5) gtt/min.

Since 39 gtt/min is outside the acceptable range of roughly 16–26 gtt/min, this change is not within the guidelines, and the adjustment may not be made. You must contact the prescriber.

## Fluid Balance: Intake/Output

To work well, the various body systems need a stable environment in which their tissues and cells can function properly. For example, the body requires somewhat constant levels of temperature, salts, glucose, and in particular, adequate hydration to maintain homeostasis.

Part of hydration management involves the monitoring of a patient's fluid intake and output. This is especially important with pediatric, geriatric, and critical-care patients.

**Fluid intake** is the amount of fluid that enters the body (oral and parenteral fluids), while **fluid output** is the amount of fluid that leaves the body (urine, liquid stool, emesis, perspiration, and drainage).

Fluid replacement is sometimes necessary to avoid dehydration. If (as in Example 10.20) a physician provides an order with a specific ratio comparing the necessary replacement fluid with the patient's fluid output, and if the patient's fluid output is known, then a proportion could be used to determine the volume of replacement fluid to give the patient.

**EXAMPLE 10.20**

Order: *For every 100 mL of urine output, replace with 40 mL of water via PEG tube q4h.* **The patient's urine output is 300 mL. What is the replacement volume?**

Think of the problem as:

$$100 \text{ mL (output)} = 40 \text{ mL (input)} \quad (order)$$
$$300 \text{ mL (output)} = x \text{ mL (input)} \quad (patient)$$

The proportion could be set up as

$$\frac{Out}{In} = \frac{Out'}{In'}$$

Substituting, you get

$$\frac{100 \text{ mL}}{40 \text{ mL}} = \frac{300 \text{ mL}}{x \text{ mL}}$$

$$12{,}000 = 100x$$
$$120 = x$$

So, the replacement volume is 120 mL.

# Summary

In this chapter, the basic concepts and standard equipment used in intravenous and enteral therapy were introduced.

- Fluids can be given to a patient slowly over a period of time through a vein (*intravenous*) or through a tube inserted into the alimentary tract (*enteral*).
- Enteral and IV fluids can be administered continuously or intermittently.
- There is a wide variety of commercially prepared enteral and IV solutions.
- In IV solutions, *letters* indicate solution compounds, whereas *numbers* indicate solution concentration.
- Care must be taken to eliminate the air from, and maintain the sterility of, IV tubing.

- An intravenous infusion can flow solely by the force of gravity or by an electronic infusion pump.
- Flow rates are usually given as either mL/h or gtt/min.
- The drop factor of the IV administration set must be known in order to calculate flow rates.
- *Microdrops/minute* are equivalent to *milliliters/hour.*
- For microdrops, the drop factor is 60 microdrops per milliliter.
- For macrodrops, the usual drop factors are 10, 15, or 20 drops per milliliter.
- The *Flow Rate Conversion Number (FC)* is the quotient of 60 and the *Drop Factor (DF); that is, $FC = \frac{60}{DF}$.*

■ *Use the FC technique to convert between the flow rates:* $\frac{mL}{h}$ *and* $\frac{gtt}{min}$:

   To get **D**rops, **D**ivide by FC.
   To get **M**illilitres, **M**ultiply by FC.

■ To calculate the duration of an IV solution, first determine the flow rate in mL/h.

■ Know the policy of the facility regarding readjustment of flow rates.

## Case Study 10.1

Read the Case Study and answer the questions. The answers are found in Appendix A.

A 54-year-old female is transferred from a nursing home and admitted to the hospital with a diagnosis of right-upper-lobe pneumonia. She has a past medical history of lung cancer, hypertension, depression, and anxiety disorder. Her vital signs are as follows: B/P 150/86; P 90; R 30; T 101°F. Her orders include the following:

■ IV fluids: D5/0.45 NaCl 1,000 mL q8h

■ Zithromax (azithromycin) 500 mg IVPB daily

■ Sustacal $\frac{3}{4}$ strength 800 mL via PEG to run 0100 to 0800 daily

■ alprazolam 0.5 mg via PEG t.i.d.

■ Zoloft (sertraline) 50 mg PO at bedtime

■ Cozaar (losartan potassium) 25 mg via PEG daily

■ fluconazole 200 mg, oral suspension, via PEG stat, then 100 mg daily for 7 days

■ Colace (docusate sodium) 100 mg, oral suspension, via PEG b.i.d.

■ furosemide 40 mg, oral suspension via PEG b.i.d.

■ Tylenol (acetaminophen) 600 mg, oral suspension, via PEG q4h prn temperature above 101.8 °F

   Read the labels in ● **Figure 10.13**, when necessary, to answer the following questions.

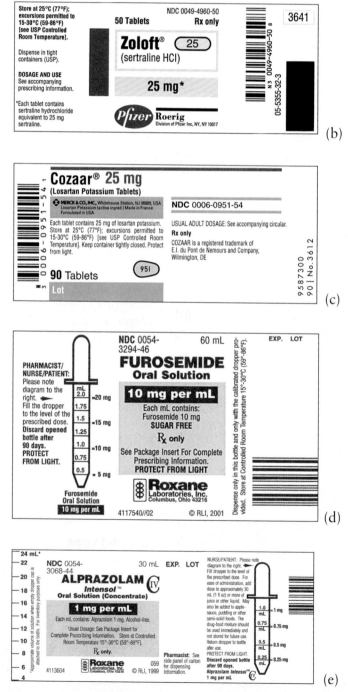

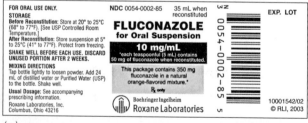

● **Figure 10.13**
**Drug labels for Case Study 10.1.** *(10-13a Courtesy of Roxane Laboratories Inc. 10-13b Reg. Trademark of Pfizer Inc. Reproduced with permission. 10-13c The labels for the products Cozaar 25 mg are reproduced with permission of Merck & Co., Inc., copyright owner. 10-13d Courtesy of Roxane Laboratories Inc. 10-13e Courtesy of Roxane Laboratories Inc.)*

1. What is the rate of flow for the IV solution in mL per hour?

2. What is the rate of flow for the IV in drops/min? Drop factor is 15 gtt/mL.

3. The IV infusion was started at 1900h. When will it be completed?

4. What is the amount of dextrose and sodium chloride in the IV solution?

5. The directions printed on the azithromycin IV bag label read "500 mg in D5W 100 mL, infuse via pump over 60 minutes." What is the pump setting in mL/h?

6. Sustacal is available in 10-ounce cans.
   (a) How many cans will you need to prepare the strength ordered?
   (b) Calculate the rate of flow in mL/h.

7. How many milliliters of alprazolam will you administer?

8. How many milliliters of fluconazole will you prepare for the stat dose?

9. The label on the docusate sodium reads 60 mg/15 mL. How many milliliters contain the prescribed dose?

## Practice Sets

The answers to *Try These for Practice, Exercises,* and *Cumulative Review Exercises* are found in Appendix A. Ask your instructor for the answers to the *Additional Exercises.*

### Try These for Practice

Test your comprehension after reading the chapter.

1. The prescriber ordered:

   *500 mL 5% D/W IV for 8h*

   Calculate the flow rate in gtt/min when the drop factor is 10 drops per milliliter.

   _____

2. The prescriber ordered:

   *1,000 mL 0.9% NaCl IV in 8h*

   The flow rate is 31 drops per minute. When the nurse assessed the infusion, 425 mL had infused in 4 hours. Calculate the new flow rate in gtt/min if the drop factor is 15 drops per milliliter. _____

3. Order: *For every 200 mL of urine output, replace with 75 mL of water via PEG tube q6h.* If the patient's urine output for the last six hours is 1 L, what is the replacement volume of water needed?

   _____

4. An IV of D/5/0.45% NaCl is infusing at a rate of 27 drops per minute. The drop factor is 15 gtt/mL. How many milliliters per hour is the patient receiving? _____

5. Order: *Pulmocare 400 mL over 6 hours via PEG.* Determine the pump setting in mL/h. _____

Workspace

**Workspace**

## Exercises

Reinforce your understanding in class or at home.

1. The physician ordered *750 mL of NS IV for 8 hours*. Calculate the flow rate in drops per minute. The drop factor is 10 gtt = 1 mL.

   _____

2. The patient is to receive *375 mL of RL over 3 hours*. Set the rate on the infusion pump in milliliters per hour.

   _____

3. Order: *For every 100 mL of urine output, replace with 30 mL of water via nasogastric tube q4h*. If the patient's urine output for the last four hours is 550 mL, what is the replacement volume of water needed?

   _____

4. Order: *1,000 mL $D_5W$ to infuse at 125 mL/h*. The tubing is calibrated at 15 gtt/mL. How long will this infusion take to finish?

   _____

5. A patient is to receive 500 mL 5%D/0.45%NaCl IV in 3 hours. Calculate the flow rate in microdrops per minute.

   _____

6. The order reads *1,500 mL $D_5W$ IV over 12 hours*. The drop factor is 20 gtt/mL.
   (a) Find the flow rate in gtt/min for this infusion.
   (b) If after 3 hours 1,200 mL remain to be infused, how must the flow rate be adjusted so that the infusion will finish on time?
   (c) If the facility has a policy that flow rate adjustments must not exceed 25% of the original rate, is the adjustment required in part (b) within the guidelines?

   _____

7. Order: *750 mL Ringer's Lactate IV in 8 hours*. Calculate the flow rate in drops per minute if the drop factor is 15 gtt/mL.

   _____

8. An IV infusion of 750 mL Ringer's Lactate began at noon. It has been infusing at the rate of 125 mL/h. At what time is it scheduled to finish?

   _____

9. A patient has an order for a total parenteral nutrition (TPN) solution 1,000 mL in 24 hours. At what rate in mL/h should the pump be set?

   _____

10. An IV is infusing at 90 mL/h. The IV tubing has a drop factor of 20 gtt/mL. Calculate the flow rate in gtt/min.

   _____

11. Order: *1,000 mL NS IV over 6 hours*. Calculate and set the flow rate in mL/h for the electronic controller.

   _____

Workspace

12. Calculate the infusion time for an IV of 500 mL that is ordered to run at 40 mL/h.

_____

13. The order reads *750 mL of NS IV. Infuse over a 24 h period.* Set the flow rate on the infusion pump in milliliters per hour.

_____

14. An IV of 800 mL is to infuse over 8 hours at the rate of 20 gtt/min. After 4 hours and 45 minutes, only 300 mL had infused. Recalculate the flow rate in gtt/min. The set calibration is 15 gtt/mL.

_____

15. The order reads *10 AM: 1,000 mL D₅W IV in 8 hours.* The IV was stopped at 4:30 P.M. for 45 minutes with 90 mL of fluid remaining. Determine the new flow rate setting for the infusion pump in mL/h so that the infusion finishes on time.

_____

16. An IV bag has 350 mL remaining. It is infusing at 35 gtt/min, and a 15 gtt/mL set is being used. How long will it take to finish?

_____

17. An IV solution is infusing at 32 microdrops per minute. How many milliliters of this solution will the patient receive in 6 hours?

_____

18. A patient must have a tube feeding of 1,000 mL Ensure for 10 hours. The drop factor is 15 gtt/mL. After 5 hours, a total of 650 mL has infused. Recalculate the new gtt/min flow rate to complete the infusion on schedule.

_____

19. An IV is infusing at a rate of 30 drops per minute. The drop factor is 15 gtt/mL. Calculate the flow rate in milliliters per hour.

_____

20. A patient is to receive 1 unit (500 mL) of packed red blood cells over 4 hours. For the first 15 minutes, infuse at 50 mL/h. At what rate would you set the pump to complete the infusion?

_____

# Additional Exercises

Now, test yourself!

1. The physician ordered *3,000 mL of 5% Dextrose and Lactated Ringer's solution IV q24h.* Calculate the flow rate in drops per minute. The drop factor is 10 gtt = 1 mL.

_____

2. The order reads: *D5W 250 mL per 8 hours IV.* Calculate the flow rate in microdrops per minute.

_____

3. The patient is to receive *1,000 mL of 0.9% NaCl IV.* The infusion begins at 0600h. It is infusing at 45 gtt/min, and the drop factor is 10 gtt/mL. At what time will the infusion finish?

_____

4. The physician ordered the enteral solution *Sustacal via feeding tube 75 milliliters per hour.* The drop factor is 18 drops per milliliter. Calculate the flow rate in drops per minute.

_____

5. A patient is to receive *100 mL D5/0.45% NaCl IV in 60 minutes.* Calculate the flow rate in microdrops per minute.

_____

6. The order reads *650 mL D5W q8h IV.* Set the flow rate on the infusion pump in milliliters per hour.

_____

7. The medication order is *300 mL D5W IV in 3 hours.* Calculate the flow rate in drops per minute. The drop factor is 12 gtt/mL.

_____

8. A patient is to receive *500 mL of D10W over 5 hours.* After 2 hours there is 200 mL remaining in the bag. Recalculate the flow rate in microdrops per minute so that the infusion finishes on time.

_____

9. A patient has an order for a solution of *2,500 mL of 5% D/W in 24 hours.* Set the rate on the infusion pump in milliliters per hour.

_____

10. The order reads *850 mL D5/0.45% NaCl q6h IV.* The drop factor is 15 gtt/mL. Calculate the flow rate in drops per minute.

_____

11. There is 550 mL of normal saline in an IV bag. It is 0800h. If the flow rate is 53 drops per minute, and the drop factor is 30 gtt/mL, at what time should this IV finish?

_____

12. An intravenous solution is infusing at a rate of 17 drops per minute. The drop factor is 10 drops per milliliter. How many milliliters per hour is the patient receiving?

_____

13. The order reads *250 mL of 2½% D/W IV. Infuse over a 24 h period.* After 12 hours, there is 150 mL left in the bag. Reset the flow rate on the infusion pump in milliliters per hour.

_____

14. An IV solution is infusing at a rate of 50 microdrops per minute.
    (a) How many milliliters per hour is the patient receiving? _____
    (b) How many milliliters will the patient receive in 24 hours? _____

15. The order reads *1,000 mL D5/W IV in 8 h*. The infusion pump is set at 125 mL/h. The IV was stopped for 1 h with 625 mL remaining. Calculate the new flow rate.

16. The flow rate for an intravenous solution of 750 mL is 150 microdrops per minute. How long will this infusion take to finish?

17. The patient has an order for *1,250 mL D5/0.45% NaCl in 15 hours IV*. The drop factor is 10 gtt/mL, and the flow rate is 14 drops per minute. Seven hours later, 500 mL remained in the IV bag. If it is necessary to recalculate the flow rate, what will the new flow rate be in milliliters per hour?

18. A patient must have a tube feeding of 1,000 mL Ensure for 10 hours. The drop factor is 20 gtt/mL.
    (a) Calculate the setting for the pump in milliliters per hour.

    (b) If each can of Ensure contains 200 mL, how many cans of Ensure will you need?

19. Order: *For every 200 mL of urine output, replace with 50 mL of water via nasogastric tube q4h*. If the patient's urine output for the last four hours is 1,000 mL, what is the replacement volume of water needed?

20. An IV solution is infusing at 40 microdrops per minute. How many milliliters of this solution will the patient receive in 18 hours?

## Cumulative Review Exercises

Review your mastery of previous chapters.

1. You have a sodium chloride solution with a concentration of 0.45%. How many milligrams of sodium chloride are in 1 mL?

2. The order reads *Compleat-B 480 mL via PEG q12h*. At how many mL/h will you set the pump?

3. The prescriber orders *2,500 mL of 20% D/W to infuse in 16 hours*. Set the rate on the infusion pump at milliliters per hour.

4. An IV of 1,000 mL of 5% D/W is to infuse at a rate of 30 drops per minute for 10 hours. After 4 hours, the patient had received 600 mL. The drop factor is 15 drops per milliliter. Recalculate the flow rate in gtt/min.

   _____

5. Use the nomogram to calculate the BSA of a patient who is 5 feet 10 inches and weighs 200 pounds.

   _____

6. The patient has a BSA of 1.6 m$^2$. The medication order is 0.8 mg/m$^2$. The drug is supplied in 1.2 mg capsules. How many capsules will you prepare?

   _____

7. An intravenous solution is infusing at 80 microdrops per minute. How many milliliters per hour is the patient receiving? _____

8. You are to prepare 0.75 g of cefuroxime IM stat for your patient. The label reads 250 mg/mL. How many milliliters will you prepare for your patient?

   _____

9. Your patient weighs 101 pounds. The prescriber has ordered 6.6 mg per kilogram of a drug PO t.i.d. The label reads 300 mg per capsule. How many capsules will you prepare?

   _____

10. The order reads *1,500 mL lactated Ringer's solution IV for 24h.* How many milliliters per hour will the patient receive?

   _____

11. The order is *cefotaxime sodium 500 mg IM q6h.* The directions on the package insert for the 1 g vial state that 3 mL of diluent be added to the vial to get a concentration of 300 mg/mL. How many milliliters would you administer? _____

12. Using the formula, find the BSA of a patient who is 5 feet 10 inches tall and weighs 200 pounds. _____

13. 10 mL = _____ mcgtt

14. $\frac{1}{2}$ lb = _____ oz

15. 1 oz = _____ mL

**MediaLink**

www.prenhall.com/giangrasso

Animated examples, interactive practice questions with animated solutions, and challenge tests for this chapter can be found on the Pearson Dosage Calculation Tutor that accompanies this text. Additional, unique, interactive resources and activities can be found on the Companion Web site.

# Calculating Flow Rates for Intravenous Medications

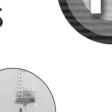

## Learning Outcomes

After completing this chapter, you will be able to

1. Describe intravenous medication administration.
2. Convert from dosage rates (drug/time) to IV rates (volume/time).
3. Convert from IV rates (volume/time) to dosage rates (drug/time).
4. Calculate infusion rates when medication must be added to the IVPB bag.
5. Calculate infusion rates based on the size (weight or BSA) of the patient.
6. Calculate flow rates for IV push medications.
7. Calculate the duration of an IVPB infusion.
8. Calculate flow rates for medication requiring titration.

T his chapter extends the discussion of intravenous infusions to include administration of intravenous medications.

# Intravenous Administration of Medications

Intravenous administration of medications provides rapid access to a patient's circulatory system, thereby presenting potential hazards. Errors in medications, dose, or dosage strength can prove fatal. Therefore, *caution must be taken in the calculation, preparation, and administration of IV medications.*

Typically, a **primary** IV line provides continuous fluid to the patient. **Secondary** lines can be attached to the primary line at injection ports, and these lines are often used to deliver *continuous or intermittent* medication intravenously. A secondary line is referred to as a **piggyback** or **intravenous piggyback (IVPB)**. With intermittent IVPB infusions, the bags hold generally 50–250 mL of fluid containing dissolved medication and usually require 20–60 minutes to infuse. Like a primary line, an IVPB infusion may use a manually controlled gravity system or an electronic pump.

A **heplock**, or **saline lock**, is an infusion port attached to an indwelling needle or cannula in a peripheral vein. Intermittent IV infusions can be administered through these ports via IV lines connected to these ports. An **IV push,** or **bolus (IVP)**, is a direct injection of medication either into the heplock/saline lock or directly into the vein.

*Syringe pumps* can also be used for intermittent infusions. A syringe with the medication is inserted into the pump. The medication is delivered at a set rate over a short period of time.

A *volume-control* set is a small container, called a burette, that is connected to the IV line. Burettes are often used in pediatric or geriatric care, where accurate volume control is critical. The danger of overdose is limited because of the small volume of solution in the burette. Burettes will be discussed in Chapter 12.

> **ALERT**
>
> Whenever two different medications are infused via the same IV line, consult the proper resource to be sure that the drugs are compatible.

# Intravenous Piggyback Infusions

Patients can receive a medication through a port in an existing IV line. This is called *intravenous piggyback (IVPB)*; ● **Figure 11.1**. The medication is in a secondary bag. Notice in Figure 11.1 that the secondary bag is higher than the primary bag so that the pressure in the secondary line will be greater than the pressure in the primary line. Therefore, the secondary medication infuses first. Once the secondary infusion is completed, the primary line begins to flow. Be sure to keep both lines open. If you close the primary line, when the secondary IVPB is completed the primary line will not flow into the vein.

A typical IVPB order might read: *cimetidine 300 mg IVPB q6h in 50 mL NS infuse over 20 min.* This is an order for an IV piggyback infusion in which 300 mg of the drug cimetidine diluted in 50 mL of a normal saline solution must infuse in 20 minutes. So, the patient receives 300 mg of cimetidine in 20 minutes via a secondary line, and this dose is repeated every 6 hours.

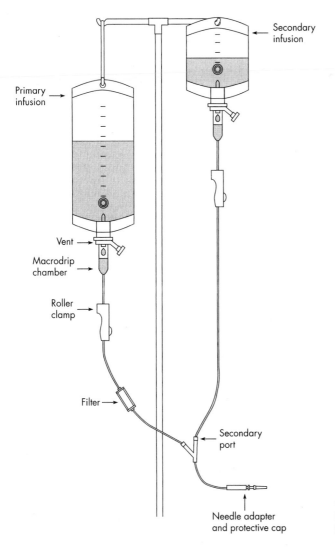

Primary infusion

Secondary infusion

Vent

Macrodrip chamber

Roller clamp

Filter

Secondary port

Needle adapter and protective cap

● **Figure 11.1**
**Primary and secondary (IVPB) infusion setup.**

## EXAMPLE 11.1

Order: *cimetidine 300 mg IVPB q6h in 50 mL NS infuse in 20 min.* Find the

(a) **IV flow rate measured in milliliters/min.**

(b) **Dosage rate measured in milligrams/min.**

(a) Because 50 mL of solution must infuse in 20 minutes, the IV flow rate is

$$\frac{50\ mL}{20\ min}$$

Because $\frac{50}{20} = 2.5$

$$\frac{50\ mL}{20\ min} = 2.5\frac{mL}{min}$$

So, the IV flow rate is 2.5 mL/min, which means that the patient receives a volume of 2.5 mL of solution every minute.

(b) Because 300 mg of cimetidine must infuse in 20 minutes, the dosage rate is

$$\frac{300 \; mg}{20 \; min}$$

Because $\frac{300}{20} = 15$

$$\frac{300 \; mg}{20 \; min} = 15 \frac{mg}{min}$$

So, the dosage rate is 15 mg/min, which means that the patient receives 15 mg of cimetidine every minute.

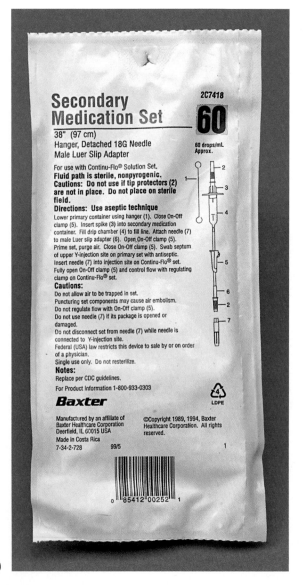

(a)                                                                     (b)

● **Figure 11.2**

**Packages of secondary IV tubing: (a) 60 drops per mL, (b) 10 drops per mL.**

*(Courtesy of Baxter Healthcare Corporation. All rights reserved. Photos by Al Dodge.)*

# Converting Dosage Rates to IV Flow Rates

Each of the next four examples (11.2 through 11.5) converts rates from dosage rates (*amount of medication per time*) to IV flow rates (*volume of solution per time*).

## EXAMPLE 11.2

Order: *cefoxitin 1 g IVPB q6h over 30 minutes*. Read the drug label in ● Figure 11.3 and find the IV flow rate measured in

(a)  milliliters per hour.

(b)  drops per minute, if the drop factor is 10 gtt/mL.

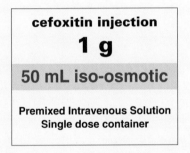

**cefoxitin injection**

**1 g**

**50 mL iso-osmotic**

**Premixed Intravenous Solution**
**Single dose container**

● **Figure 11.3**
**Drug label for cefoxitin.**

(a)  The dosage rate in the order is $\frac{1\,g}{30\,min}$, and this rate must be changed to mL/h. So the problem is

$$\frac{1\,g}{30\,min} = ?\,\frac{mL}{h}$$

The strength of the solution stated on the IV bag is *1 g = 50 mL*. Substituting 50 mL for 1 g, the problem becomes

$$\frac{50\,mL}{30\,min} = ?\,\frac{mL}{h}$$

Change $\frac{50\,mL}{30\,min}$ to $\frac{mL}{h}$ by multiplying by $\frac{2}{2}$ as follows:

$$\frac{50\,mL}{30\,min} \times \frac{2}{2} = \frac{100\,mL}{60\,min} = \frac{100\,mL}{1\,h}$$

So, the IV flow rate is 100 mL/h.

(b)  Now, change the rate 100 *mL/h* to gtt/min, using the FC technique.

DF = 10 and $FC = \frac{60}{10} = 6$. You want <u>D</u>rops per minute, so <u>D</u>ivide.

$$\frac{100}{6} \approx 16.7$$

Therefore,

$$100\frac{mL}{h} \approx 16.7\frac{gtt}{min}$$

So, the IV flow rate is 17 gtt/min.

## EXAMPLE 11.3

The medication order reads: *1,000 mL of D/5/W with 1,000 mg of a drug at 1 mg/min*. The drop factor is 15 gtt/mL. Find the IV flow rate in

(a) gtt/min.

(b) mL/h.

(a) The problem is

$$\frac{1\ mg}{min} = ?\frac{gtt}{min}$$

In this example, change 1 mg to mL and then to gtt.

Change the mg to mL by using the strength of the solution which is

$$1,000\ mg = 1,000\ mL\ \text{(strength)}$$

Dividing both sides of this equivalence yields

$$1\ mg = 1\ mL\ \text{(strength)}$$

Therefore, 1 mL may be substituted for 1 mg, and the problem becomes

$$\frac{1\ mL}{min} = ?\frac{gtt}{min}$$

The drop factor is 15 gtt = 1 mL. Therefore 15 gtt may be substituted for 1 mL and you have

$$\frac{1\ mL}{min} = \frac{15\ gtt}{min}$$

So, the IV flow rate is 15 gtt/min.

(b) Change 15 gtt/min to mL/h by using the FC technique.

DF = 15 and $FC = \frac{60}{15} = 4$. Because you want <u>M</u>illiliters per hour, <u>M</u>ultiply.

$$15\frac{gtt}{min} = (15 \times 4)\frac{mL}{H} = 60\frac{mL}{h}$$

So, the IV flow rate is 60 mL/h.

## EXAMPLE 11.4

The medication order reads: *heparin 1,250 units/hour IV*. The IV solution has 10,000 units of heparin in 1,000 mL of 5% D/W. Calculate the infusion rate in

(a)  mL/h.

(b)  gtt/min if the drop factor is 10 gtt/mL.

(a)  The problem is

$$\frac{1,250\ units}{1\ h} = \frac{?\ mL}{h}$$

In the numerator change 1,250 units to mL of solution.

Think:

$$1,250\ units = x\ mL$$
$$10,000\ units = 1,000\ mL\ \text{(strength of the solution)}$$

Use the proportion

$$\frac{1,250\ units}{x\ mL} = \frac{10,000\ units}{1,000\ mL}$$
$$10,000x = 1,250,000$$
$$x = 125$$

This means that 1,250 units are contained in 125 mL and therefore,

$$\frac{1,250\ units}{1\ h} = \frac{125\ mL}{h}$$

So, the IV flow rate is 125 mL/h.

(b)  Now, change 125 *mL/h* to gtt/min, using the FC technique.

DF $= 10$ and $FC = \frac{60}{10} = 6$. You want <u>D</u>rops per minute, so <u>D</u>ivide.

$$125\frac{mL}{h} = \frac{125}{6}\frac{gtt}{min} \approx 20.8\frac{gtt}{min}$$

So, the IV flow rate is 21 gtt/min.

**NOTE**

1 unit = 1,000 milliunits (mU)

## EXAMPLE 11.5

The prescriber writes an order for 1,000 mL of 5% D/W with 10 units of a drug. Your patient must receive 30 mU of this drug per minute. Calculate the flow rate in milliliters per hour.

The problem is

$$\frac{30\ mU}{min} = ?\frac{mL}{h}$$

In the numerator, change 30 mU to 0.03 units by moving the decimal point three places to the left. Now the problem is

$$\frac{0.03\ units}{min} = ?\frac{mL}{h}$$

Change 0.03 units of the drug to mL of solution.

Think:

$$0.03\ units = x\ mL$$
$$10\ units = 1,000\ mL \text{ (strength)}$$

Use the proportion

$$\frac{0.03\ units}{x\ mL} = \frac{10\ units}{1,000\ mL}$$
$$10\ x = 30$$
$$x = 3$$

So, 0.03 units $= 3$ mL and the problem becomes

$$\frac{3\ mL}{min} = ?\frac{mL}{h}$$

Change 3 mL/min to mL/h by multiplying by $\frac{60}{60}$

$$\frac{3\ mL}{min} \times \frac{60}{60} = \frac{180\ mL}{60\ min} = \frac{180\ mL}{1\ h}$$

So, the IV flow rate is 180 mL/h.

# Converting IV Flow Rates to Dosage Rates

Each of the next three examples (11.6 through 11.8) converts infusion rates from IV flow rates (*volume of solution per time*) to dosage rates (*amount of medication per time*).

## EXAMPLE 11.6

Calculate the number of units of Regular insulin a patient is receiving per hour if the order is *500 mL NS with 300 units of Regular insulin and it is infusing at the rate of 12.5 mL per hour via the pump.*

The problem is

$$\frac{12.5 \ mL}{h} = ? \frac{units}{h}$$

In the numerator, change 12.5 mL of solution to units of insulin.

Think:

$$12.5 \ mL = x \ units$$

$$300 \ mL = 500 \ units = \ \text{(strength of the solution)}$$

Use the proportion

$$\frac{12.5 \ mL}{x \ units} = \frac{500 \ mL}{300 \ units}$$

$$500 \ x = 3{,}750$$

$$x = 7.5$$

This means that 7.5 units of insulin are contained in 12.5 mL of the solution and therefore

$$\frac{12.5 \ mL}{h} = \frac{7.5 \ units}{h}$$

So, the patient is receiving 7.5 units/h.

## EXAMPLE 11.7

**An IV bag contains 1,000 mL of NS with 1,000 mg of a drug. It is infusing at 12 gtt/min. The drop factor is 10 gtt/mL. How many mg/min is the patient receiving.**

The problem is

$$\frac{12 \ gtt}{min} = \frac{x \ mg}{min}$$

Change 12 gtt to mL and then to mg.

In the numerator, first change 12 gtt of solution to milliliters of solution.

Think:

$$12 \ gtt = x \ mL$$

$$10 \ gtt = 1 \ mL \ \text{(drop factor)}$$

Use the proportion

$$\frac{12 \ gtt}{x \ mL} = \frac{10 \ gtt}{1 \ mL}$$

$$10 \ x = 12$$

$$x = 1.2$$

So, 12 gtt = 1.2 mL and the problem becomes

$$\frac{12 \ gtt}{min} = \frac{1.2 \ mL}{min}$$

Now change 1.2 mL of solution to mg of drug. The strength of the solution is

$$1,000 \; mL = 1,000 \; mg.$$

Divide both sides by 1,000 to obtain the equivalent strength of

$1 \; mL = 1 \; mg$ [This means mg and mL are interchangeable in this example because each 1 mL of solution in the IV bag contains 1 mg of the drug.]

Substitute 1.2 mg for 1.2 mL to obtain

$$\frac{1.2 \; mL}{min} = \frac{1.2 \; mg}{min}$$

So, the patient is receiving 1.2 milligrams of the drug per minute.

### EXAMPLE 11.8

Order: *heparin 40,000 units continuous IV in 1,000 mL of D5W infuse at 30 mL/h.* Find the dosage rate in units/day and determine if it is in the safe dose range—the normal heparinizing range is between 20,000 to 40,000 units per day.

The problem is

$$\frac{30 \; mL}{h} = ? \frac{units}{d}$$

In the numerator, change 30 mL of solution to units of heparin. A proportion may be used to do this by thinking:

$$30 \; mL = x \; units$$
$$1,000 \; mL = 40,000 \; units = \text{(strength)}$$

Use the proportion

$$\frac{30 \; mL}{x \; units} = \frac{1,000 \; mL}{40,000 \; units}$$

$$1,000x = 1,200,00$$
$$x = 1,200$$

This means that 1,200 units of heparin are contained in 30 mL of the solution and

$$\frac{30 \; mL}{h} = \frac{1,200 \; units}{h}$$

Change $1,200 \frac{units}{h}$ to $\frac{units}{day}$ by multiplying by $\frac{24}{24}$

$$\frac{1,200 \; units}{1 \; h} \times \frac{24}{24} = \frac{28,800 \; units}{24 \; h} = \frac{28,800 \; units}{1 \; day}$$

So, the dosage rate is 28,800 units/d. This rate is within the safe dosage range of 20,000–40,000 units per day.

# IV Push

To infuse a small amount of medication in a short period of time, a syringe can be inserted directly into a vein, or a saline lock or heparin lock can be attached to an IV catheter. For patients who have a primary IV line, the medication should be administered through the port closest to the patient. The medication can then be "pushed" directly into the vein. This route of medication administration is referred to as **IV Push (IVP)**. See ● **Figure 11.4.**

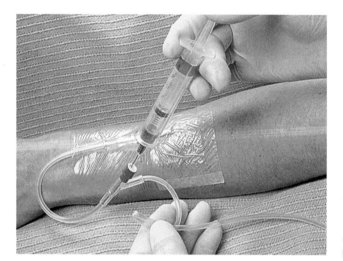

● **Figure 11.4**
**IV push administration.**

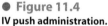

> ### ALERT
>
> An IV push generally involves medications administered over a short period of time. Be sure to verify the need for the drug, route, concentration, dose, expiration date, and clarity of the solution. It is also essential to verify the rate of injection with the package insert. Some medications (e.g., adenosine) require very rapid administration, whereas others (e.g., verapamil) are administered more slowly.

Because the IVP flow rate is determined by the speed at which the plunger of the syringe is manually pushed, it is important to control that speed. It is difficult to maintain the desired flow rate over the entire infusion. Therefore, the infusion may be mentally divided into smaller pieces in order to make the flow rate easier to control.

For example, suppose that 16 mL of solution must be infused in 2 minutes (120 seconds). Because the total infusion volume (16 mL) and duration (120 sec) are known, you may divide both of them by a convenient number and then determine the equivalent infusion rate using these smaller quantities.

- If you divide the flow rate of $\frac{16\ mL}{2\ min}$ by $\frac{8}{8}$, you obtain

$$\frac{16\ mL}{120\ sec} \div \frac{8}{8} = \frac{16 \div 8}{120 \div 8}\ \frac{mL}{sec} = \frac{2\ mL}{15\ sec}$$

And the flow rate of $\frac{16\ mL}{2\ min}$ is equivalent to $\frac{2\ mL}{15\ sec}$. So, you would push 2 mL every 15 seconds until the 16 mL of medication in the syringe are infused.

- If you divide the flow rate of $\frac{16\ mL}{2\ min}$ by $\frac{4}{4}$, you obtain

$$\frac{16\ mL}{120\ sec} \div \frac{4}{4} = \frac{16 \div 4}{120 \div 4}\ \frac{mL}{sec} = \frac{4\ mL}{30\ sec}$$

The flow rate of $\frac{16\ mL}{2\ min}$ is equivalent to $\frac{4\ mL}{30\ sec}$. So, you would push 4 mL every 30 seconds until the 16 mL of medication in the syringe are infused.

## EXAMPLE 11.9

750 mg of a drug is ordered IVP stat over 5 minutes, and the concentration of the drug is 75 mg/mL.

(a) Find the total number of milliliters you will administer.

(b) Determine the IVP flow rate if you divide the infusion into 5 equal segments.

(c) Determine the IVP flow rate if you divide the infusion into 10 equal segments.

(a) Think:

$$750 \, mg = ? \, mL \; (dose)$$

$$75 \, mg = 1 \, mL \; (strength)$$

Use the proportion

$$\frac{750 \, mg}{x \, mL} = \frac{75 \, mg}{1 \, mL}$$

$$75x = 750$$

$$x = 10$$

So, you would administer a total of 10 mL over 5 minutes.

(b) From part (a), the rate of infusion is $\frac{10 \, mL}{5 \, min}$. Because you want to cut the infusion into 5 equal segments, divide the flow rate by $\frac{5}{5}$.

$$\frac{10 \, mL}{5 \, min} \div \frac{5}{5} = \frac{2 \, mL}{1 \, min}$$

So, 2 mL will be pushed during every 1 minute interval. If a 10 mL syringe is used, each tick represents 1 mL, and the plunger will move 2 ticks each minute.

(c) In part (a) the flow rate was determined to be 10 milliliters in 5 minutes. Because you want to cut the infusion into 10 equal segments, divide the flow rate by $\frac{10}{10}$.

$$\frac{10 \, mL}{5 \, min} \div \frac{10}{10} = \frac{1 \, mL}{0.5 \, min}$$

Substitute 30 seconds for 0.5 minutes to obtain

$$\frac{1 \, mL}{0.5 \, min} = \frac{1 \, mL}{30 \, sec}$$

So, each milliliter is administered in 30 seconds. If a 10 mL syringe is used, the plunger will move one tick on the syringe every 30 seconds.

## EXAMPLE 11.10

Order: *Cefizox (ceftizoxime sodium) 1,500 mg IVP stat over 4 min.* The 2 g Cefizox vial has strength of 1 g/10 mL.

(a) Find the total number of milliliters you will administer.

(b) Determine the number of mL you will push during each 30 second interval.

(c) Determine the number of seconds needed to deliver each 1 mL of the solution.

(a) Think:

$$1,500 \ mg = ? \ mL \ (dose)$$
$$1,000 \ mg = 10 \ mL \ (strength)$$

Use the proportion

$$\frac{1500 \ mg}{x \ mL} = \frac{1,000 \ mg}{10 \ mL}$$
$$1,000x = 15,000$$
$$x = 15$$

So, you would administer a total of 15 mL of Cefizox over 4 minutes.

(b) From part (a), the rate of infusion is $\frac{15 \ mL}{4 \ min}$. Because 4 min = 240 sec, the flow rate is $\frac{15 \ mL}{240 \ sec}$. You want to divide the 240 second infusion time into 30-second segments and

$$\frac{240 \ sec}{30 \ sec} = 8$$

So, divide the flow rate by $\frac{8}{8}$

$$\frac{15 \ mL}{240 \ sec} \div \frac{8}{8} = \frac{1.875 \ mL}{30 \ sec}$$

So, 1.9 mL of Cefizox should be pushed during every 30-second interval. This amount cannot be accurately measured on a 20 mL syringe; it is only a guideline. Because each tick on a 20 mL syringe represents 1 mL, the plunger will move about 2 ticks on the syringe each 30 seconds.

(c) In part (a) the flow rate was determined to be $\frac{15 \ mL}{240 \ sec}$

You want to divide the 15 mL into 1 mL pieces and

$$\frac{15 \ mL}{1 \ mL} = 15$$

So, the IVP rate must be divided by $\frac{15}{15}$

$$\frac{15 \ mL}{240 \ sec} \div \frac{15}{15} = \frac{1 \ mL}{16 \ sec}$$

So, 1 mL is administered each 16 seconds. If a 20 mL syringe is used, the plunger will move 1 tick on the syringe every 16 seconds.

# Compound Rates

In Chapter 6, you calculated dosages based on the *size of the patient,* measured in either kilograms or meters squared. For example, if a patient weighing 100 *kg* has an order to receive a drug at the rate of *2 micrograms per kilogram (2 mcg/kg),* the dose would be obtained by multiplying the size of the patient by the rate in the order, as follows:

$$\text{Size of the patient} \times \text{Order} = \text{Dose}$$

$$100\,kg \times \frac{2\ mcg}{kg} = 200\ mcg$$

So, the dose is 200 mcg, and the single unit of measurement (*100 kg*) was converted to another single unit of measurement (200 *mcg*).

In this chapter, some IV medications are prescribed not only based on the patient's *size,* but the amount of drug the patient receives also depends on *time.* For example, an order might indicate that a drug is to be administered at the rate of *2 micrograms per kilogram per minute (2 mcg/kg/min).* This means that, *each minute,* the patient is to receive 2 mcg of the drug for every kg of body weight. Therefore, the amount of medication the patient receives depends on two things, body weight and time.

This new type of rate, called a **compound rate,** for computational purposes is written as follows:

$$\frac{2\ mcg}{kg \cdot min}$$

where the dot in the denominator stands for multiplication.

Suppose a patient weighing 100 *kg* has an order to receive a drug at the compound rate of *2 mcg/kg/min.* The dosage rate would be obtained by multiplying the size of the patient by the compound rate in the order as follows:

$$\text{Size of the patient} \times \text{Order} = \text{Dosage Rate}$$

$$100\ kg \times \frac{2\ mcg}{kg \cdot min} = \frac{200\ mcg}{min}$$

So, the dosage rate is 200 mcg/min, and the single unit of measurement (*100 kg*) was converted to a dosage rate (200 *mcg/min*).

## EXAMPLE 11.11

The prescriber ordered: *250 mL 5% D/W with 60 mg Aredia (pamidronate disodium) 0.006 mg/kg/min IVPB.* The patient weighs 75 kg. Calculate the flow rate for this antihypercalcemic drug in mL/h.

Notice that this order involves a compound rate of 0.006 mg/kg/min. Multiply the size of the patient by the order as follows:

$$75\ kg \times \frac{0.006\ mg}{kg \cdot min} = \frac{0.45\ mg}{min}$$

This dosage rate of 0.45 mg/min must be changed to mL/h.

$$\frac{0.45\ mg}{min} = \frac{?\ mL}{h}$$

In the numerator, change 0.45 mg of Aredia to mL of solution. Think:

$$0.45\ mg = x\ mL$$

$$60\ mg = 250\ mL\ \text{(strength of the solution)}$$

Use the proportion

$$\frac{0.45\ mg}{x\ mL} = \frac{60\ mg}{250\ mL}$$

$$60\ x = 112.5$$

$$x = 1.875$$

This means that 0.45 mg of Aredia are contained in 1.875 mL of the solution. The problem becomes

$$\frac{1.875\ mL}{min} = \frac{?\ mL}{h}$$

Change $\frac{1.875\ mL}{min}$ to $\frac{mL}{h}$ by multiplying by $\frac{60}{60}$

$$\frac{1.875\ mL}{min} \times \frac{60}{60} = \frac{112.5\ mL}{60\ min} = \frac{112.5\ mL}{1h}$$

So, the flow rate is 113 mL/h.

## EXAMPLE 11.12

The prescriber ordered: *Ifex (ifosfamide) 1.2 g/m²/d IVPB for 5 consecutive days, administer slowly over 30 min.* The IV solution strength is 50 mg/mL. The patient has BSA of 1.50 m². Find the flow rate in mL/h.

Notice that the order contains the compound rate of *1.2 g/m²/d*. Multiply the size of the patient by this compound rate as follows:

$$1.50\ m^2 \times \frac{50\ mg}{m^2 \cdot d} = \frac{75\ mg}{d}$$

This means that the patient should receive 75 mg of Ifex once per day. Because the drug must be administered over 30 minutes, the dose rate is $\frac{75\ mg}{30\ min}$, and it must be changed to $\frac{mL}{h}$.

$$\frac{75\ mg}{30\ min} = ?\frac{mL}{h}$$

Change $\frac{75\ mg}{30\ min}$ to $\frac{mg}{h}$ by multiplying by $\frac{2}{2}$ as follows:

$$\frac{75\ mg}{30\ min} \times \frac{2}{2} = \frac{150\ mg}{60\ min} = \frac{150\ mg}{1\ h}$$

The problem becomes

$$\frac{150\ mg}{h} = \frac{x\ mL}{h}$$

Think:

$$150\ mg = x\ mL \text{ (dose)}$$
$$50\ mg = 1\ mL \text{ (strength of the solution in the bag)}$$

Use the proportion

$$\frac{150\ mg}{x\ mL} = \frac{50\ mg}{1\ mL}$$
$$50\ x = 150$$
$$x = 3$$

Therefore,

$$\frac{150\ mg}{h} = \frac{3\ mL}{h}$$

So, the flow rate is 3 mL/h.

The next example, 11.13, shows how to determine the time it would take a patient to receive a given amount of drug when the dosage rate is known.

## EXAMPLE 11.13

**The patient weighs 80 kg and must receive a drug at the rate of 0.025 mg/kg/min.**

**(a)  How many mg/min should the patient receive?**

**(b)  How long will it take for the patient to receive 50 mg of the drug?**

(a)  Multiply the size of the patient by the order as follows:

$$80\ kg \times \frac{0.025\ mg}{kg \cdot min} = \frac{2\ mg}{min}$$

So, the patient should receive the drug at the rate of 2 mg/min.

(b)  The problem is to find the time (minutes) it will take for the patient to receive 50 mg of the drug.

Think:

$$50\ mg = x\ min$$
$$2\ mg = 1\ min \text{ (dosage rate)}$$

The proportion is

$$\frac{50\ mg}{x\ min} = \frac{2\ mg}{1\ min}$$

$$2x = 50$$

$$x = 25$$

So, it will take 25 minutes for the patient to receive 50 mg of the drug.

Although premixed IVPB bags are generally supplied, sometimes the drug must be added to the bag at the time of administration. The next three examples (11.14–11.16) illustrate this.

## EXAMPLE 11.14

A patient must receive a drug at the recommended rate of 15 mg/kg/d.

(a) If the patient weighs 100 kg, how many mg/d must the patient receive?

(b) The drug is to be administered IVPB in 200 mL D/5/W over 60 min. The vial contains 1.5 g of the drug in powdered form. This vial is used with a reconstitution device similar to that shown in ● Figure 11.5. Find the IV flow rate in mL/h.

(c) How many mg/min will the patient receive?

(a) Multiply the size of the patient by this compound rate as follows:

$$100\,kg \times \frac{15\ mg}{kg \cdot d} = \frac{1{,}500\ mg}{d}$$

This means that the patient should receive the dosage rate of 1,500 milligrams per day.

(b) Because the drug is dissolved in 200 mL and the infusion time is 60 minutes, the IV flow rate is

$$\frac{200\ mL}{60\ min}$$

Replace 60 minutes by 1 hour.

$$\frac{200\ mL}{60\ min} = \frac{200\ mL}{1\ h}$$

So, the IV flow rate is 200 mL/h.

(c) The problem is to find the dosage rate in mg/min.

Because the patient is receiving 1,500 mg in 60 min, the dosage rate is

$$\frac{1{,}500\ mg}{60\ min} = \frac{1{,}500}{60}\frac{mg}{min} = 25\frac{mg}{min}$$

So, the dosage rate is 25 mg/min.

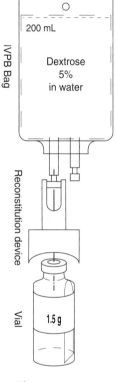

● **Figure 11.5**
**Reconstitution system.**

There are reconstitution systems that enable the healthcare provider to re-constitute a powdered drug and place it into an IVPB bag without using a syringe. One such device is shown in Figure 11.5. With this device, when the IVPB bag is squeezed, fluid is forced into the vial, dissolving the powder. The system is then placed in a vertical configuration with the vial on top and the IVPB bag on the bottom. The IVPB bag is then squeezed and released, thereby creating a negative pressure, which allows the newly reconstituted drug to flow into the IVPB bag.

Another reconstitution device is the ADD-Vantage system, which employs an IV bag containing intravenous fluid. The bag is designed with a special port, which will accept a vial of medication. When the vial is placed into this port, the contents of the vial and the fluid mix to form the desired solution. See ● Figure 11.6.

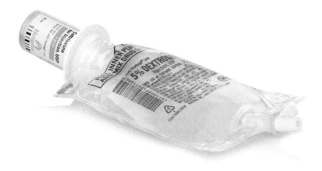

● **Figure 11.6**
**ADD-Vantage System.**

### EXAMPLE 11.15

A patient is to receive 150 mg of a drug IVPB in 200 mL NS over 1 hour. The vial of medication has strength of 75 mg/mL.

(a) How many milliliters must be withdrawn from the vial and added to the IV bag?

(b) At what rate in mL/h should the pump be set?

(a) Think:

$$150 \ mg = ? \ mL \ (dose)$$

$$75 \ mg = 1 \ mL \ (strength \ in \ the \ vial)$$

Use the proportion

$$\frac{150 \ mg}{x \ mL} = \frac{75 \ mg}{1 \ mL}$$

$$75x = 150$$

$$x = 2$$

So, 2 mL of the drug must be withdrawn from the vial and added to the IVPB bag.

(b) *Method 1: Include the volume of drug added to the IV bag.*

After 2 mL of drug are withdrawn from the vial and added to the 200 mL of NS, the IVPB bag will then contain (200 + 2) 202 mL of solution. Because the infusion will last 1 hour, the pump rate would be set at 202 *mL/h.*

*Method 2: Do not include the volume of drug added to the IV bag.*

When the 2 mL of drug from the vial are added to the 200 mL of NS, the volume of the bag increases by $\left(\frac{Change}{Old} = \frac{2}{200}\right)$ 1%. Because this increase in volume is relatively small, some institutional guidelines permit it to be excluded in IV flow rate calculation. If the increase in volume is excluded, the pump rate would be set at 200 *mL/h.*

Consult facility protocols to determine which calculation method to use.

## EXAMPLE 11.16

The order is: *Taxol (paclitaxel) 100 mg/m² IVPB in 250 mL NS infuse over 3 h q2wk.* The patient's BSA is 1.65 m², and the drug is available in a vial labeled 6 mg/mL.

(a) How many milligrams of Taxol must the patient receive?

(b) How many milliliters must be withdrawn from the vial and added to the IV bag?

(c) The order indicates that the Taxol should be added to 250 mL of NS. At what rate in mL/h should the pump be set?

(a) Multiply the size of the patient by the order.

$$1.65 \ m^2 \times \frac{100 \ mg}{m^2} = 165 \ mg$$

So, the patient should receive 165 mg of Taxol.

(b) Think:

$$165 \ mg = ? \ mL \ (dose)$$

$$6 \ mg = 1 \ mL \ (strength \ in \ the \ vial)$$

Use the proportion

$$\frac{165 \ mg}{x \ mL} = \frac{6 \ mg}{1 \ mL}$$

$$6 \ x = 165$$

$$x = 27.5$$

So, 27.5 mL of the drug must be withdrawn from the vial and added to the bag.

(c) If the additional volume of the Taxol is added to the volume of the IVPB bag, the bag will contain (250 + 27.5) 277.5 mL, and the pump rate would be set at $\frac{277.5\ mL}{3\ h} = 92.5\ \frac{mL}{h}$. So, the pump would be set at the rate of 93 mL/h.

   If only the volume of the IV solution (250 mL) is considered, the pump rate would be set at $\frac{250\ mL}{3\ h} \approx 83.3\ \frac{mL}{h}$. So, the pump would be set at the rate of 83 mL/h.

## EXAMPLE 11.17

**A patient who weighs 55 kg is receiving a medication at the rate of 30 mL/h. The concentration of the medication is 400 mg in 500 mL of D5W. The recommended dose range for the drug is 2–5 mcg/kg/min. Is the patient receiving a safe dose?**

First use the *minimum* recommended dose of *2 mcg/kg/h* to determine the minimum IV rate in mL/h that the patient may receive. Multiply the size of the patient by the order.

$$55\ kg \times \frac{2\ mcg}{kg \cdot min} = \frac{110\ mcg}{min}$$

Change the dosage rate of 110 *mcg/min* to an IV rate in *mL/h*.

$$\frac{110\ mcg}{1\ min} = ?\ \frac{mL}{h}$$

Multiply $\frac{110\ mcg}{1\ min}$ by $\frac{60}{60}$ to change to mcg/h as follows:

$$\frac{110\ mcg}{1\ min} \times \frac{60}{60} = \frac{6{,}600\ mcg}{60\ min} = \frac{6{,}600\ mcg}{1\ h}$$

Convert 6,600 *mcg* to 6.6 *mg* by moving the decimal point 3 places to the left, and the problem becomes:

$$\frac{6.6\ mg}{h} = ?\ \frac{mL}{h}$$

Think:

$$6.6\ mg = x\ mL$$
$$400\ mg = 500\ mL\ \text{(strength of the solution)}$$

Use the proportion

$$\frac{6.6\ mg}{x\ mL} = \frac{400\ mg}{500\ mL}$$
$$400x = 3{,}300$$
$$x = 8.25$$

So, the *minimum IV flow rate* is 8 mL/h.

   Now, use the *maximum* recommended dose of *5 mcg/kg/h* to determine the maximum IV rate in mL/h the patient should receive.

You could follow a procedure similar to what was done for the minimum, but it is easier to use a single proportion, as follows:

Think:

$$2 \text{ mcg/kg/h} \quad \text{results in} \quad 8.3 \text{ mL/h}$$

$$5 \text{ mcg/kg/h} \quad \text{results in} \quad x \text{ mL/h}$$

Use the proportion

$$\frac{2 \text{ } mcg/kg/min}{8.3 \text{ } mL/h} = \frac{5 \text{ } mcg/kg/min}{x \text{ } mL/h}$$

$$41.5 = 2x$$

$$20.75 = x$$

So, the *maximum flow rate* is 21 mL/h.

The safe dose range of 2–5 mcg/kg/min is equivalent to the flow rate range of *8–21 mL/h* for this patient. The patient is receiving an IV rate of 30 mL/h. Because 30 mL/h is larger than the maximum allowable flow rate of 21 mL/h, the patient is not receiving a safe dose. The patient is receiving an overdose. Turn off the IV and contact the prescriber.

> **ALERT**
>
> Whenever your calculations indicate that the prescribed dose is not within the safe range, you must verify the order with the prescriber.

## Titrated Medications

The process of adjusting the dosage of a medication based on patient response is called **titration**. Orders for titrated medications are often prescribed for critical-care patients. Such orders require that therapeutic effects, such as pain reduction, be monitored. The dose of the medication must be adjusted accordingly until the desired effect is achieved.

An order for a titrated medication generally includes a purpose for titrating and a maximum dose. If either the initial dose or directions for subsequent adjustments of the initial dose are not included in the order, the medication cannot be given, and you must contact the prescriber.

Dosage errors with titrated medications can quickly result in catastrophic consequences. Therefore, a thorough knowledge of the particular medication and its proper dosage adjustments is crucial. Dosage increment choices are medication-specific, and depend on many factors that go beyond the scope of this book.

Suppose an order indicates that a certain drug must be administered with an initial dosage rate of 10 mcg/min, and that the rate should be increased by 5 mcg/min every 3–5 min for chest pain until response, up to a maximum rate of 30 mcg/min. The IV bag has a strength of 50 mg/250 mL.

To administer the drug, first determine the IV rate in *mL/h* for the initial dose rate of 10 *mcg/min*.

The problem is

$$\frac{10 \text{ } mcg}{min} = ? \frac{mL}{h}$$

Change 10 mcg to 0.01 mg by moving the decimal 3 places to the left, and the problem becomes

$$\frac{0.01 \text{ } mg}{min} = ? \frac{mL}{h}$$

> **ALERT**
>
> Drugs that are titrated are administered according to protocol. Therefore, it is imperative to know the institution's protocols.

Multiplying $\frac{0.01\ mg}{min}$ by $\frac{60}{60}$ will convert the minutes to hours.

$$\frac{0.01\ mg}{min} \times \frac{60}{60} = \frac{0.6\ mg}{60\ min} = \frac{0.6\ mg}{1\ h}$$

The problem becomes

$$\frac{0.6\ mg}{h} = \frac{?\ mL}{h}$$

Now convert 0.6 mg in the numerator to mL.

Think:

$$0.6\ mg = x\ mL$$
$$50\ mg = 250\ mL \quad \text{(strength of the solution)}$$

Use the proportion

$$\frac{0.6\ mg}{x\ mL} = \frac{50\ mg}{250\ mL}$$
$$50\ x = 150$$
$$x = 3$$

So, the initial IV rate is 3 mL/h.

After the initial dose is administered, the patient is monitored. If the desired response is not achieved, the order indicates to increase the dose rate by 5 mcg/min. This requires that you find the corresponding IV rate in mL/h for the new dosage rate. This titration may also require other dosage changes. Every time the dose rate is changed, recalculation of the corresponding IV rate is necessary. Rather than performing such calculations each time a dose is modified, it is useful to compile a *titration table* that will quickly provide the IV rate for any possible drug dosage rate choice.

Construction of the titration table for each incremental dose change of 5 mcg/min, up to the maximum rate of 30 mcg/min, could be accomplished by repeating a procedure similar to that which was used to determine the initial flow rate. Instead, however, the table can be quickly compiled by first using a proportion to determine the incremental IV flow rate for a dosage rate change of 5 mcg/min.

Think:

$$10\ \frac{mcg}{min} = 3\ \frac{mL}{h} \quad \text{(\textit{initial rate})}$$

$$5\ \frac{mcg}{min} = x\ \frac{mL}{h} \quad \text{(\textit{incremental rate})}$$

The proportion is

$$\frac{10\ mcg/min}{3\ mL/h} = \frac{5\ mcg/min}{x\ mL/h}$$
$$10\ x = 15$$
$$x = 1.5$$

So, for each change of 5 mcg/min, the incremental IV flow rate is 1.5 mL/h.

Table 11.1 shows the titration table for the order. It contains the various dosage rates in mcg/min and their corresponding flow rates. As you move down the columns, the dosage rate increases in 5 mcg/min increments, while the corresponding flow rate increases in 1.5 mL/h increments.

| Table 11.1 **Titration Table** | |
| --- | --- |
| **Dosage Rate (mcg/min)** | **Flow Rate (mL/h)** |
| 10 mcg/min (initial) | 3   mL/h |
| 15 mcg/min | 4.5 mL/h |
| 20 mcg/min | 6   mL/h |
| 25 mcg/min | 7.5 mL/h |
| 30 mcg/min (maximum) | 9   mL/h |

## EXAMPLE 11.18

The order is: Pitocin (oxytocin) start at 1 mU/min IV, may increase by 1 mU/min q 15 min to a max of 20 mU/min. The IV strength is 10 mU/mL.

(a)  Calculate the initial pump setting in mL/h.

(b)  Construct a titration table for this order.

(a)  Determine the flow rate in *mL/h* for the initial dosage rate of 1 *mU/min*.

The problem is

$$\frac{1 \; mU}{min} = ? \frac{mL}{h}$$

Multiplying $\frac{1 \; mU}{min}$ by $\frac{60}{60}$ will convert the minutes to hours.

$$\frac{1 \; mU}{min} \times \frac{60}{60} = \frac{60 \; mU}{60 \; min} = \frac{60 \; mU}{1 \; h}$$

The problem becomes

$$\frac{60 \; mU}{h} = \frac{? \; mL}{h}$$

Convert 60 mU in the numerator to mL using a proportion. Think:

$$60 \; mU = x \; mL$$
$$10 \; mU = 1 \; mL \text{ (strength)}$$

The proportion is

$$\frac{60\ mU}{x\ mL} = \frac{10\ mU}{1\ mL}$$

$$10x = 60$$

$$x = 6\ mL$$

Therefore,

$$1\ \frac{mU}{min} = 6\ \frac{mL}{h}$$

and the initial flow rate is 6 mL/h.

(b) The order indicates that the dosage rate may be changed in $1\ \frac{mU}{min}$ increments. Because in part (a) it was shown that $1\ \frac{mU}{min} = 6\ \frac{mL}{h}$, the flow rate increments are also 6 mL/h.

Table 11.2 shows the entire titration table. Notice that the dose rates increase in 1 mU/min increments, while the flow rates increase in 6 mL/h increments.

| Table 11.2 **Titration Table for Example 11.18** | |
|---|---|
| **Dosage Rate (mU/min)** | **Flow Rate (mL/h)** |
| 1 mU/min (initial) | 6 mL/h |
| 2 mU/min | 12 mL/h |
| 3 mU/min | 18 mL/h |
| 4 mU/min | 24 mL/h |
| 5 mU/min | 30 mL/h |
| 6 mU/min | 36 mL/h |
| 7 mU/min | 42 mL/h |
| 8 mU/min | 48 mL/h |
| 9 mU/min | 54 mL/h |
| 10 mU/min | 60 mL/h |
| 11 mU/min | 66 mL/h |
| 12 mU/min | 72 mL/h |
| 13 mU/min | 78 mL/h |
| 14 mU/min | 84 mL/h |
| 15 mU/min | 90 mL/h |
| 16 mU/min | 96 mL/h |
| 17 mU/min | 102 mL/h |
| 18 mU/min | 108 mL/h |
| 19 mU/min | 114 mL/h |
| 20 mU/min (maximum) | 120 mL/h |

# Summary

In this chapter, the IV medication administration process was discussed. IVPB and IVP infusions were described, and orders based on body weight and body surface area were illustrated.

- A secondary line is referred to as an IV piggyback.
- IV push, or bolus, medications can be injected into a heplock/saline lock or directly into the vein.
- In a gravity system, the IV bag that is hung highest will infuse first.

- An order containing a compound rate of the form *mg/kg/min* directs that each minute, the patient must receive the stated number of milligrams of medication for each kilogram of the patient's body weight.
- For calculation purposes, write mg/kg/min as $\dfrac{mg}{kg \cdot min}$.
- When the size of the patient is multiplied by a compound rate, the dosage rate is obtained.
- When titrating medications, the dose is adjusted until the desired therapeutic effect is achieved.

## Case Study 11.1

Read the Case Study and answer the questions. The answers are found in Appendix A.

A woman is admitted to the labor room with a diagnosis of preterm labor. She states that she has not seen a physician because this is her third baby and she "knows what to do while she is pregnant." Her initial workup indicates a gestational age of 32 weeks, and she tests positive for Chlamydia and Strep-B. Her vital signs are: T 100 °F; P 98; R 18; B/P 140/88; and the fetal heart rate is 140–150. The orders include the following:

- NPO
- IV fluids: D5/RL 1,000 mL q8h
- Electronic fetal monitoring
- Vital signs q4h
- dexamethasone 6 mg IM q12h for 2 doses
- Brethine (terbutaline sulfate) 0.25 mg subcutaneous q30 minutes for 2h
- Rocephin (ceftriaxone sodium) 250 mg IM stat

- Penicillin G 5 million units IVPB stat; then 2.5 million units q4h
- Zithromax (azithromycin) 500 mg IVPB stat and daily for 2 days

1. Calculate the rate of flow for the D5/RL in mL/h.
2. The label on the dexamethasone reads 8 mg/mL. How many milliliters will you administer?
3. The label on the terbutaline reads 1 mg/mL. How many milliliters will you administer?
4. The label on the ceftriaxone states to reconstitute the 1 g vial with 2.1 mL of sterile water for injection, which results in a strength of 350 mg/mL. How many milliliters will you administer?
5. The instructions state to reconstitute the penicillin G (use the minimum amount of diluent), add to 100 mL D5W, and infuse in one hour. The drop factor is 15. What is the rate of flow of the stat dose in gtts/min? See the label in ● Figure 11.7.

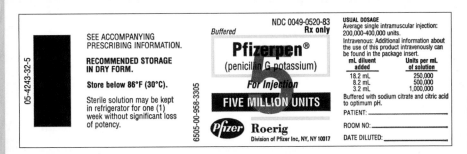

● Figure 11.7
Drug label for penicillin G.

*(Reg. Trademark of Pfizer Inc. Reproduced with permission.)*

6. The instructions for the azithromycin state to reconstitute the 500 mg vial with 4.8 mL until dissolved to yield a strength of 100 mg/mL, and add to 250 mL of D5W and administer over at least 60 minutes. What rate will you set the infusion pump if you choose to administer the medication over 90 minutes?

7. The patient continues to have uterine contractions, and a new order has been written: *magnesium sulfate 4g IV bolus over 20 minutes, then 1g/h.*

   The label on the IV bag states magnesium sulfate 40 g in 1,000 mL.
   (a) What is the rate of flow in mL/h for the bolus dose?
   (b) What is the rate of flow in mL/h for the maintenance dose?

The patient continues to have contractions and her membranes rupture. The following orders are written:
- Discontinue the magnesium sulfate.
- Pitocin (oxytocin) 10 units/1,000 mL RL, start at 0.5 mU/min increase by 1 mU/min q20 minutes.
- Stadol (butorphanol tartrate) 1 mg IVP stat.

8. What is the rate of flow in mL/h for the initial dose of Pitocin?

9. The Pitocin is infusing at 9 mL/h. How many mU/h is the patient receiving?

10. The vial of butorphanol tartrate is labeled 2 mg/mL. How many milliliters will you administer?

## Practice Sets

The answers to *Try These for Practice*, *Exercises*, and *Cumulative Review Exercises* are found in Appendix A. Ask your instructor for the answers to the *Additional Exercises.*

### Try These for Practice

Test your comprehension after reading the chapter.

1. Order: *Tagamet (cimetidine) 300 mg IVPB q6h in 50 mL NS infuse over 30 min.* The drop factor is 15 gtt/mL. Find the flow rate in gtt/min.

2. The order is for a continuous infusion of theophylline at a rate of 25 mg/h. It is diluted in 5% dextrose to produce a concentration of 500 mg per 500 mL. Determine the rate of the infusion in mL/h.

3. A 500 mL D5W solution with 2 g of Pronestyl (procainamide HCl) is infusing at 15 mL/h via a volumetric pump. How many mg/h is the patient receiving?

4. Order: *Dobutrex (dobutamine) 250 mg in 250 mL of D5W at 3.5 mcg/kg/min.* Determine the flow rate in mcgtt/min for a patient who weighs 120 pounds.

5. A patient is receiving heparin 1,200 units/hour. The directions for the infusion are, add *"25,000 units of heparin in 250 mL of solution."* Determine the flow rate in mL/h.

### Exercises

Reinforce your understanding in class or at home.

1. The patient is to receive 20 mEq of KCl (potassium chloride) in 100 mL of IV fluid at the rate of 10 mEq/h. What is the flow rate in microdrops per minute?

2. A maintenance dose of *Levophed (norepinephrine bitartrate) 2 mcg/min* IVPB has been ordered to infuse using 8 mg in 250 mL of D5W solution. What is the pump setting in mL/h?

3. The patient is receiving lidocaine at 40 mL/h. The concentration of the medication is 1 g per 500 mL of IV fluid. How many mg/min is the patient receiving?

4. Order: *dopamine 400 mg in 250 mL D5W at 3 mcg/kg/min IVPB*. Calculate the flow rate in mL/h for a patient who weighs 91 kg.

5. A drug is ordered 180 mg/m$^2$ in 500 mL NS to infuse over 90 minutes. The BSA is 1.38 m$^2$. What is the flow rate in mL/h?

6. How long will a 550 mL bag of fluid take to infuse at the rate of 25 mL/h?

7. The patient is receiving heparin at 1,000 units/hour. The IV has been prepared with 24,000 units of heparin per liter. Find the flow rate in mL/h.

8. Order: *Humulin R 50 units in 500 mL NS infuse at 1 mL/min IVPB*. How many units per hour is the patient receiving?

9. An IVPB of 50 mL is to infuse in 30 minutes. After 15 minutes, the IV bag contains 40 mL. If the drop factor is 20 gtt/mL, recalculate the flow rate in gtt/min.

10. A drug is ordered to start at a rate of 4 mcg/min IV. This rate may, depending on the patient's response, be increased by 2 mcg/min q 15 min to a max of 12 mcg/min. The IV strength is 5 mcg/mL.

    (a) Calculate the initial pump setting in mL/h.

    (b) Construct a titration table for this order.

11. Order: *digoxin 0.5 mg IVP stat over 5 min*. The digoxin vial has a concentration of 0.1 mg/mL. Find the

    (a) total number of milliliters you will administer.

    (b) number of mL you will push during each 30-second interval.

    (c) number of seconds needed to deliver each mL of the solution.

12. The patient is to receive Aldomet (methyldopa) 500 mg IVPB dissolved in 100 mL of IV fluid over 60 minutes. If the drop factor is 15 gtt/mL, determine the rate of flow in gtt/min.

13. The patient is to receive Isuprel (isoproterenol) at a rate of 4 mcg/min. The concentration of the Isuprel is 2 mg per 500 mL of IV fluid. Find the pump setting in mL/h.

14. The patient is receiving aminophylline at the rate of 20 mL/h. The concentration of the medication is 500 mg/1,000 mL of IV fluid. How many mg/h is the patient receiving?

15. Nipride 3 mcg/kg/min has been ordered for a patient who weighs 82 kg. The solution has a strength of 50 mg in 250 mL of D5W. Calculate the flow rate in mL/h.

16. A medication is ordered at 75 mg/m$^2$ IVP. The patient has BSA of 2.33 m$^2$. How many milliliters of the medication will be administered if the vial is labeled 50 mg/mL?

17. A liter of D5/NS with 10 units of Regular insulin is started at 9:55 A.M. at a rate of 22 gtt/min. If the drop factor is 20 gtt/mL, when will the infusion finish?

18. Mefoxin 2 g in 100 mL NS IVPB. Infuse in 1 hour. After 30 minutes, 70 mL remain in the bag. Reset the flow rate on the pump in mL/h.

19. Order: *heparin sodium 40,000 units IV in 500 mL of $\frac{1}{2}$ NS to infuse at 1,200 units/hour.* What is the flow rate in mL/h?

20. A patient who weighs 150 pounds is receiving medication at the rate of 100 mL/h. The concentration of the IVPB solution is 200 mg in 50 mL NS. The recommended dosage range is 0.05–0.1 mg/kg/min. Is the patient receiving a safe dose?

## Additional Exercises

Now, test yourself!

1. Physician's order:

   *Dobutamine (Dobutrex) 500 mg in 500 mL D$_5$W, 6 mcg/kg/min IVPB. Weight 145 lb.*

   (a) Set the flow rate on the infusion pump in milliliters per hour. _____

   (b) If the above infusion begins at 6 A.M., when will it be completed? _____

2. Order: *Amiodarone 160 mg in 20 mL D$_5$W IVPB; infuse over 10 minutes.* The label on the vial reads 50 mg/mL. Calculate the flow rate in mcgtt/min. _____

3. A drug is ordered to start at a rate of 15 mg/min IV. This rate may, depending on the patient's response, be increased by 5 mg/min q 20 min to a max of 60 mg/min. The IV strength is 30 mg/mL.

   (a) Calculate the initial pump setting in mL/h. _____

   (b) Construct a titration table for this order. _____

4. Order: *furosemide 20 mg IVP stat over 2 min.* The furosemide vial has a strength of 10 mg/mL. Find

   (a) the total number of milliliters you will administer. _____

   (b) the number of mL you will push during each 30 second interval. _____

   (c) the number of seconds needed to deliver each mL of the solution. _____

5. Order: *lidocaine HCl IV drip 0.75 mg/kg in 500 mL D5W.* The patient weighs 150 pounds.

   (a) How many milliliters of lidocaine 2% will be needed to prepare the IV solution? _____

   (b) Calculate the flow rate in mL/h in order for the patient to receive 5 mg/h. _____

6. Order: *Diltiazem (Cardizem) 0.25 mg/kg IV push over 2 min.* The label on the vial reads 5 mg/mL. The patient weighs 210 pounds.

   (a) How many milligrams of Cardizem will the patient receive? _____

   (b) How many milliliters contain the dose of medication? _____

7. Physician's order:

   *Phenytoin (Dilantin) 500 mg IV push over 10 min*

   The label on the vial reads 50 mg/mL.

   (a) How many milliliters will you prepare? _____

   (b) Calculate the flow rate in microdrops per minute. _____

8. The loading dose of digoxin is 0.25 mg IV push q6h for 4 doses. The label on the ampule reads 0.5 mg/mL. How many milliliters contain this dose? _____

9. The prescriber ordered cefuroxime 18 mg/kg IVPB in 200 mL NS. Infuse in 1.5 hours. The patient weighs 80 kg. The label on the vial states that after reconstitution the strength is 3 g/32 mL.

   (a) How many milligrams of cefuroxime will the patient receive? _____

   (b) How many milliliters of cefuroxime will you add to the 200 mL of NS? _____

   (c) Calculate the flow rate in milliliters per hour. _____

10. Adenocor, (adenosine) 6 mg IV push over 1–2 seconds has been prescribed for your patient. The label on the vial reads 3 mg/mL. How many milliliters will you prepare? _____

11. The order for *cefuroxime is 500 mg in 100 mL D₅W IVPB q8h; infuse in 20 min.* The vial states: "add 77 mL of sterile water, and the concentration is 750 mg/8mL."

   (a) How many milliliters of cefuroxime contain this dose? _____

   (b) Calculate the flow rate in milliliters per minute. _____

12. A patient who weighs 75 pounds is receiving medication at the rate of 150 mL/h. The concentration of the IVPB solution is 500 mg in 100 mL NS. The recommended dosage range is 0.5–1 mg/kg/min. Is the patient receiving a safe dose? _____

13. The patient weighs 72 kg and must receive a drug at the rate of 0.05 mg/kg/min.

   (a) How many mg/min should the patient receive? _____

   (b) How long will it take for the patient to receive 720 mg of the drug? _____

14. A patient has been admitted to the ER with a diagnosis of lead poisoning. The physician orders edetate calcium disodium (calcium EDTA) 1.5 g/m² IV. The BSA is 2.0 m². The label on the vial reads 200 mg/mL. Add the prescribed amount of drug to 250 mL D₅W and infuse at a rate of 11 mL/h. At what time will the infusion finish if it begins at 10 A.M.? _____

15. The order is *cefuroxime 1.5 g added to 100 mL NS infuse in 60 minutes IVPB*. The strength of the cefuroxime is 750 mg per 8 mL.

    (a) How many milliliters of cefuroxime will you add to the normal saline solution? _____

    (b) Calculate the milligrams per minute the patient is receiving. _____

16. The order is *Narcan maxolone (a narcotic antidote) 2 mg IV push*. The vial reads 0.4 mg/mL. How many milliliters will you give the patient? _____

17. Prescriber order:

    *Sufentanil 6 mcg/kg IVPB in 100 mL D$_5$W, infuse over 30 minutes. Weight 172 lb.* The label states that the concentration is 50 mcg/mL. Each ampule contains 1 mL.

    (a) How many milliliters contain the prescribed dose? _____

    (b) How many ampules of this drug will you need? _____

    (c) How many microdrops are infused per minute? _____

18. The prescriber ordered *morphine sulfate 50 mg to be added to 250 mL of NS IVPB. Infuse in 5 hours.* The strength of the morphine is 1 mg/mL.

    (a) How many milliliters contain the prescribed dose? _____

    (b) Calculate the flow rate in milliliters per hour. _____

    (c) After 90 minutes, the patient had breakthrough pain, and the physician increased the morphine to 15 mg/h. Recalculate the flow rate in mL/h. _____

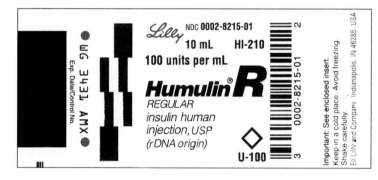

● **Figure 11.8**
**Drug label for Regular insulin.**

*(Copyright Eli Lilly and Company. Used with permission.)*

19. The prescriber ordered a continuous IV insulin drip of *500 units of Regular insulin added to 250 mL 0.45% NaCl q12h*. Read the information on the label in ● **Figure 11.8.**

    Calculate the flow rate in units per hour. _____

20. You have an infusion of heparin 50,000 units in 500 mL D$_5$W. The patient is receiving 1,500 units/h. What is the setting on the pump? _____

# Cumulative Review Exercises

Review your mastery of previous chapters.

1. The patient weighs 130 pounds. The medication order for a drug is 150 mcg/kg of body weight. The label reads 2 mg/mL. How many milliliters of solution are equal to the medication order? _____

2. The prescriber ordered 0.04 mg of Methergine (methylergonovine maleate) PO q6h. How many tablets will you prepare if the label reads 0.02 mg/tab? _____

3. The patient must receive 1,500,000 units of penicillin IM, and the vial contains 20,000,000 units (in powdered form). The directions are as follows: Add 38.7 mL to vial; 1 mL = 500,000 units. How many milliliters will you administer? _____

4. A patient must receive 0.5 mg of scopolamine IM, a parasympathetic antagonist. The label on the ampule reads 0.3 mg/mL. How many milliliters will you administer to this patient? _____

5. The prescriber ordered *cefprozil 200 mg PO q12h for 10 days*. The bottle is labeled 100 mg/5 mL. How many milliliters of this antibiotic will you give your patient? _____

6. If you have a vial labeled 120 mg/mL, how many milliliters would equal 1.2 g? _____

7. If tablets are 250 mg each, how many tablets equal 0.5 g? _____

8. The prescriber has requested that you give 40 mEq of potassium chloride (K-Lor) PO to a patient from a bottle labeled 10 mEq/5 mL. How many milliliters are needed? _____

9. An IV is running at 120 mL/h. The IV solution has a strength of 50 mg/250 mL. How many mg/min is the patient receiving? _____

10. A patient is to receive a drug at the rate of 30 mg/min. At what rate would you set the pump (in mL/h) if the IV solution has a strength of 50 mg/mL? _____

11. A patient weighs 120 lb. Find the dose in milligrams if the patient is to receive 20 mg/kg. _____

12. A patient weighs 120 lb. Find the dosage rate in milligrams per minute if the patient is to receive 20 mg/kg/min. _____

13. Find the body surface area of a person who is 150 cm and 80 kg. _____

14. A 2-gram vial has a strength of 500 mg/mL. How many milliliters of solution are in the vial? _____

15. A 10-mL vial has a strength of 500 mg/mL. How many grams of the drug are in the vial? _____

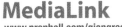

**MediaLink**
www.prenhall.com/giangrasso

Animated examples, interactive practice questions with animated solutions, and challenge tests for this chapter can be found on the Pearson Dosage Calculation Tutor that accompanies this text. Additional, unique, interactive resources and activities can be found on the Companion Web site.

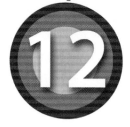

# Chapter

# 12

# Calculating Pediatric Dosages

## Learning Outcomes

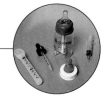

After completing this chapter, you will be able to

1. Determine if a pediatric dose is within the safe dose range.
2. Calculate pediatric oral and parenteral dosages based on body weight.
3. Calculate pediatric oral and parenteral dosages based on body surface area.
4. Perform calculations necessary for administering medications using a volume control chamber.
5. Calculate daily fluid maintenance.

B ecause the metabolism and body mass of children are different from those of adults, children are at greater risk of experiencing adverse effects of medications. Therefore, with pediatric and high-risk medications, it is essential to *carefully calculate* the dose, determine if the dose is in the *safe dose range* for the patient, and *validate your calculations* with another healthcare professional. As always, before administering any medication it is imperative to know its *indications, uses, side effects,* and possible *adverse reactions.*

In this chapter, you will be applying many of the techniques that you have already learned in the previous chapters to the calculation of pediatric dosages.

Pediatric dosages are generally based on the weight of the child. It is important to *verify* that the dose ordered is safe for the particular child. Pediatric dosages are generally rounded down, instead of rounded off, because of the danger that overdose poses to infants and children.

# Pediatric Drug Dosages

Most pediatric doses are based on body weight. Body surface area is also used, especially in pediatric oncology and critical care. You must be able to determine whether the amount of a prescribed pediatric dosage is within the recommended range. In order to do this, you must compare the child's ordered dosage to the recommended safe dosage as found in a reputable drug resource. The recommended dose or dosage range found can be on the package insert, hospital formulary, *Physician's Desk Reference (PDR)*, or *United States Pharmacopeia*.

# Administration of Oral Medications

When prescribing medications for the pediatric population, the oral route is preferred. However, if a child cannot swallow, or the medication is ineffective when given orally, the parenteral route is used.

The developmental age of the child must be taken into consideration when determining the device needed to administer oral medication. For example, an older child may be able to swallow a pill or drink a liquid medication from a cup. Children younger than five years of age, however, generally are not able to swallow tablets and capsules. Therefore, most medications for these children are in the form of elixirs, syrups, or suspensions. An *oral syringe, calibrated dropper, or measuring spoon* can be selected when giving medication to an infant or younger child. An oral syringe is different from a parenteral syringe in two ways. Generally, an **oral syringe** does not have a Luer-Lok™ hub and has a cap on the tip that must be removed before administering a medication. Since a needle does not fit on an oral syringe, the chance of administering a medication via a wrong route is decreased. See ● **Figures 12.1** and **12.2**.

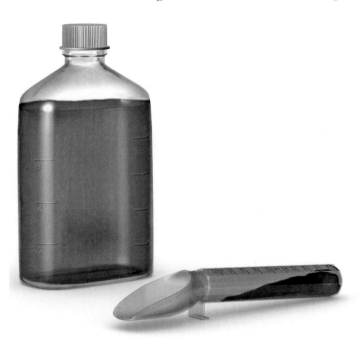

● **Figure 12.1**
**A Bottle of Oral Medication and a Measuring Spoon.**

### NOTE

Many oral pediatric medications are suspensions. Remember to shake them well immediately before administering.

**ALERT**

Currently, devices used to measure oral doses are not standardized. Therefore, in order to prevent overdosing or underdosing, never use a measuring device supplied with one medication for a different medication.

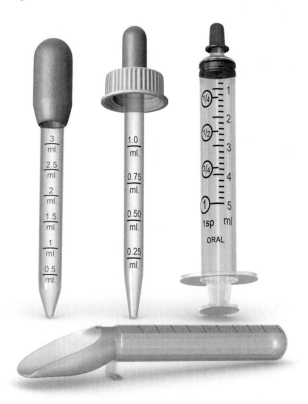

● **Figure 12.2**
**Liquid medication administration devices: Two droppers, an oral syringe, and a measuring spoon.**

## Administration of Parenteral Medications

Subcutaneous or intramuscular routes may be necessary, depending on the type of medication to be administered. For example, many childhood immunizations are administered via subcut or IM. Intramuscular injections are rarely ordered on a routine basis for children because of: limited sites, developmental considerations, and the possibility of trauma. Because of the small muscle mass of children, usually not more than 2 mL is injected. You should consult a current pediatric text for the equipment, injection sites, and procedure.

## Calculating Drug Dosages Based on Body Size

Drug manufacturers can recommend pediatric dosages based on patient size, as measured by either body weight (kg) or body surface area (m²). Body weight in particular is frequently used when prescribing drugs for infants and children.

**EXAMPLE 12.1**

The order is for *Ceftin (cefuroxime) 15mg/kg PO q12h.* How many milligrams of this antibiotic would you administer to a child who weights 25 kg?

The patient's weight is 25 kg, and the order is for 15 mg/kg. *Multiply the size of the patient by the order* to determine how many milligrams of Ceftin to give the patient.

$$25 \ \cancel{kg} \times \frac{15 \ mg}{\cancel{kg}} = 375 \ mg$$

So, the child should receive 375 mg of Ceftin.

## EXAMPLE 12.2

The medication order reads: *erythromycin 10mg/kg PO q8h*. Read the label in ● Figure 12.3. The child weighs 40 kg. How many milliliters of the drug will you administer to this child?

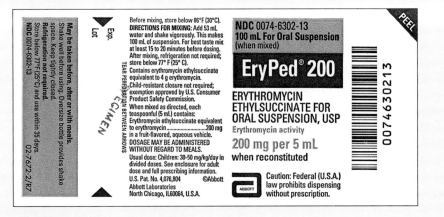

● **Figure 12.3**
**Drug label EryPed 200.**

*(Reproduced with permission of Abbott Laboratories.)*

The patient's weight is 40 kg, and the order is 10 mg/kg. Multiply the *size of the patient by the order* to determine how many milligrams of Ceftin to give the child.

$$40 \ \cancel{kg} \times \frac{10 \ mg}{\cancel{kg}} = 400 \ mg$$

Think:

$$400 \ mg = ? \ mL \quad \text{(dose)}$$
$$200 \ mg = 5 \ mL \quad \text{(strength)}$$

One way to set up the proportion is

$$\frac{400 \ mg}{x \ mL} = \frac{200 \ mg}{5 \ mL}$$
$$200x = 2,000$$
$$x = 10$$

So, the child should receive 10 mL of erythromycin.

## EXAMPLE 12.3

The prescriber ordered: *Zithromax (azithromycin) 10 mg/kg PO stat, then give 5 mg/kg/day for 4 days*. The child weighs 18 kg. Read the information on the label in ● Figure 12.4 and determine the number of milliliters that would contain the stat dose.

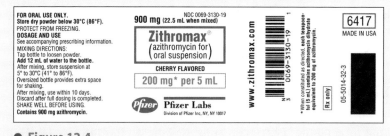

● **Figure 12.4**
**Drug label for Zithromax.**

*(Reg. Trademark of Pfizer Inc. Reproduced with permission.)*

The patient's weight is 18 kg, and the stat dose is 10 mg/kg. Multiply the *size of the patient by the order* to determine how many milligrams of Zithromax to give the child.

$$18 \; kg \times \frac{10 \; mg}{kg} = 180 \; mg$$

Think:

$$180 \; mg = ? \; mL \quad \text{(dose)}$$
$$200 \; mg = 5 \; mL \quad \text{(strength)}$$

One way to set up the proportion is

$$\frac{180 \; mg}{x \; mL} = \frac{200 \; mg}{5 \; mL}$$
$$200x = 900$$
$$x = 4.5$$

So, the child should receive 4.5 mL of Zithromax.

## EXAMPLE 12.4

The recommended dosage for neonates receiving *Tazidime (ceftazidime)* is 30mg/kg IM every 12 hours. If an infant weighs 2,600 grams how many milligrams of Tazidime would the neonate receive in one day?

The patient's weight is 2,600 g. Convert this weight to kilograms by moving the decimal point *three places to the left*. Therefore, the neonate weighs 2.6 kg, and the order is 30 mg/kg. Multiply the *size of the neonate by the order* to determine how many milligrams of Tazidime are needed.

$$2.6 \; kg \times \frac{30 \; mg}{kg} = 78 \; mg \; per \; dose$$

Because the neonate receives two doses per day, the total daily dose is 156 mg.

The following example illustrates that pediatric dosage orders should always be compared with recommended dosages, as found in reputable drug references such as the PDR and drug package inserts.

**ALERT**

Both overdoses and underdoses are dangerous. Too much medication results in the risk of possible life-threatening effects, while too little medication risks suboptimal therapeutic effects.

### EXAMPLE 12.5

The order reads: *morphine sulfate 2 mg IM q4h*. **The recommended dose is 0.1–0.2 mg/kg q4h (max 15 mg/dose). Is the ordered dose safe for the child who weighs 30 kg?**

Use the *minimum* recommended dose of *0.1 mg/kg* to determine the minimum number of milligrams the child should receive q4h.

Multiply the size of the patient by the order.

$$30 \; \cancel{kg} \times \frac{0.1 \; mg}{\cancel{kg}} = 3 \; mg$$

So, the *minimum safe dose is 3 mg q4h*.

Now, use the *maximum* recommended dose of *0.2 mg/kg* to determine the maximum number of milligrams the child may receive q4h.

Multiply the size of the patient by the order.

$$30 \; \cancel{kg} \times \frac{0.2 \; mg}{\cancel{kg}} = 6 \; mg$$

So, the *maximum safe dose is 6 mg q4h*.

The safe dose range of *0.1–0.2 mg/kg q4h* is equivalent to a dose range of *3–6 mg q4h* for this child. The ordered dose of *2 mg* is smaller than the minimum recommended dose of 3 mg. Therefore, the ordered dose is not in the safe dose range, and it should not be administered. The healthcare provider must contact the prescriber.

### EXAMPLE 12.6

The order reads *Kantrex (kanamycin sulfate) 41 mg IM q8h for a two-week-old infant who weighs 9 lb*. **The recommended dosage is 30 mg/kg/day, in three equally divided doses. The vial is labeled 75 mg/2 mL.**

(a) **What is the recommended dosage in mg/day, and is the order safe?**

(b) **How many milliliters would you administer for one dose?**

(a) The patient's weight is 9 lb. Divide by 2.2 to convert this weight to kg.

$$\frac{9 \; lb}{2.2} = 4.09 \; kg$$

Multiply the *weight of the child by the order* to determine how many milligrams per day of Kantrex are needed.

$$4.09 \; \cancel{kg} \times \frac{30 \; mg}{\cancel{kg} \cdot d} = \frac{122.7 \; mg}{d}$$

The recommended daily dose for this child is 122.7 mg. Because the ordered dosage is 41 mg q8h, the infant will receive three doses per day for a total of 123 mg/d. Therefore, the ordered dose is safe.

(b)  Think:

$$41 \ mg = ? \ mL \quad \text{(dose)}$$
$$75 \ mg = 2 \ mL \quad \text{(strength on the label)}$$

One way to set up the proportion is

$$\frac{41 \ mg}{x \ mL} = \frac{75 \ mg}{2 \ mL}$$
$$75x = 82$$
$$x = 1.09$$

So, the child should receive 1 mL of Kantrex IM q8h.

Pediatric dosages may also be based on body surface area (BSA). For example, antineoplastic agents used in the treatment of cancer are often ordered using the BSA. To calculate the BSA accurately, it is important that the *actual* height and weight be assessed, not just estimated. In most instances, the prescriber will calculate the BSA. However, it is the responsibility of the person who administers the drug to verify that the BSA is correct, and that the dose is within the safe dosage range.

**ALERT**

When calculating BSA, be sure to check your calculations with another professional.

### EXAMPLE 12.7

A child who has BSA of 0.75 m$^2$ is to receive Cosmegen (dactinomycin) 2.5 mg/m$^2$ IVP daily for 5 days. Calculate the dose of this antineoplastic drug in milligrams.

The child's BSA is 0.75 m$^2$. Multiply the *BSA of the child by the order* to determine how many milligrams of Cosmegen are needed per day.

$$0.75 \ m^2 \times \frac{2.5 \ mg}{m^2} = 1.875 \ mg$$

So, the child should receive 1.8 mg of Cosmegen daily.

### EXAMPLE 12.8

Order: *Platinol (cisplatin) 30 mg/m$^2$ PO once every week.* The child weighs 40 kg and is 45 inches tall. The strength of the Platinol is 1 mg/mL. How many milliliters should this child receive?

Convert 45 inches to centimeters.

Think:

$$45 \ in = ? \ cm$$
$$1 \ in = 2.5 \ cm$$

One way to set up the proportion is

$$\frac{45 \ in}{x \ cm} = \frac{1 \ in}{2.5 \ cm}$$

$$1x = 112.5$$

So, the child's height is 112.5 cm.

Calculate the BSA using the formula:

$$BSA = \sqrt{\frac{40 \times 112.5}{3600}} \approx 1.118 \ m^2$$

Multiply the size of the patient by the order.

$$1.118 \ m^2 \times \frac{30 \ mg}{m^2} = 33.54 \ mg$$

Because

$$1 \ mg = 1 \ mL \qquad \text{(strength on the label)},$$

$$33.54 \ mg = 33.54 \ mL$$

No calculations were necessary for the last step, and the child should receive 33.5 mL of Platnol.

## EXAMPLE 12.9

Valium (diazepam) 3.75 mg IVP slowly stat was ordered for a child who has status epilepticus. The package insert says that the recommended dose is 0.2–0.5 mg/kg IVP slowly every 2–5 minutes up to a maximum of 5 mg. The child weighs 33 lbs, and the label on the vial reads 5 mg/mL.

(a) Is the ordered dose within the safe range?

(b) How many milliliters would you administer?

(a) The child's weight is 33 lb. Divide by 2.2 to convert this weight to kg.

$$\frac{33 \ lb}{2.2} = 15 \ kg$$

Multiply the *weight of the child* by the *minimum and maximum recommended doses* to determine the *safe dose range for this child in milligrams.*

$$15 \ kg \times \frac{0.2 \ mg}{kg} = 3 \ mg \qquad \text{(min)}$$

$$15 \ kg \times \frac{0.5 \ mg}{kg} = 7.5 \ mg \quad \text{(max)}$$

But 7.5 mg is above the recommended maximum of 5 mg as stated in the example, therefore the *safe dose range for this child is 3–5 mg*. Because the ordered dose of 3.75 mg is between 3 mg and 5 mg, the ordered dose is safe.

(b) Convert the ordered dose of 3.75 mg to milliliters.

Think:

$$3.75 \ mg = ? \ mL \quad \text{(dose)}$$
$$5 \ mg = 1 \ mL \quad \text{(strength on the label)}$$

One way to set up the proportion is

$$\frac{3.75 \ mg}{x \ mL} = \frac{5 \ mg}{1 \ mL}$$
$$5x = 3.75$$
$$x = 0.75$$

So, the child should receive 0.75 mL of Valium IVP slowly.

# Administration of Intravenous Medications

When a child is NPO, needs pain relief, or needs a high concentration of a medication, the intravenous route is the most effective route to use. In addition, when the duration of the therapy is long term, or when gastrointestinal absorption is poor, the IV route is indicated.

Methods of intravenous infusions include peripheral intravenous catheters, peripherally inserted central catheters (PICC line), central lines, and long-term central venous access devices (VAD) or ports. The method chosen is based on the age and size of the child and the duration of therapy.

Most IV medications must be further diluted once the correct dose is calculated. Follow the directions precisely for the reconstitution process. An electronic infusion device and a volume control chamber should always be used to administer IV fluids and IVPB medications, especially high-alert drugs, to infants and children.

## Using a Volume Control Chamber

To avoid fluid overload, pediatric intravenous medications are frequently administered using a volume control chamber (VCC) (burette, Volutrol, Buretrol, Soluset).

A VCC is calibrated in 1 mL increments and has a capacity of 100–150 mL. It can be used as a primary or secondary line. When administering IVPB medications, the medication is added to the top injection port of the VCC. Fluid is then added from the IV bag to further dilute the medication. After the infusion is complete, additional IV fluid is added to the VCC to flush any remaining medication left in the tubing. See ● **Figure 12.5**.

The following example illustrates the use of such a device.

## ALERT

An excessively high concentration of an intravenous drug can cause irritation to the vein and have potentially life-threatening toxic effects. Read the manufacturer's directions very carefully.

## NOTE

Know the facility's policy concerning the amount of fluid used to flush the VCC tubing.

## Volume Control Chamber

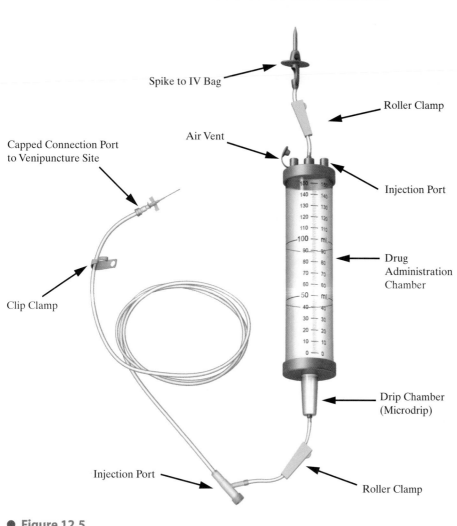

Spike to IV Bag

Roller Clamp

Air Vent

Capped Connection Port
to Venipuncture Site

Injection Port

140
130
120
110
100  ml
90
80
70
60
50  ml
40
30
20
10
0

Drug
Administration
Chamber

Clip Clamp

Drip Chamber
(Microdrip)

Injection Port

Roller Clamp

● **Figure 12.5**
**Volume control chamber.**

---

## EXAMPLE 12.10

Order: *Chloromycetin (chloramphenicol) 500 mg in 50 mL of* D₅W
*IVPB q6h*. The recommended dose is 50–75 mg/kg/day divided every
6 hours. The child weighs 34.6 kg.

(a) Is the ordered dose in the safe dose range?

(b) The strength on the vial is 1 g/10 mL. How many mL will you
withdraw from the vial and add to the VCC?

(c) How would you dilute the medication in the VCC?

(a) Multiply the *weight of the child* by the *minimum and maximum
recommended doses* to determine the daily *safe dosage range for
this child in milligrams*.

**NOTE**

In Example 12.10 following the infusing of the 50 mL, the tubing must be flushed; be sure to follow the institutions policy.

$$34.6 \; \cancel{kg} \times \frac{50 \; mg}{\cancel{kg} \cdot d} = 1{,}730 \; \frac{mg}{d} \quad (\text{min})$$

$$34.6 \; \cancel{kg} \times \frac{75 \; mg}{\cancel{kg} \cdot d} = 2{,}595 \; \frac{mg}{d} \quad (\text{max})$$

So, the safe dose range for this child is 1,730–2,595 mg daily. The ordered dose is 500 mg every six hours (4 times per day). Therefore, the ordered dose is (500 × 4) 2,000 mg daily. Because 2,000 is between 1,730 and 2,595, the child is receiving a safe dose.

(b)  Convert the ordered dose of 500 mg to milliliters.

Think:

$$500 \; mg = ? \; mL \quad (\text{dose})$$
$$1{,}000 \; mg = 10 \; mL \quad (\text{strength in the vial})$$

One way to set up the proportion is

$$\frac{500 \; mg}{x \; mL} = \frac{1{,}000 \; mg}{10 \; mL}$$

$$1{,}000x = 5{,}000$$

$$x = 5$$

So, 5 mL will be withdrawn from the vial and added to the VCC.

(c)  Because the medication is to be delivered in 50 mL D5W, add D5W from the IV bag to the VCC until the level of 50 mL is reached.

### EXAMPLE 12.11

The physician orders *Garamycin (gentamycin) 25 mg IVPB q8h for a child.*

(a)  If the label on the Garamycin vial reads 10 mg/mL, how many milliliters will you withdraw from the vial to add to the volume control chamber?

(b)  If the recommended concentration of the solution for infusion is 2 mg/mL, how would you then dilute the medication in the VCC?

(a)  Think: *in the vial*

$$25 \; mg = ? \; mL \quad (\text{dose})$$
$$10 \; mg = 1 \; mL \quad (\text{strength in the vial})$$

One way to set up the proportion is

$$\frac{25 \; mg}{x \; mL} = \frac{10 \; mg}{1 \; mL}$$

$$10x = 25$$

$$x = 2.5$$

So, 2.5 mL will be withdrawn from the vial and added to the VCC.

(b) The amount of drug in the VCC is 25 mg. It must be diluted with IV fluid to a concentration of 2 mg/mL.

Think: *in the VCC*

$$25 \ mg = ? \ mL \quad \text{(dose)}$$
$$2 \ mg = 1 \ mL \quad \text{(strength in the VCC)}$$

One way to set up the proportion is

$$\frac{25 \ mg}{x \ mL} = \frac{2 \ mg}{1 \ mL}$$
$$2x = 25$$
$$x = 12.5$$

So, IV fluid must be added to the VCC to the level of 12.5 mL.

In summary, in Example 12.11, you would add *2.5 mL from the vial of Garamycin* to the top injection port of the volume control chamber, and then add additional *(10 mL) IV solution from the bag to obtain the required total of 12.5 mL,* which would contain the recommended safe medication concentration.

# Calculating Daily Fluid Maintenance

The administration of pediatric intravenous medication requires careful and exact calculations and procedures. Infants and severely ill children are not able to tolerate extreme levels of hydration and are quite susceptible to dehydration, and fluid overload. Therefore, you must closely monitor the amount of fluid a child receives. The fluid a child requires over a 24-hour period is referred to as *daily fluid maintenance needs.* Daily fluid maintenance includes both oral and parenteral fluids. The amount of maintenance fluid required depends on the weight of the patient (see the formula in Table 12.1). The daily maintenance fluid does not include body fluid losses through vomiting, diarrhea, or fever. Additional fluids referred to as *replacement fluids* (usually Lactated Ringer's or 0.9% NaCl) are utilized to replace fluid losses and are based on each child's condition (e.g., if 20 mL are lost, then 20 mL of replacement fluids are usually added to the daily maintenance).

**Table 12.1  Daily Fluid Maintenance Formula**

| Pediatric Daily Fluid Maintenance Formula | | |
|---|---|---|
| For the *first* | *10 kg* of body weight: | *100 mL/kg* |
| For the *next* | *10 kg* of body weight: | *50 mL/kg* |
| For *each kg above* | *20 kg* of body weight: | *20 mL/kg* |

### EXAMPLE 12.12

**If the order is *half maintenance* for a child who weighs 25 kg, at what rate should the pump be set in mL/h?**

Because the child weighs 25 kg, this weight would be divided into three portions following the formula in Table 12.1 as follows:

$$25 \text{ kg} = 10 \text{ kg} + 10 \text{ kg} + 5 \text{ kg}$$

For each of these three portions, the number of milliliters must be calculated. A table will be useful for organizing the calculations (Table 12.2). The daily "maintenance" was determined to be 1,600 mL. "Half maintenance" ($\frac{1}{2}$ of maintenance) is, therefore, $\frac{1}{2}$ of 1,600 mL, or 800 mL.

Now, you must change $\frac{800 \ mL}{1 \ day}$ to $\frac{mL}{h}$.

Replace 1 day with 24 hours to obtain

$$\frac{800 \ mL}{1 \ day} = \frac{800 \ mL}{24 \ h} = 33.3\frac{mL}{h}$$

So, the pump would be set at the rate of 33 mL/h.

---

**Table 12.2 Daily Fluid Maintenance Computations for Example 12.12**

| | | | | | |
|---|---|---|---|---|---|
| 1st Portion | 10 kg | × | $\dfrac{100 \text{ mL}}{\text{kg}}$ | = | 1,000 mL |
| 2nd Portion | 10 kg | × | $\dfrac{50 \text{ mL}}{\text{kg}}$ | = | 500 mL |
| 3rd Portion | 5 kg | × | $\dfrac{20 \text{ mL}}{\text{kg}}$ | = | 100 mL |
| *Total* | 25 kg | | | | 1,600 mL |

## Summary

In this chapter, you learned to calculate oral and parenteral dosages for pediatric patients. Some dosages were based on the size of the patient: body weight (kg) or BSA (m²). The calculations needed for the use of the volume control chamber, as well as the method for determining daily fluid maintenance were explained.

- Taking shortcuts in pediatric medication administration can be fatal to the child.
- Check to see if the order is in the safe dose range.
- Consult a reliable source when in doubt about a pediatric medication order.

- Question the order or check your calculations if the ordered dose differs from the recommended dose.
- Pediatric dosages are generally rounded down (truncated) to avoid the danger of an overdose.
- IV bags of no more than 500 mL should be hung for pediatric patients.
- No more that 2 mL should be given IM to a pediatric patient.
- Because accuracy is crucial in pediatric infusions, electronic control devices or volume control chambers should always be used.

- Minimal and maximal dilution volumes for some IV drugs are recommended in order to prevent fluid overload, minimize irritation to veins, and reduce toxic effects.
- When preparing IV drug solutions, the smallest added volume (minimal dilution) results in the strongest concentration; the largest added volume (maximal dilution), results in the weakest concentration.

- For a volume control chamber, a flush is always used to clear the tubing after the medication is infused.
- Know the facility policy regarding the inclusion of medication volume as part of the total infusion volume.
- Daily fluid maintenance depends on the weight of the child and includes both oral and parenteral fluids.

## Case Study 12.1

Read the Case Study and answer the questions. The answers are found in Appendix A.

A 4-year-old girl is admitted to the hospital with a diagnosis of cystic fibrosis and pneumonia. Her parents say that she has been very irritable, has had a chronic cough, decreased appetite, and diarrhea for almost a week. Chest auscultation revealed labored breathing with the presence of rhonchi in the right upper lobe (RUL) of the lung, and inspection revealed mild circumoral cyanosis. She is small in stature for a child of her age (38 inches tall) and underweight (30 pounds). She is allergic to milk products. Vital signs are: T 102°F; BP 88/64; P 100; R 26. Throat culture returned positive for Group A streptococcus. Her orders include the following:

- Bed rest
- Diet as tolerated, encourage PO fluids
- Peptamin Junior Supplement 600 mL HS via pump to GT over 6 hours
- Ventolin (albuterol) 1 mg with Intal (cromolyn sodium) $\frac{1}{2}$ ampule (20 mg in a 2 mL ampule) via nebulizer q6h

- Pulmozyme (deoxyribonuclease) $\frac{1}{2}$ ampule (2.5 mg in a 1 mL ampule) q12h via nebulizer
- Tobramycin $\frac{1}{2}$ ampule (300 mg in a 5 mL ampule) q12h via nebulizer for 28 days
- CPT and postural drainage q4h following nebulization therapy
- Penicillin G 600,000 units in 50 mL D$_5$W IVPB q6h
- Tylenol (acetaminophen) 180 mg PO q4h prn temp over 101°F
- Vitamin ADEK 2 mL once daily in A.M.

1. Calculate the child's 24-hour fluid requirement.
2. The recommended dose for penicillin G is 25,000–400,000 units/kg/day divided in equal doses every 4–6 hours. Is the ordered dose safe?
3. The penicillin G is available in a 5,000,000 units vial (● Figure 12.6 for a portion of package insert). How many milliliters of diluent will you use to obtain a concentration of 750,000 units/mL,

● **Figure 12.6**
**Portion of penicillin G package insert.**

*(Reg. Trademark of Pfizer Inc. Reproduced with permission.)*

**Buffered**
# PFIZERPEN®
**(penicillin G potassium)**
**for Injection**

**Reconstitution**
The following table shows the amount of solvent required for solution of various concentrations:

| Approx. Desired Concentration (units/mL) | Approx. Volume (mL) 1,000,000 units | Solvent for Vial of 5,000,000 units | Infusion Only 20,000,000 units |
|---|---|---|---|
| 50,000 | 20.0 | – | – |
| 100,000 | 10.0 | – | – |
| 250,000 | 4.0 | 18.2 | 75.0 |
| 500,000 | 1.8 | 8.2 | 33.0 |
| 750,000 | – | 4.8 | – |
| 1,000,000 | – | 3.2 | 11.5 |

and how many mL of penicillin G will you withdraw from the vial?

4. Calculate the setting in mL/h on the infusion pump to administer the penicillin G if it were given over 30 minutes.

5. If the usual dose range of albuterol is 0.1 to 0.15 mg/kg per dose, is the albuterol dose safe for this child?

6. How many milligrams of Pulmozyme is the patient receiving per dose?

7. How many milligrams of the cromolyn sodium will you administer with the albuterol?

8. If the Ventolin is supplied 1.25 mg/3 mL, what is the total amount of solution (in milliliters) in the nebulizer containing the combination of the Ventolin and the Intal?

9. How many milliliters of Pulmozyme will you administer?

10. How many milligrams of Tobramycin will you administer?

Workspace

# Practice Sets

The answers to *Try These for Practice, Exercises,* and *Cumulative Review Exercises* are found in Appendix A. Ask your instructor for the answers to the *Additional Exercises*.

## Try These for Practice

Test your comprehension after reading the chapter.

1. The following order has been given for a child who weighs 45 kilograms: *Humulin R insulin 0.1 unit/kg subcutaneously b.i.d. ac breakfast and dinner* How many units of insulin will this child receive in 24 h? _____

2. Order: *Retrovir (azidothymidine) 90 mg IVPB q6h.* The patient is a two-year-old child with BSA of 0.62 m². If the recommended safe dose range is 100–180 mg/m² q6h, is the prescribed dose safe?

3. The order is *Amoxil (amoxicillin) 250 mg PO q12h.* The label reads 125 mg/ 5 mL. How many milliliters would you administer?

4. Read the information on the label in ● **Figure 12.7**. Calculate the number of milliliters you would administer to a child who weighs 40 kg. The order is *Codeine 0.3 mg/kg PO q12h.*

5. Order: *IV D5/$\frac{1}{3}$ NS at maintenance and one half for a 42 kg child.* How many mL/h does the child need?

## Exercises

Reinforce your understanding in class or at home.

1. The prescriber ordered gentamicin 50 mg IVPB q8h for a child who weighs 40 lb. The recommended dosage is 6–7.5 mg/kg/day divided in three equal doses. Is the prescribed dose within the safe range?

2. The prescriber ordered Vancocin (vancomycin) 10 mg/kg q12h, IVPB for a neonate who weighs 4,000 g. What is the dose in milligrams?

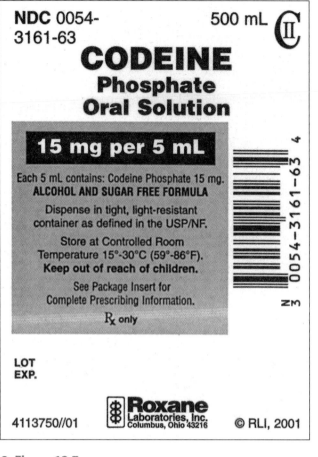

● **Figure 12.7**
**Drug label for codeine.**

*(Courtesy of Roxane Laboratories Inc.)*

3. The prescriber ordered methotrexate 2.9 mg PO weekly for a child who is 42 inches tall and weighs 50 pounds. The package insert states that the recommended dosage is 7.5–30 mg/m² q1–2 weeks. Is the order a safe dose?

4. Order: *Panadol (acetaminophen) 10 mg/kg PO q4h prn* for a child who weighs 32 kg. How many milligrams will you administer?

5. A manufacturer recommends giving from a minimum of 350 mg/m²/day to a maximum of 450 mg/m²/day for a certain drug. A child has a BSA of 1.2 m². Calculate the safe dose range (in milligrams per day) for this child.

6. Order: *Ceclor (cefaclor) suspension 30 mg/kg/day q8h*. The child weighs 77 pounds. The label reads 187 mg/mL. How many milliliters will you administer?

7. Order: *1,000 mL D5/RL infuse at 65 mL/h*. Calculate the infusion rate in microdrops per minute.

8. Order: *Zantac (ranitidine) 30 mg IV q8h*. The patient weighs 52 pounds. The package insert states that the recommended dose for pediatric patients is 2–4 mg/kg/day, to be divided and administered every 6 to 8 hours, up to a maximum of 50 mg per dose. Is the prescribed dose safe?

9.  Order: Daily fluid maintenance IV D5/0.33% NS.

    (a) The child weighs 55 lb. If the child is NPO, what is the daily IV fluid maintenance?

    (b) What is the rate of flow in mL/h?

10. A child has a BSA of 0.82 m². The recommended dose of a drug is 2 million units/m². How many units will you administer?

11. Order: *Claforan (cefotamine sodium) 1.2 g IVPB q8h*. The safe dose range for the solution concentration is 20–60 mg/mL to infuse over 15 to 30 minutes. What is the minimal amount of IV fluid needed to safely dilute this dosage? [HINT: The minimal amount of IV fluid is the maximal safe concentration.]

12. Calculate the daily fluid maintenance for an infant who weighs 7 lb.

13. Order: *Retrovir (zidovudine) 160 mg/m² q8h PO*. The child has a BSA of 1.1 m². Read the label in ● **Figure 12.8**. How many milliliters will you prepare?

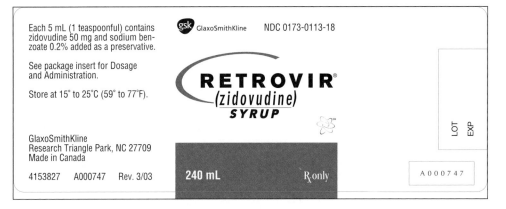

Each 5 mL (1 teaspoonful) contains zidovudine 50 mg and sodium benzoate 0.2% added as a preservative.

See package insert for Dosage and Administration.

Store at 15° to 25°C (59° to 77°F).

gsk GlaxoSmithKline    NDC 0173-0113-18

GlaxoSmithKline
Research Triangle Park, NC 27709
Made in Canada

4153827    A000747    Rev. 3/03

**RETROVIR®**
*(zidovudine)*
*SYRUP*

240 mL                ℞ only

LOT   EXP

A 000 747

● **Figure 12.8**
**Drug label for Retrovir.**

*(Reproduced with permission of GlaxoSmithKline.)*

14. Order: D5/½NS with KCl 20 mEq per liter, infuse at 30 mL/h. The child is 60 cm and weighs 9.1 kg.

    (a) How many mEq of KCl would you add to a 500 mL IV bag?

    (b) The label on the KCl vial reads 2 mEq/mL. How many milliliters will you add to the IV?

    (c) How many mEq/h will the child receive?

15. Order: *erythromycin estolate* 125 mg PO q4h. The child weighs 14.5 kg. The recommended dosage is 30–50 mg/kg/day in equally divided doses. The label reads 125 mg/mL.

    (a) Is the ordered dose safe?

    (b) How many milliliters would you administer?

16. Order: Vancocin (vancomycin) 40 mg/kg/d IVPB q6h to infuse over 90 minutes in 200 mL NS. The child weighs 41 kg. The Vancocin vial has a concentration of 50 mg/mL. At what rate in mL/h will you set the pump?

17. A medication of 100 mg in 1 mL is diluted to 15 mL and administered IVP over 20 minutes. How many mg/min is the patient receiving?

18. 40 mL of IV fluid is to infuse over 60 minutes. What is the rate of flow in microdrops per minute?

19. Order: *Pediaprophen (ibuprofen) 10 mg/kg PO q4h*. The label reads 100 mg/2.5 mL. The child weighs 35 pounds. How many milliliters will you administer?

20. Order: *ampicillin 125 mg PO q6h*. A child weighs 22 pounds. The package insert states that the recommended dose is 50 mg/kg/24 h. Is the prescribed dose safe?

## Additional Exercises

Now, test yourself!

1. The antiretroviral medication Videx (didanosine) 180 mg/m$^2$ PO q12h has been prescribed for a child with a BSA 0.9 m$^2$. The concentration is 10 mg/mL. How many milliliters will you administer to the child? _____

2. Physician's order:

   *Epivir (lamivudine) 4 mg/kg PO b.i.d.*

   The label reads 10 mg/mL. How many milliliters will you prepare for an infant who weighs 16 pounds? _____

3. *Lanoxin (digoxin) 20 mcg/kg IV push as a loading dose, give 10 mcg stat and 5 mcg IVP q8h for 2 doses.*

   The label reads 0.1 mg/mL, and the infant weighs 7 pounds. How many milliliters will you prepare for the stat dose?

4. Order:

   *Rocaltrol (calcitriol) 0.01 oral solution mcg/kg PO daily*

   The label reads 1 mcg/mL. How many milliliters will you prepare for a child who weighs 35 kg?

5. Physician's order:

   *Diamox (acetazolamide) 8 mg/kg IV push q6h*

   The label reads 500 mg in 5 mL. How many milliliters will you prepare for a child with acute angle-closure glaucoma who weighs 56 pounds? _____

6. Physician's order: *Vistaril (hydroxyzine) 20 mg IM q4h prn anxiety*. The safe dose is 0.5–1 mg/kg/dose q 4–6h as needed. Is the prescribed dose safe for a 44-pound child? _____

7. Order: *Havrix (hepatitis A vaccine, inactivated) 720 Elisa units (EL. units) IM stat*. The label reads 1,440 EL. units/mL. How many milliliters will you prepare? _____

8. The physician ordered 120 mg of guaifenesin PO q4h prn cough. The label reads 100 mg in 5 mL. How many milliliters will you prepare? _____

9. The order for Regular insulin is 0.1 units per kilogram IV bolus stat. The child weighs 18 kg. How many units will you administer? _____

10. Physician's order:

    *Add 100 units of Regular insulin to 100 milliliters of normal saline. Infuse at a rate of 0.1 units per kilogram per hour IV.*

    The child weighs 50 pounds; how many milliliters per hour will the child receive? _____

11. Lorabid (loracarbef) has been prescribed for a 2-year-old child with acute otitis media. The order is 30 milligrams per kilogram PO, q12h and the child weighs 21 pounds. The oral suspension is labeled 100 mg in 5 mL. How many milliliters will you give this child? _____

12. Biaxin (clarithromycin) 7.5 mg/kg PO q12h has been ordered for a child who weighs 23 kg. The label reads 125 milligrams in 5 milliliters. How many milliliters will you prepare? _____

13. Order: *Augmentin (amoxicillin) oral suspension 200 mg PO q12h.* The label reads 125 mg/5 mL. How many milliliters will you administer? _____

14. The BSA of a child is 0.5 m$^2$, and the order is 400 mg/m$^2$ of a drug PO. The label reads 250 mg in 5 mL. How many milliliters will you prepare for this child? _____

15. The normal dose range for erythromycin, is 30–50 mg/kg PO in divided doses q6h. The physician ordered 250 mg PO q6h for a child who weighs 30 kg. Is this a safe dose for this child? _____

16. Prescriber's order:

    *Mefoxin (cefoxitin) 35 mg/kg IVPB 60 minutes before surgery. The post-operative order is 35 mg/kg q6h for 24h.*

    The child weighs 35 kg. What is the total amount in grams that the child will receive preoperatively and postoperatively? _____

17. Order:

    *150 mg Vantin (cefpodoxime) PO q12h*

    The label reads 50 mg/5 mL. How many milliliters will you prepare? _____

18. The prescriber ordered 1.0 g of Rocephin (ceftriaxone) IVPB stat. The label on the vial reads 1 g in 10 mL of D/5/W. Add to 90 mL D$_5$W. Infuse total amount in 30 minutes. Calculate the amount in microdrops per minute. _____

19. Order: *D5/0.3 NaCl at maintenance for a 19 kg child.* How many mL/d does the child need? _____

20. Ampicillin 25 mg/kg PO q.i.d. has been prescribed for a child who weighs 42 pounds. The label reads 250 mg = 5 mL. Calculate the dose in milliliters for this child. _____

# Cumulative Review Exercises

Review your mastery of previous chapters.

1. How many milligrams of Myambutal (ethambutol HCl), an antitubercular drug, would you administer if the prescribed dose is 15 milligrams per kilogram PO daily and the child weighs 35 kg? _____

2. How many units of Regular insulin subcutaneously would you prepare for a child who weighs 30 kg if the order is 1 unit per kilogram subcutaneously stat? _____

3. Order: *Suprax (cefixime) 8 mg/kg PO once daily.*

   (a) How many milligrams of this antibiotic would you administer to a child whose weight is 25 kg? _____

   (b) What is the dose in grams? _____

4. The order reads:

   *Lente insulin 50 units subcutaneously ac breakfast*

   The vial is labeled 100 units per milliliter. How many units would you administer to the patient? _____

5. The prescriber has ordered 10 million units of penicillin G IVPB q12h. The 20-million-unit vial of powder has these instructions: add 40 mL of sterile water. How many milliliters will you administer? _____

6. The order is Zantac (ranitidine HCl) 300 mg PO daily. The label indicates that each capsule contains 150 mg.

   (a) How many capsules equal the prescribed dose? _____

   (b) Calculate the dose in grams. _____

7. Physician's order:

   *Apply 0.025% vitamin A acid (tretinoin) solution to affected skin once daily at hour of sleep.*

   How many milligrams of vitamin A acid are in 4 mL of solution? _____

8. The prescriber ordered 900 mL of 5% D/W IV to infuse in 5 hours. Calculate the flow rate in drops per minute. The drop factor is 20 drops per milliliter. _____

9. The order reads:

   *Tagamet (cimetidine) 300 mg IVPB q12h in 50 mL of 5% D/W. Infuse in 20 minutes.*

   Calculate the flow rate in milliliters per minute for this histamine-2 receptor antagonist drug. _____

10. The prescriber ordered 1,000 mL 5% D/W q12h. At what rate will you set the pump in milliliters per hour? _____

11. Physician's order: *naproxen 12 mg/kg PO daily*. The patient weighs 50 kg. How many 200 mg tablets will you administer? _____

12. How many tablets of a drug would you administer PO to an adult with a BSA of 1.9 square meters if the order is 200 mg/m$^2$ and each tablet contains 375 mg? _____

13. A child who has BSA of 1.2 m$^2$ is to receive 175 mg/m$^2$ of a drug by mouth stat. The label on the drug vial reads 200 mg/5 mL. How many milliliters should the child receive? _____

14. The order is verapamil 80 mg PO q8h. Each tablet contains 40 mg. How many tablets will you administer of this calcium channel blocker drug? _____

15. Order: *Zithromax (azithromycin) 10 mg/kg PO once daily for 3 days.* The child weighs 20 kg. The strength in the vial is 100 mg/5 mL. How many milliliters will you administer? _____

**MediaLink**
www.prenhall.com/giangrasso

Animated examples, interactive practice questions with animated solutions, and challenge tests for this chapter can be found on the Pearson Dosage Calculation Tutor that accompanies this text. Additional, unique, interactive resources and activities can be found on the Companion Web site.

# Comprehensive
# Self-Tests

# Comprehensive Self-Test 1

Answers to *Comprehensive Self-Tests* 1–4 can be found in Appendix A at the back of the book.

1. Calculate the dosage of calcium EDTA for a patient who has a BSA of 1.47 m². The recommended dose is 500 mg/m².

2. Order:

    *Tikosyn 1 mg PO q8h*

    Read the label in ● **Figure S.1** to determine how many capsules you will give the patient.

● **Figure S.1**
**Drug label for Tikosyn.**
*(Reg. Trademark of Pfizer Inc. Reproduced with permission.)*

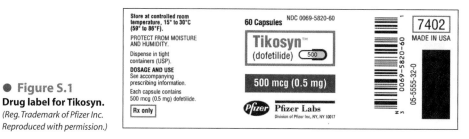

3. How would you prepare 400 mL of 10% Clorox solution from a 100% solution?

4. Kineret (anakinra) 100 mg subcut daily has been prescribed for a patient with rheumatoid arthritis. The prefilled syringe is labeled 100 mg/mL. Calculate the dose in grams.

5. An IV of 1,000 mL D5W is infusing at a rate of 40 gtt/min. How long will it take to finish if the drop factor is 20 gtt/mL?

6. Calculate the number of grams of dextrose in 250 mL of D5W.

7. Order:

    *Humulin Regular insulin U-100 6 units and Humulin NPH insulin 14 units subcutaneous ac breakfast*

    Read the labels in ● **Figure S.2** and place an arrow on the syringe indicating the total amount of insulin you will give.

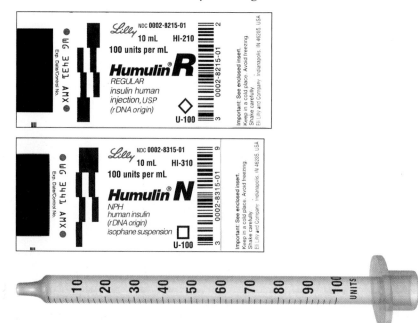

● **Figure S.2**
**Drug labels for Humulin R and Humulin N and syringe.**
*(Copyright Eli Lilly and Company. Used with permission.)*

8. The prescriber ordered Cordarone (amiodarone HCl) 400 mg PO b.i.d. Each tablet contains 200 mg. How many tablets will you give the patient?

9. The prescriber ordered Cefobid (cefoperazone) 1g IVPB q12h to infuse in 30 minutes. The label on the 1 gram premixed IV bag reads cefoperazone 50 mL, 50 mg/mL.
   (a) Calculate the flow rate in milliliters per hour.
   (b) How many milligrams will the patient receive?

10. Your patient is to receive morphine sulfate 5 mg subcutaneously stat. The 20 mL multiple dose vial is labeled morphine 15 mg/mL. Calculate the dose in milliliters and place an arrow on the syringe indicating the dose.

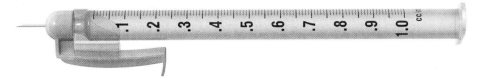

11. A dosage of 300 mcg has been ordered. The solution strength is 0.4 mg/mL. Calculate in milliliters the volume of medication needed.

12. A prescriber ordered a premixed solution of nitroglycerine 25 mg in 250 mL D5W to be titrated at a rate of 5 mcg/min, increase q 5–10 min until pain subsides. The medication is to be infused via pump. How many mL/h will you set the pump to begin the infusion?

13. Order:

    *Humulin R insulin 100 units in 100 mL NS, infuse at 0.1 unit/kg/h*

    The patient weighs 68 kg. How many units per hour is the patient receiving?

14. The prescriber ordered Claforan (cefotaxime) 750 mg IM q12h. The 1 g vial of Claforan is in a powder form. The package insert states for IM injection, add 3 mL of sterile water for injection for an approximate volume of 3.4 mL containing 300 mg/mL. How many milliliters will you give the patient?

15. Rebif (interferon beta-1a) 44 mcg subcutaneous three times a week is prescribed for a patient with multiple sclerosis. How many milligrams will the patient receive in one week?

16. Order:

    *Lanoxin (digoxin) elixir 0.15 mg PO q12h*

    The child weighs 70 lb and the recommended maintenance dose is 7–10 mcg/kg/day.
    (a) What is the minimum daily maintenance dosage in mg/day?
    (b) What is the maximum daily maintenance dosage in mg/day?
    (c) Is the dose ordered safe?

17. Vibramycin (doxycycline hyclate) 4.4 mg/kg IVPB daily is ordered for a child who weighs 80 pounds. The premixed IV solution bag is labeled Vibramycin 200 mg/250 mL D5W to infuse in 4 hours.
    (a) How many milligrams of Vibramycin will the patient receive?
    (b) Calculate the flow rate in mL/h.

18. Order:

    *Levaquin (levofloxacin) 500 mg in 100 mL D5W IVPB daily for 14 days to infuse in 1 h*

    Calculate the flow rate in drops per minute if the drop factor is 15 gtt/mL.

19. Calculate the BSA of a child who is 44 inches and weighs 72 pounds.

20. Order:

*heparin 5,000 units subcutaneous q12h*

The multidose vial label reads 10,000 units/mL. How many milliliters will you give the patient?

21. Order:

*D10W 1,000 mL to infuse at 75 mL/h*

The drop factor is 20 gtt/mL.
(a) What is the rate of flow in $\frac{mL}{min}$?
(b) How many drops per minute will you set the IV to infuse?
(c) How long will it take for the infusion to be complete?

22. Calculate the total daily fluid maintenance for a child who weighs 45 kg.

23. Order:

*Keflex (cephalexin) oral suspension 50 mg/kg PO q6h*

The label reads 125 mg/5 mL. The patient weighs 33 pounds. How many milliliters will you give?

24. Read the label in ● **Figure S.3**.

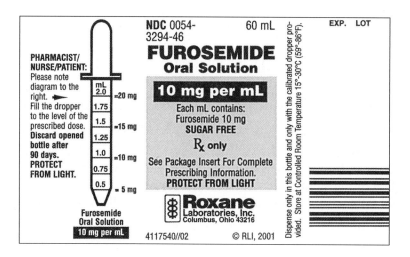

● **Figure S.3**
**Drug label for furosemide.**
*(Courtesy of Roxane Laboratories Inc.)*

(a) How many milligrams of furosemide are in 1 mL?
(b) How many milliliters of furosemide are in the bottle?

25. The prescriber ordered ReoPro (abciximab) 0.125 mcg/kg/min IV in 250 mL NS to be infused in 12 hours for a patient who weighs 75 kg. The abciximab label reads 2 mg/mL. Calculate the flow rate in milliliters per hour.

## Comprehensive Self-Test 2

1. A patient has an IV of 250 mL D5RL with 25,000 units of heparin infusing at 20 mL/h. How many units of heparin is the patient receiving each hour?

2. Order:

> *Alkeran (melphalan HCl) 16 mg/m² 100 mL NS IV q2 weeks*
> *for four doses infuse in 20 min*

The package insert states to rapidly inject 10 mL of supplied diluent into a 50 mg vial and shake vigorously until a clear solution results (5 mg/mL). The patient has a BSA of 1.2 m².
(a) How many milligrams contain the dose?
(b) How many milliliters of Alkeran will you add to 100 mL of NS?
(c) Determine the flow rate in mL/h.

3. A patient is receiving Zantac (ranitidine HCl) 150 mg PO b.i.d. The label reads 150 mg tablets. How many tablets will the patient receive in 24 hours?

4. Order:

> *Lanoxicaps (digoxin solution in capsules) 0.1 mg PO b.i.d.*

The label on the bottle reads 50 mcg/capsule. How many capsules will you give the patient?

5. Order:

> *protamine sulfate 22 mg IVP over 10 min*

The label reads 50 mg/5 mL. Dilute with 20 mL of NS or D5W. How many milliliters of protamine sulfate will you prepare?

6. Order:

> *Garamycin (gentamicin sulfate) 9 mg IM q12h*

The package insert states that the recommended dose for neonates is 2.5 mg/kg q 12–24h. The label on the vial reads Pediatric Injectable Garamycin 10 mg/mL. The infant weighs 10 lb.
(a) Is the dose safe?
(b) How many milliliters will you give?

7. An IV of D5/NS (1,000 mL) is infusing at 50 mL/h. The infusion started at 1300h; what time will it finish?

8. The prescriber ordered Dilantin (phenytoin sodium) 250 mg/m² per day in three divided doses for a child who has a BSA of 1.25 m². The bottle is labeled 125 mg/5 mL oral suspension. How many milliliters will you give for each dose?

9. Order:

> *Lasix (furosemide) 20 mg IM stat*

The label reads 40 mg/4 mL.
(a) How many milliliters will you give the patient?
(b) Place an arrow on the syringe that indicates the dose.

10. The recommended dose of Cleocin (clindamycin) pediatric oral solution is 8 to 25 mg/kg/day in three to four equally divided doses. A child weighs 60 pounds.
    (a) Calculate the minimum safe daily dose in mg/d.
    (b) Calculate the maximum safe daily dose in mg/d.

11. Calculate how many grams of sodium chloride are in 250 mL of a 0.9% NaCl solution.

12. A patient has an IV infusing at 25 gtt/min. How many mL/h is the patient receiving? The drop factor is 15 gtt/mL.

13. Calculate the total volume and hourly IV flow rate for a 10-pound infant who is receiving maintenance fluids.

14. Order:

    *nitroprusside sodium 50 mg in 250 mL D$_5$W infuse at 1 mL/h*

    The recommended dosage range is 0.1 to 5 mcg/kg/min. The patient weighs 154 pounds. Is this a safe dose?

15. A patient with aspiration pneumonia has an order for aminophylline IVPB 250 mg in 250 mL D5W to Infuse at 0.5 mg/kg/h. The patient weighs 80 kg. What is the flow rate in mL/h?

16. Your patient has an IV of Humulin R insulin 50 units in 500 mL of NS infusing at 12 units per hour. Calculate the flow rate in mL/h.

17. Order:

    *Ticar (ticarcillin disodium) 1 g IM q6h*

    The package insert states to reconstitute each 1g vial with 2 mL of sterile water for injection. Each 2.5 mL = 1g. How many milliliters will you administer?

18. Order:

    *Indocin SR (indomethacin) 150 mg PO t.i.d. for 7 days*

    The label reads Indocin SR 75 mg capsules.
    (a) How many capsules will you give the patient for each dose?
    (b) Calculate the entire 7 day dosage in grams.

19. Order:

    *Colace (docusate sodium) syrup 100 mg via PEG t.i.d.*

    The label reads 50 mg/15 mL. How many mL will you give?

20. Order:

    *theophylline 0.8 mg/kg/h IV via pump*

    The premixed IV bag is labeled theophylline 800 mg in 250 mL D$_5$W. The patient weighs 185 pounds. How many mL/h will you set the pump?

21. Order:

    *cefazolin 1 g IVPB q6h, add to 50 mL D5W and infuse over 20 minutes*

    Read the reconstitution information from the cefazolin label in ● **Figure S.4.**

| Total Amount of Diluent | Approximate Concentration |
|---|---|
| 45 mL | 1 g/5 mL |
| 96 mL | 1 g/10 mL |

● **Figure S.4**
**Reconstitution information from the cefazolin label.**

(a) How many milliliters of diluent will you add to the vial, so that 1 gram of cefazolin is contained in 5 mL of the solution?

(b) Based on the answer in part (a), calculate the flow rate in milliliters per minute.

22. The nurse has prepared 7 mg of dexamethasone for IV administration. The label on the vial reads 10 mg/mL. How many milliliters did the nurse prepare?

23. Order:

   *Cogentin (benztropine mesylate) 2 mg IM stat and then 1 mg IM daily*

   The label reads 2 mg/2 mL.
   (a) How many milliliters will you administer daily?
   (b) What size syringe will you use?

24. Order:

   $\frac{2}{3}$ *strength Sustacal 900 mL via PEG, give over 8h*

   How will you prepare this solution?

25. An IV of 250 mL NS is infusing at 25 mL/h. The infusion began at 1800h. What time will it be completed?

# Comprehensive Self-Test 3

1. An IV is infusing at 35 gtt/min. How many milliliters will the patient receive in 6 hours? The drop factor is 10 gtt/mL.

2. Order:

   *Augmentin (amoxicillin clavulanate potassium)*
   *200 mg oral suspension PO q12h*

   The label reads 125 mg/5 ml. How many milliliters will you administer?

3. The prescriber ordered neomycin sulfate 8.75 mg/kg PO q6h for an infant with infectious diarrhea. The vial is labeled 125 mg/5 mL. The infant weighs 8 pounds. How many milliliters will you administer?

4. Order:

   *heparin 40,000 units in 1,000 mL NS, infuse at 40 mL/h*

   The normal heparinizing range is 20,000–40,000 units q24h. Calculate the units/h and determine if the dose is safe.

5. Order:

>   *Amicar (aminocaproic acid) 3g/m² IV,*
>       *add to 250 mL NS and infuse via pump over 1h*

The patient weighs 30 pounds and is 32 inches tall.
(a) How many mg is the child receiving?
(b) At what rate will you set the pump in mL/h?

6. A prescriber ordered 1,350 mg of a drug q2h prn pain. The label reads 675 mg/5 mL. What is the maximum number of milliliters that the patient may receive in 24 hours?

7. A patient is to receive 3,500 units of heparin subcutaneously. The label reads 10,000 units/mL.
(a) How many milliliters will you administer?
(b) What type of syringe will you use?

8. Order:

>   *Epivir (lamivudine) oral solution 150 mg PO b.i.d.*

The recommended safe dose is 4 mg/kg b.i.d. Is this a safe dose for a child who weighs 42 pounds?

9. Order:

>   *Mandol (cefamandole nafate)750 mg IM q8h*

The instructions on the 1g vial state reconstitute with 3 mL of sterile water for injection. The resulting solution is 285 mg/mL.
(a) How many milliliters will you administer?
(b) What size syringe will you use?

10. Order:

>   *potassium chloride 40 mEq PO daily*

The label reads potassium chloride 20 mEq per 15 mL. How many milliliters will you administer?

11. Calculate the hourly IV flow rate and total daily IV fluid volume for a child who is NPO, weighs 15 pounds, and is receiving maintenance fluids.

12. Order:

>   *Novolin R regular insulin 24 units and Novolin N NPH*
>       *insulin 17 units subcutaneous ac breakfast*

Draw an arrow on the syringe indicating the dose of each of the insulins.

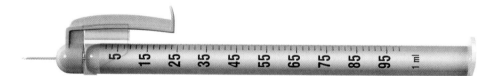

13. A patient who is 160 cm tall and weighs 60 kg is to receive Intron A (interferon alpha-2b) 20,000 units/m². How many units contain this dose?

14. Order:

>   *Unipen (nafcillin sodium) oral solution 500 mg PO q4h*

The label reads 250 mg/5 mL. How many milliliters will you give the patient?

15. A patient is receiving an IV of 1,000 mL of D5W with 15 mEq of KCL for 24 hours. Calculate the flow rate in mL/h.

16. A patient is receiving TPN 1,500 mL at a rate of 65 mL/h via pump. The infusion began at 0600. What time will it be finished?

17. Order:

    *Myambutol (ethambutol HCl)15 mg/kg PO daily*

    The label reads 400 mg tablets. How many tablets will you give the patient who weighs 178 pounds?

18. A patient is receiving Zyloprim (allopurinol) 300 mg PO daily. What is the total number of grams per day?

19. Order:

    *Pitocin (oxytocin) 20 units IV in LR 1,000 mL via pump*

    Start at *1* milliunit/min, increase by *1* milliunit q *15–30* min to a maximum of *20* milliunits/min. What rate will you set the infusion pump in mL/h to begin the infusion?

20. Calculate how many grams of sodium chloride are contained in 1,000 mL of $D_5$ 1/3 NS.

21. Order:

    *heparin 750 units subcutaneously daily*

    The vial is labeled 1,000 units/mL. What size syringe will you use?

22. A patient has an IV of 0.9% sodium chloride infusing at 75 mL/h. Calculate the flow rate in microdrops per minute.

23. Order:

    *Decadron (dexamethasone) 1.5 mg PO daily*

    The label reads 0.75 mg tablets. How many tablets will you give?

24. Calculate the body surface area for a child who is 28 inches tall and weighs 30 pounds.

25. Calculate the daily fluid maintenance needs for a child who weighs 13.6 kg.

# Comprehensive Self-Test 4

1. Order:

    *Adriamycin PFS (doxorubicin HCl) 80 mg IV once q21days*

    The package insert states that the recommended dose for use as a single agent is 60–75 mg/m$^2$ repeat every 3 weeks. Is this a safe dose for a patient who weighs 39 kg and is 51 inches tall?

2. Order:

    *Biaxin (clarithromycin) oral suspension 7.5 mg/kg PO q12h*

    The label reads 250 mg/5 mL. How many milliliters will you give a child who weighs 40 pounds?

3. Order:

*nitroglycerine 0.6 mg SL stat*

The label reads 0.3 mg tablets. How many tablets will you give the patient?

4. A patient has an IV of 1,000 mL LR infusing at 125 mL/h. How many hours will it take to infuse?

5. Calculate the daily fluid maintenance needs for an infant who weighs 2,500 g.

6. Order:

*Dilaudid-HP (hydromorphone HCl) 4 mg IM stat*

The label reads 10 mg/mL.
(a) How many milliliters will you administer?
(b) What size syringe will you use?

7. Order:

*Synthroid (levothroxine sodium) 50 mcg PO daily*

How many milligrams is the patient receiving?

8. Order:

*Procardia (nifedipine) 20 mg PO t.i.d.*

Read the label in ● **Figure S.5** and calculate how many capsules of this calcium channel-blocker drug the patient is receiving daily.

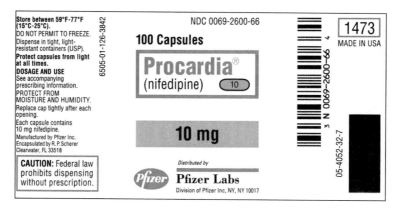

● **Figure S.5**
**Drug label for Procardia.**
*(Reg. Trademark of Pfizer Inc. Reproduced with permission.)*

9. Order:

*atropine sulfate 0.4 mg IM on call to OR*

The label reads 1 mg/mL. How many milliliters will you give the patient?

10. Order:

*Sandostatin (octreotide acetate) 200 mcg subcutaneously q.i.d*

The label reads 1 mg/mL. How many milliliters will you administer?

11. Order:

    *Normodyne (labetalol HCl) 20 mg IVP slowly over 2 min*

    The label reads 5 mg/mL. How many milliliters of this antihypertensive drug will the patient receive per minute?

12. Order:

    *lidocaine 1 g in 250 mL D5W infuse at 3 mg/min*

    Calculate the pump setting in mL/h.

13. Order:

    *Zantac (ranitidine) 50 mg in 100 mL D$_5$ W IVPB q8h, infuse in 20 min*

    Calculate the flow rate in milliliters per minute.

14. Calculate the flow rate in mL/h if heparin is to be infused at the rate of 2,000 units per hour. The solution strength is heparin 50,000 units in 1,000 mL D5W.

15. Order:

    *Pfizerpen (penicillin G potassium) 350,000 units IM b.i.d.*

    The label reads 500,000 units/1.8 mL.
    (a) How many milliliters will you give the patient?
    (b) What size syringe will you use?

16. Calculate the amount of dextrose and sodium chloride in 500 mL of D5/$\frac{1}{3}$ NS.

17. An infusion of D$_5$W has 800 milliliters left in the bag. The flow rate is 31 drops per minute, and the drop factor is 15 gtt/mL. How long will it take for the remainder of this IV fluid to infuse?

18. Order:

    *Mutamycin (mitomycin-C) 20 mg/m$^2$ IV once q6weeks*

    Calculate the dose for a patient who has a BSA of 1.62 m$^2$.

19. Calculate the total daily fluid maintenance for a child who weighs 26 pounds.

20. Order:

    *Tagamet (cimetidine) 250 mg IVPB q6h*

    The recommended dose is 5 to 10 mg/kg q6h. Is this a safe dose for a child who weighs 80 pounds?

21. Order:

    *Humulin R regular insulin 300 units in 150 mL NS infuse at 10 mL/h*

    How many units/h is the patient receiving?

22. Order:

    *heparin 5,000 units subcutaneous q12h*

    The label reads 10,000 units/mL. How many milliliters will you give the patient?

23. Order:

*Ancef (cefazolin) 500 mg IM q8h*

The directions for the 1 g vial state: reconstitute with 2.5 mL of sterile water for injection and 330 mg/mL. How many milliliters will you give the patient?

24. Order:

*Proventil (albuterol) syrup 4 mg daily*

The label reads Proventil (albuterol sulfate) syrup 2 mg per 5 mL. How many milliliters will you administer?

25. A prescriber ordered Vancocin (vancomycin HCl) 500 mg PO q6h for a child who weighs 110 pounds. The package insert states that the recommended child's dose is 40 mg/kg/d in three or four divided doses. Is the prescribed dose safe?

# Appendices

# Appendix A

## Diagnostic Test of Arithmetic

1. $\frac{3}{8}$  

2. 0.285  

3. 6.5  

4. 0.83

5. 3.2  

6. 3.8  

7. 0.0639  

8. 500

9. 2  

10. $\frac{1}{4}$ and 0.25  

11. $2\frac{1}{3}$  

12. $\frac{1}{25}$

13. $\frac{9}{20}$  

14. 0.025  

15. $\frac{18}{7}$  

16. 12

17. 7.6  

18. 6  

19. 0.4  

20. $\frac{3}{4}$

## Chapter 1

### Try These for Practice

1. 0.3125  

2. 74.4  

3. 0.4 and $\frac{2}{5}$

4. $\frac{1}{3}$  

5. 2

### Exercises

1. $0.85 = \dfrac{85 \div 5}{100 \div 5} = \dfrac{17}{20}$

2. $2\dfrac{1}{2} + 3\dfrac{1}{4} = 2\dfrac{2}{4} + 3\dfrac{1}{4} = 5\dfrac{3}{4}$

3. $\dfrac{\overset{5}{\cancel{40}}}{1} \times \dfrac{1}{2} \times \dfrac{9}{\underset{2}{\cancel{16}}} = \dfrac{45}{4} = 11\dfrac{1}{4}$

4. $2\dfrac{3}{5} \div \dfrac{2}{1} = \dfrac{13}{5} \times \dfrac{1}{2} = \dfrac{13}{10} = 1\dfrac{3}{10}$

5. $\dfrac{15}{1} \div \dfrac{11}{3} = \dfrac{15}{1} \times \dfrac{3}{11} = \dfrac{45}{11} = 4\dfrac{1}{11}$

6. $9.6 \div \dfrac{3}{7} = \dfrac{9.6}{1} \times \dfrac{7}{3} = \dfrac{67.2}{3} = 22.4 = 22\dfrac{2}{5}$

7. $\dfrac{\overset{14}{\cancel{42}}}{1} \times \dfrac{1}{\underset{3150}{\cancel{9450}}} \times \dfrac{3}{0.02} = \dfrac{42}{63} = \dfrac{2}{3}$

8.
$$
\begin{array}{r}
.125 \\
8\overline{)1.000} \\
\underline{8\phantom{.000}} \\
20 \\
\underline{16} \\
40 \\
\underline{40} \\
0
\end{array}
\approx 0.12
$$

9.
$$
\begin{array}{r}
.56 \\
25\overline{)14.00} \\
\underline{12\,5} \\
1\,50 \\
\underline{1\,50} \\
0
\end{array}
\quad 0.56
$$

10. $5\dfrac{3}{10} = 5.3$

11. 
$$200\overline{)1.000}$$ 
.005
  
1 000
  
0   0.005

12. 
$$75\overline{)1.000}$$ 
.013 ≈ 0.01
  
75
  
250
  
225
  
25

13. $\dfrac{870}{1000} = 8\underset{\smile\smile\smile}{7\,0} = 0.87$

14. $\dfrac{2.73}{100} = \underset{\smile\smile}{273} = 0.0273$

15. 
$$7\overline{)14.36}$$ 
2.05 ≈ 2.0
  
14
  
0 3
  
0
  
36
  
35
  
1

16. 
$$0.9\overline{)0.63}$$ 
.7   0.7
  
63
  
0

17. 
$$0.09\overline{)0.063}$$ 
.7   0.7
  
63
  
0

18. $5\frac{1}{2}\% = 5 \cdot 5\% = \underset{\shortmid\;\shortmid}{5 \cdot 5} = 0.055$

19. $55\% = \underset{\smile}{5\,5} = 0.55$

20. 
```
      4.63
   ×  6.21
   ───────
      4 63
      92 6
     2778
   ────────
    28.7523  ≈ 28.75
```

21. $0.\underset{\smile\smile}{0\,0\,4} = 0.4$

22. $2 . \underset{\smile\smile\smile}{3\,4\,5\,6} = 2{,}345.6$

23. 
$$0.03\overline{).8500}$$ 
28.33 ≈ 28.3
  
6
  
25
  
24
  
10
  
9
  
10
  
9
  
1

24. 
$$0.12\overline{)8.50000}$$ 
70.833 ≈ 70.83
  
8 4
  
10
  
0
  
100
  
96
  
40
  
36
  
40
  
36
  
4

25. $0.72 \times \dfrac{1}{0.7} = \dfrac{0.72}{0.7} \Rightarrow$ 
$$.7\overline{).720}$$ 
1.02 ≈ 1.0
  
7
  
02
  
0
  
20
  
14
  
6

$\dfrac{0.72 \times 100}{0.7 \times 100} = \dfrac{72}{70} = 1\dfrac{2}{70}$

$1\dfrac{2}{70}$ and 1.0

26. $\dfrac{\frac{2}{3}}{8} = 2 \div \dfrac{3}{8} = \dfrac{2}{1} \times \dfrac{8}{3} = \dfrac{16}{3} = 5\dfrac{1}{3}$

$\begin{array}{r} 5.33 \\ 3\overline{)16.00} \end{array} \approx 5.3$

$\underline{15}$

$1\ 0$

$\underline{\ \ 9}$

$10$

$\underline{\ \ 9}$

$1$

$5\dfrac{1}{3}$ and 5.3

27. $\dfrac{\frac{2}{5}}{100} \times \dfrac{\cancel{500}}{6} = \dfrac{\frac{2}{5} \times \frac{\cancel{5}}{1}}{6} = \dfrac{2}{6} = \dfrac{1}{3}$

$\begin{array}{r} .33 \\ 3\overline{)1.00} \end{array} \approx 0.3$

$\underline{\ \ 9}$

$10$

$\underline{\ \ 9}$

$1$

$\dfrac{1}{3}$ and 0.3

28. $\dfrac{26 \times \frac{5}{13}}{\frac{9}{100}} = \dfrac{26}{1} \times \dfrac{5}{13} \div \dfrac{9}{100} = \dfrac{\overset{2}{\cancel{26}}}{1} \times \dfrac{5}{\underset{1}{\cancel{13}}} \times \dfrac{100}{9} = \dfrac{1{,}000}{9}$

$\begin{array}{r} 111 \\ 9\overline{)1{,}000} \end{array} \Rightarrow 111\dfrac{1}{9}$

$\underline{\ \ 9}$

$10$

$\underline{\ \ 9}$

$10$

$\underline{\ \ 9}$

$1$

$\begin{array}{r} .11 \\ 9\overline{)1.00} \end{array}$  $111\dfrac{1}{9} \approx 111.11 \approx 111.1$

$\underline{\ \ 9}$

$10$

$\underline{\ \ 9}$

$1$

$111\dfrac{1}{9}$ and 111.1

29. $10.3\% = 10.3 = 0.103 \approx 0.1$

$0.103 = \dfrac{103}{1{,}000}$

$\dfrac{103}{1{,}000}$ and 0.1

30. $99.5\% = 99.5 = 0.995 \approx 1.0$

$0.995 = \dfrac{995 \div 5}{1{,}000 \div 5} = \dfrac{199}{200}$

$\dfrac{199}{200}$ and 1.0

31. $\dfrac{25}{40} = \dfrac{25 \div 5}{40 \div 5} = \dfrac{5}{8}$ 

32. $\dfrac{60}{90} = \dfrac{6\cancel{0}}{9\cancel{0}} = \dfrac{6 \div 3}{9 \div 3} = \dfrac{2}{3}$

33. $\dfrac{3}{7} = \dfrac{3 \times 3}{7 \times 3} = \dfrac{9}{21}$   answer is 9

34. $\dfrac{6}{11} = \dfrac{6 \times 5}{11 \times 5} = \dfrac{30}{55}$   answer is 30

35.  $\begin{array}{r} 0.30 \\ 2.00 \\ +2.55 \\ \hline 4.85 \end{array}$

36.  $\begin{array}{r} 2.56 \\ -1.93 \\ \hline 0.63 \end{array}$

37. $\left.\begin{array}{l} 0.370 \\ 0.244 \end{array}\right\}$ answer is 0.37

38. $0.30 \times 500 = 150$

39. $\dfrac{\text{change}}{\text{old}} = \dfrac{1}{4} = 25\%$ increase

40. $\dfrac{\text{change}}{\text{old}} = \dfrac{60}{300} = \dfrac{1}{5} = 20\%$ decrease

# Chapter 2

## Try These for Practice

1. PO (orally)
2. 1,000
3. 400 mg
4. Depakene
5. lopinavir 80 mg and ritonavir 20 mg

## Exercises

1. lopinavir/ritonavir
2. Singulair
3. 160 mL
4. 400 mg/5 mL
5. 40 mg per tablet
6. (a) Anusol supp
   (b) 6 A.M.
   (c) 4
   (d) Bonivar, Humulin N, Humulin R
   (e) December 16
7. (a) digoxin, Lasix
   (b) Reglan
   (c) 10 mg PO
   (d) transdermal
   (e) Omnicef
8. (a) 2 mg to 10 mg, 3 or 4 times daily
   (b) periodic blood counts and liver function tests
   (c) 5 mg/5 mL
   (d) 0054-3185-44
9. 9 A.M.–0900h
   3 P.M.–1500h
   Noon–1200h
   6 P.M.–1800h
   8:15 P.M.–2015h

2:30 A.M.–0230h

4:45 P.M.–1645h

6 A.M.–0600h

Midnight–0000h

10. (a) digoxin twenty-five hundredths milligram, by mouth daily, do not give if the heart rate is less than 60

   (b) Toradol (ketorolac) 15 milligrams intravenous push every six hours for four doses

   (c) Milk of Magnesia 30 milliliters by mouth each day whenever necessary (or as needed) for constipation

   (d) ibuprofen 800 milligrams by mouth three times a day

   (e) Novolin Regular insulin 5 units subcutaneously immediately

11. (a) Missing prescriber's name and route of administration

   (b) Missing date, and time order was written

   (c) Missing time order was written, frequency of administration, and prescriber's name

   (d) Missing date order was written, and frequency of administration

   (e) Missing dosage of medication

# Chapter 3

## Try These for Practice

1. 270 min
2. 115 oz
3. 252 h
4. 6 qt/h
5. 1.1 lb/wk

## Exercises

1. $\dfrac{1.5}{x} = \dfrac{1}{60} \Rightarrow x = 90$ sec
2. $\dfrac{5.5}{x} = \dfrac{1}{12} \Rightarrow x = 66$ mon

3. $\dfrac{4\frac{1}{4}}{x} = \dfrac{1}{24} \Rightarrow x = 102$ h
4. $\dfrac{40}{x} = \dfrac{16}{1} \Rightarrow 16x = 40 \Rightarrow x = 2.5$ lb

5. $\dfrac{\frac{3}{4}}{x} = \dfrac{1}{60} \Rightarrow x = 45$ min
6. $\dfrac{51}{x} = \dfrac{12}{1} \Rightarrow 12x = 51 \Rightarrow x = 4\frac{1}{4}$ yr

7. $\dfrac{3}{x} = \dfrac{1}{2} \Rightarrow x = 6$ pt
8. $\dfrac{3\ \text{lb}}{x} = \dfrac{1}{16} \Rightarrow x = 48$ oz

9. Since 12 in = 1 ft, $\dfrac{12\ \text{in}}{\text{sec}} = \dfrac{1\ \text{ft}}{\text{sec}}$

10. Since 1 min = 60 sec,

$\dfrac{30\ \text{pt}}{\text{min}} = \dfrac{30\ \text{pt}}{60\ \text{sec}} \Rightarrow \dfrac{1}{2}$ pt/sec

11. $\dfrac{8}{x} = \dfrac{1}{16} \Rightarrow x = 128$ oz + 10 oz = 138 oz

12. $\dfrac{6}{x} = \dfrac{1}{12} \Rightarrow x = 72$ in $+ 4$ in $= 76$ in

13. $\dfrac{4}{x} = \dfrac{1}{3} \Rightarrow x = 12$ ft

$\dfrac{12}{x} = \dfrac{1}{12} \Rightarrow x = 144$ in

14. $\dfrac{42}{x} = \dfrac{12}{1} \Rightarrow 12x = 42 \Rightarrow x = 3.5$ ft

15. $\dfrac{2700 \text{ sec}}{x \text{ min}} = \dfrac{60 \text{ sec}}{1 \text{ min}} \Rightarrow 60\,x = 2700$

$x = 45$ min

$\dfrac{45 \text{ min}}{x \text{ hr}} = \dfrac{60 \text{ min}}{1 \text{ hr}} \Rightarrow 60\,x = 45$

$x = \dfrac{3}{4}$ hr

16. $\dfrac{6 \text{ pt}}{\text{h}} = \dfrac{6 \times 24 \text{ pt}}{1 \times 24 \text{ h}} = \dfrac{144 \text{ pt}}{24 \text{ h}} = \dfrac{144 \text{ pt}}{\text{d}}$

$\dfrac{144}{x} = \dfrac{2}{1} \Rightarrow 2x = 144 \Rightarrow x = 72$ qt

$\dfrac{6 \text{ pt}}{\text{h}} = \dfrac{72 \text{ qt}}{\text{d}}$

17. $\dfrac{6}{x} \times \dfrac{1}{2} \Rightarrow x = 12$ pt

$\dfrac{6 \text{ qt}}{\text{d}} = \dfrac{12 \text{ pt}}{1 \text{ d}}$ but $1$ d $= 24$ h

$\dfrac{6 \text{ qt}}{\text{d}} = \dfrac{12 \text{ pt}}{24 \text{ h}} = \dfrac{1}{2}$ pt/h

18. $\dfrac{1680 \text{ h}}{x \text{ d}} = \dfrac{24 \text{ h}}{1 \text{ d}}$

$24x = 1680$

$x = 70$ d

$\dfrac{70 \text{ d}}{x \text{ wk}} = \dfrac{7 \text{ d}}{1 \text{ wk}}$

$7x = 70 \Rightarrow x = 10$ wk

19. $\dfrac{1{,}209{,}600 \text{ sec}}{x \text{ min}} = \dfrac{60 \text{ sec}}{1 \text{ min}}$

$60x = 1{,}209{,}600 \Rightarrow x = 20{,}160$ min

$\dfrac{20{,}160 \text{ min}}{x \text{ h}} = \dfrac{60 \text{ min}}{1 \text{ h}} \Rightarrow 60x = 20{,}160 \Rightarrow x = 336$ h

$\dfrac{336 \text{ h}}{x \text{ d}} = \dfrac{24 \text{ h}}{1 \text{ d}} \Rightarrow 24x = 336 \Rightarrow x = 14$ d

$\dfrac{14 \text{ d}}{x \text{ wk}} = \dfrac{7 \text{ d}}{1 \text{ wk}} \Rightarrow 7x = 14 \Rightarrow x = 2$ wk

20. $\dfrac{5 \text{ cases}}{x \text{ cans}} = \dfrac{1 \text{ case}}{24 \text{ cans}} \implies x = 120 \text{ cans}$

$\dfrac{120 \text{ cans}}{x \text{ oz}} = \dfrac{1 \text{ can}}{12 \text{ oz}} \implies x = 1440 \text{ oz}$

$\dfrac{1440 \text{ oz}}{x \text{ cup}} = \dfrac{60 \text{ oz}}{1 \text{ cup}} \implies 60x = 1440 \implies x = 24 \text{ cups}$

# Chapter 4

## Try These for Practice

1. (a) 1,000 mL          (f) 1,000 mcg          (k) 8 oz
   (b) 1 cc              (g) 10 mm              (l) 2 T
   (c) 1,000 cm$^3$      (h) 2 pt               (m) 3 t
   (d) 1,000 g           (i) 2 cups             (n) 12 in
   (e) 1,000 mg          (j) 8 oz               (o) 16 oz

2. 0.01 g          3. 5,000 mcg          4. 1.8 L          5. 3 pt

## Exercises

1. 400 mg = 4 0 0 . mg = 0.4 g

2. 0.003 g = 0. 0 0 3 g = 3 mg

3. 0.07 g = 0. 0 7 0 = 70 mg

4. 3 L = 3. 0 0 0 L = 3,000 mL

5. 2,500 mL = 2 5 0 0 . mL = 2.5 L

6. 600 mcg = 6 0 0 . mcg = 0.6 mg

7. 1.7 L = 1. 7 0 0 L = 1,700 mL

8. $\dfrac{1 \text{ qt}}{2 \text{ pt}} = \dfrac{4.5 \text{ qt}}{x \text{ pt}} \implies x = 9 \text{ pt}$

9. 2.5 kg = 2 . 5 0 0 kg = 2,500 g

10. $\dfrac{1 \text{ T}}{3 \text{ t}} = \dfrac{4 \text{ T}}{x \text{ t}} \implies x = 12 \text{ t}$

11. $\dfrac{5 \text{ T}}{x \text{ oz}} = \dfrac{2 \text{ T}}{1 \text{ oz}} \implies 2x = 5 \implies x = 2\frac{1}{2} \text{ oz}$

12. $\dfrac{32 \text{ oz}}{x \text{ pt}} = \dfrac{16 \text{ oz}}{1 \text{ pt}} \implies 16x = 32 \implies x = 2 \text{ pt}$

13. 125 mg = 125. 0 0 0 mg = 125,000 mcg

14. 520 mcg = 5 2 0 . mcg = 0.52 mg

15. 50 mg = 0 5 0 . mg = 0.05 g

16. $\dfrac{\frac{1}{2} \text{ pt}}{2 \text{ h}} = \dfrac{x \text{ pt}}{8 \text{ h}} \implies 2x = 4 \implies x = 2 \text{ pt} = 1 \text{ qt}$

17. 100 mg = 1 0 0 . mg = 0.1 g

18. 3,400 g = 3 4 0 0 . g = 3.4 kg

19. 2.1 cm = 2 . 1 cm = 21 mm

20. $\dfrac{5 \text{ ft}}{x \text{ in}} = \dfrac{1 \text{ ft}}{12 \text{ in}} \implies x = 60 \text{ in}$

## Cumulative Review Exercises

1. 7,800 mg
2. 250 mcg
3. 4,500 mL
4. 6 oz
5. 1.2 L
6. 7,600 g
7. 0.75 L
8. 15 t
9. 1,000 mg
10. 0.25 g
11. 650 mcg
12. 6 t
13. 15 mL
14. 0.25 L
15. 32 mg

# Chapter 5

## Try These for Practice

1. (a) 1,000 mL   (i) 8 oz   (q) 15 mL
   (b) 1,000 g   (j) 2 T   (r) 30 mL
   (c) 1,000 mg   (k) 3 t   (s) 240 mL
   (d) 1,000 mcg   (l) 16 oz   (t) 240 mL
   (e) 10 mm   (m) 12 in   (u) 500 mL
   (f) 2 pt   (n) 2.5 cm   (v) 1,000 mL
   (g) 2 cups   (o) 2.2 lb   (w) 2 T = 6 t ≈ 30 mL
   (h) 8 oz   (p) 5 mL   (x) 2 pt = 4 cups = 32 oz ≈ 1,000 mL

2. 0.025 g   3. 110 lb   4. 1 t   5. 1.6 in by 2 in

## Exercises

1. 4.5 0 0 mg = 4.5 mg

2. 1 . 5 0 0 mL = 1,500 mL

3. $\dfrac{4\ t}{x\ mL} = \dfrac{1\ t}{5\ mL} \Rightarrow x = 20\ mL$

4. $\dfrac{15\ mL}{x\ t} = \dfrac{5\ mL}{1\ t} \Rightarrow 5x = 15 \quad x = 3\ t$

5. $\dfrac{45\ kg}{x\ lb} = \dfrac{1\ kg}{2.2\ lb} \Rightarrow x = 99\ lb$

6. $\dfrac{110\ lb}{x\ kg} = \dfrac{2.2\ lb}{1\ kg} \Rightarrow 2.2x = 110 \Rightarrow x = 50\ kg$

7. $\dfrac{48\ oz}{x\ pt} = \dfrac{16\ oz}{1\ pt} \Rightarrow 16x = 48 \Rightarrow x = 3\ pt$

8. $\dfrac{3\ oz}{x\ T} = \dfrac{1\ oz}{2\ T} \Rightarrow x = 6\ T$

9. $\dfrac{10\ cm}{x\ in} = \dfrac{2.5\ cm}{1\ in} \Rightarrow 2.5x = 10 \Rightarrow x = 4\ in$

10. $\dfrac{6\ in}{x\ cm} = \dfrac{1\ in}{2.5\ cm} \Rightarrow x = 15\ cm$

11. 72 in + 2 in = 74 in   $\dfrac{74\ in}{x\ cm} = \dfrac{1\ in}{2.5\ cm} \Rightarrow x = 185\ cm$

12. 10 gm = 1 mL   $\dfrac{1\ mL}{x\ oz} = \dfrac{30\ mL}{1\ oz} \Rightarrow 30x = 1 \Rightarrow x = \dfrac{1}{30}\ oz$

13. $\dfrac{165\ lb}{x\ kg} = \dfrac{2.2\ lb}{1\ kg} \Rightarrow 2.2\ lb = 165 \Rightarrow x = 75\ kg$

14. $\dfrac{2\ t}{x\ mL} = \dfrac{1\ t}{5\ mL} \Rightarrow x = 10\ mL$   15. $\dfrac{30\ mL}{x\ T} = \dfrac{15\ mL}{1\ T} \Rightarrow 15x = 30 \Rightarrow x = 2\ T$

16. 10 mg = 5 mL = 1 t               17. $\dfrac{12 \text{ oz}}{x \text{ mL}} = \dfrac{1 \text{ oz}}{30 \text{ mL}}$     $x = 360$ mL

18. 1 blister = 250 mcg = . 2 5 0 mg = 0.25 mg

19. $\dfrac{120 \text{ sprays}}{x \text{ mcg}} = \dfrac{1 \text{ spray}}{32 \text{ mcg}}$     $x = 3{,}840$ mcg

   3840 mcg = 3 . 8 4 0 mg = 3.84 mg

20. 1 tab = 10 mg = 1 0 0 0 0 . mcg = 10,000 mcg

## Cumulative Review Exercises

1. 125 mcg                    2. 9 mg                    3. 5,650 g

4. 60 mg                      5. 7,750 mL                6. 1.25 L

7. 2,500 g = 2,500,000 mg = 2,500,000,000 mcg = 5.5 lb = 88 oz

8. 1,740 mL                   9. 15.2 in                 10. 7 qt

11. 160 mL                    12. 0.15 g                 13. 0.01 g

14. 36 doses                  15. 0.09 g

# Chapter 6

## Case Study 6.1

1. 500 mL
2. (a) 360 mL
   (b) 0.585 g
   (c) 1,415 mg
3. (a) 4 tab
   (b) 7 tab
4. 100 mEq
5. (a) 3 times per day
   (b) 150 mL
6. 3 tab
7. one 200-mcg tab and one 50-mcg tab
8. (a) 875 mg
   (b) $3\frac{1}{2}$ tab

## Practice Reading Labels

1. 750 mg/tab, 1 tab          2. 20 mg/cap, 2 cap

3. 333 mg/tab, 2 tab          4. 80 mg/mL, 0.25 mL

5. 50 mg/5 mL, 10 mL          6. 500 mcg/2 mL, 0.5 mL

7. 80 mg/mL, 1.6 mL           8. 500 mcg/2 mL, 1.6 mL

9. 25 mg/5 mL, 20 mL          10. 2.5 mg/tab, 4 tab

11. 2 mg/cap, 2 cap           12. 100 mg/5 ml, 20 mL

13. 600 mg/tab, 1 tab  
14. 100 mg/tab, 2 tab  
15. 2.5 mg/tab, 4 tab  
16. 2.5 mg/tab, 2 tab  
17. 40 mg/tab, 2 tab  
18. 200 mg/5 mL, 12.5 mL  
19. 10 mg/tab, 5 tab  
20. 8 mg/tab, 2 tab  
21. 500 mg/tab, 1 tab  
22. 20 mg/tab, 1 tab  
23. 25 mg/5 mL, 15 mL  
24. 20 mg/tab, 4 tab  
25. 250 mg/tab, 2 tab

## Try These for Practice

1. (a) 3 tablets  
   (b) 0.06 g  
2. 86 mg  
3. 40 mL  
4. 6 capsules  
5. One 50 mg and two 15 mg tablets

## Exercises

1. 20 mg + 30 mg = 50 mg  
   Administer one 20-mg and one 30-mg tablet.

2. 500 mcg = 5 0 0 . mcg = 0.5 mg  
$$\frac{0.5 \text{ mg}}{x \text{ mL}} = \frac{0.05 \text{ mg}}{1 \text{ mL}} \Rightarrow 10 \text{ mL}$$

3. 40 mg daily for 28 days = 1,120 mg  
$$\frac{1,120 \text{ mg}}{x \text{ cap}} = \frac{10 \text{ mg}}{1 \text{ cap}} \Rightarrow 112 \text{ cap}$$

4. $\dfrac{75 \text{ mg}}{x \text{ tab}} = \dfrac{25 \text{ mg}}{1 \text{ tab}} \Rightarrow$ 3 tab per dose  
   or 9 tab per 24 hours.

5. 1 tab daily for 7 days = 7 tab

6. $40 \text{ kg} \times \dfrac{50 \text{ mg}}{\text{kg}} = 2,000 \text{ mg}$  
$$\frac{2000 \text{ mg}}{x \text{ tab}} = \frac{500 \text{ mg}}{1 \text{ tab}} \Rightarrow 4 \text{ tab/d} = 2 \text{ tab per dose}$$

7. $\dfrac{600 \text{ mg}}{x \text{ mL}} = \dfrac{100 \text{ mg}}{5 \text{ mL}} \Rightarrow 30 \text{ mL}$

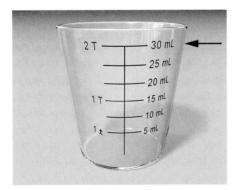

8. $0.015 \text{ g} = 0\underset{\curvearrowright}{0}1\underset{\curvearrowright}{5}. \text{ mg} = 15 \text{ mg}$

$$\frac{15 \text{ mg}}{x \text{ tab}} = \frac{7.5 \text{ mg}}{1 \text{ tab}} \Rightarrow 2 \text{ tab}$$

9. 50 mg three times per day = 150 mg per day
It is safe.

10. $\frac{25 \text{ mg}}{x \text{ mL}} = \frac{10 \text{ mg}}{5 \text{ mL}} \Rightarrow 12.5 \text{ mL}$

11. 25 mg per day = 75 mg for 3 days

$$\frac{75 \text{ mg}}{x \text{ tab}} = \frac{50 \text{ mg}}{1 \text{ tab}} \Rightarrow 1\frac{1}{2} \text{ tab}$$

12. 7.5 mg per dose = 22.5 mg per 24 hours

$$\frac{22.5 \text{ mg}}{x \text{ tab}} = \frac{15 \text{ mg}}{1 \text{ tab}} \Rightarrow 1\frac{1}{2} \text{ tab}$$

13. $\frac{75 \text{ mg}}{x \text{ cap}} = \frac{25 \text{ mg}}{1 \text{ cap}} \Rightarrow 3 \text{ cap}$

14. $\frac{300 \text{ mg}}{6 \text{ h}} = \frac{x \text{ mg}}{24 \text{ h}} \Rightarrow 1{,}200 \text{ mg}$

15. $\frac{4 \text{ mg}}{x \text{ cap}} = \frac{2 \text{ mg}}{1 \text{ cap}} \Rightarrow 2 \text{ cap}$

16. $0.25 \text{ g} = 0\underset{\curvearrowright}{2}\underset{\curvearrowright}{5}\underset{\curvearrowright}{0}. \text{ mg} = 250 \text{ mg}$

$$\frac{250 \text{ mg}}{x \text{ tab}} = \frac{500 \text{ mg}}{1 \text{ tab}} \Rightarrow \frac{1}{2} \text{ tab}$$

17. Patient receives Coumadin on Mon, Wed, Fri, and Sun, 6.5 mg per dose = 26 mg for 4 doses.

18. $\frac{200 \text{ mg}}{x \text{ mL}} = \frac{100 \text{ mg}}{5 \text{ mL}} \Rightarrow 10 \text{ mL}$

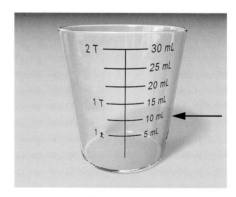

19. (a) $\text{BSA} = \sqrt{\dfrac{66 \times 140}{3131}} \approx 1.72 \text{ m}^2$

$$1.72 \text{ m}^2 \times \frac{60 \text{ mg}}{\text{m}^2} = 103 \text{ mg}$$

(b) $\dfrac{103 \text{ mg}}{x \text{ tab}} = \dfrac{50 \text{ mg}}{1 \text{ tab}} \Rightarrow 2 \text{ tab}$

20. 500 mg on day 1 and 250 mg on the next 4 days means
500 mg + 1,000 mg = 1,500 mg

## Cumulative Review Exercises

1. (a) two 0.2-mg cap
   (b) one 0.1-mg and one 0.2-mg cap
   (c) 1.2 mg

2. 10 mL                  3. 0.5 g                   4. 400 mg

5. 2,500 mL               6. 3,494 g                 7. 2 cups

8. 10 mL                  9. 2 cap                   10. one 100-mg tab

11. 3 tab                 12. 3 tab                  13. 0.2 g

14. 2 tab                 15. 5 mL

# Chapter 7

## Case Study 7.1

1. (a) $\dfrac{75 \text{ mg}}{x \text{ mL}} = \dfrac{100 \text{ mg}}{1 \text{ mL}} \Rightarrow 100x = 75 \Rightarrow x = 0.75$ mL

   (b) the 1 mL syringe

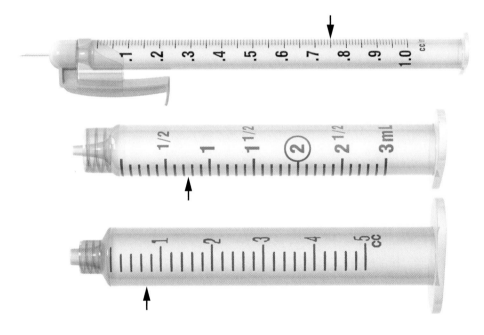

2. (a) 75 mg/mL
   (b) 1 mL of Phenergan
   (c)

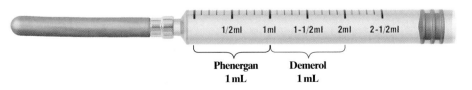

3.

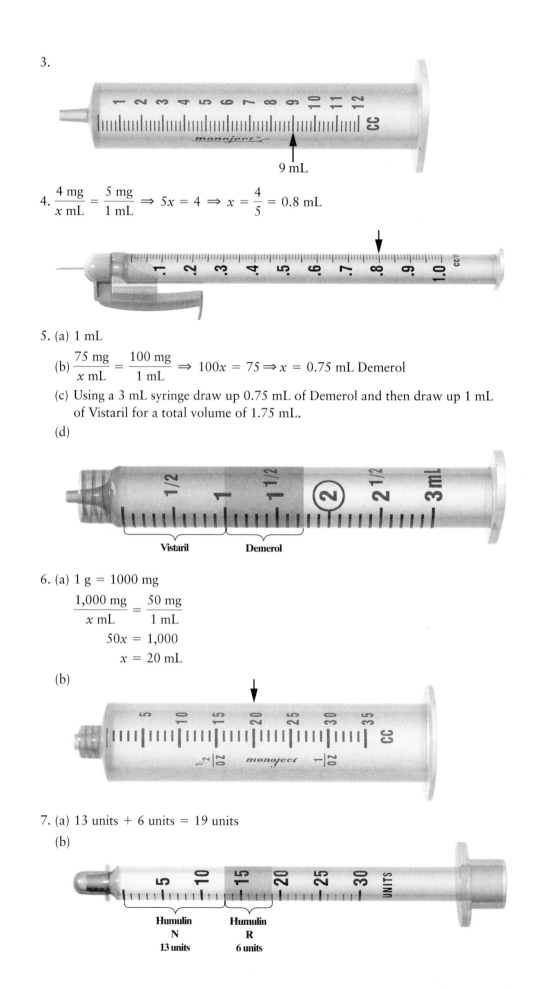

9 mL

4. $\dfrac{4 \text{ mg}}{x \text{ mL}} = \dfrac{5 \text{ mg}}{1 \text{ mL}} \Rightarrow 5x = 4 \Rightarrow x = \dfrac{4}{5} = 0.8 \text{ mL}$

5. (a) 1 mL

(b) $\dfrac{75 \text{ mg}}{x \text{ mL}} = \dfrac{100 \text{ mg}}{1 \text{ mL}} \Rightarrow 100x = 75 \Rightarrow x = 0.75 \text{ mL Demerol}$

(c) Using a 3 mL syringe draw up 0.75 mL of Demerol and then draw up 1 mL of Vistaril for a total volume of 1.75 mL.

(d)

Vistaril    Demerol

6. (a) 1 g = 1000 mg

$$\dfrac{1,000 \text{ mg}}{x \text{ mL}} = \dfrac{50 \text{ mg}}{1 \text{ mL}}$$
$$50x = 1,000$$
$$x = 20 \text{ mL}$$

(b)

7. (a) 13 units + 6 units = 19 units

(b)

Humulin    Humulin
N          R
13 units   6 units

388

# Try These for Practice

1. 1 mL tuberculin syringe; 0.72 mL

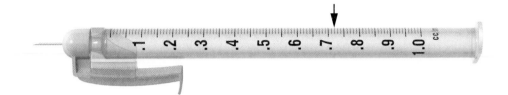

2. 12 mL syringe; 6.8 mL

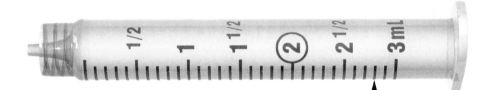

3. 3 mL syringe; 2.8 mL

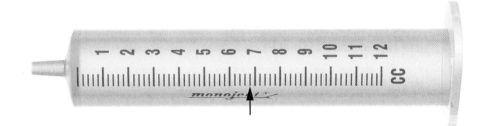

4. 5 mL syringe; 4.4 mL

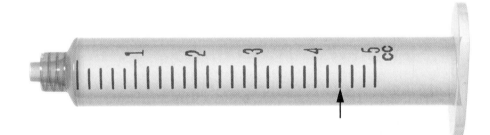

5. (a) 100 unit insulin syringe

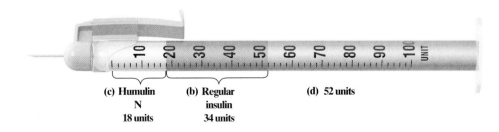

**(c) Humulin N** 18 units  **(b) Regular insulin** 34 units  **(d) 52 units**

# Exercises

1. 1 mL tuberculin syringe; 0.62 mL

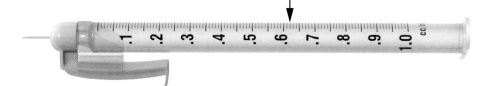

2. 30 unit Lo-Dose insulin syringe; 28 units

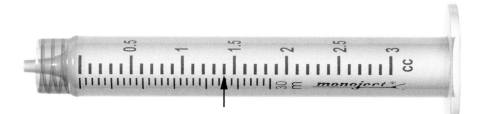

3. 5 mL syringe; 3.6 mL

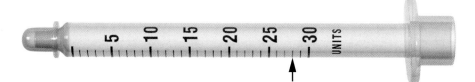

4. 3 mL syringe; 1.4 mL

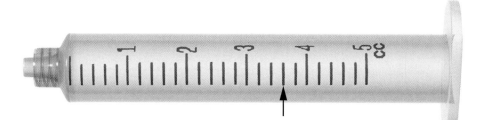

5. 35 mL syringe; 13 mL

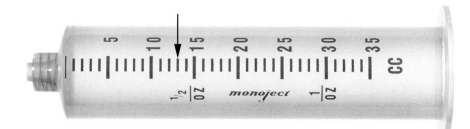

6. 12 mL syringe; 9.6 mL

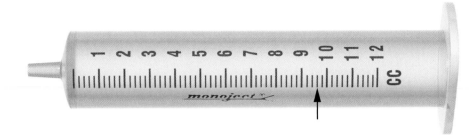

7. 50 unit Lo-Dose insulin syringe; 32 units

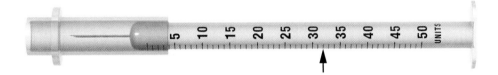

8. 100 unit insulin syringe; 56 units

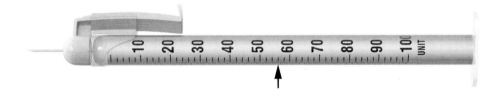

9. 0.5 mL syringe; 0.37 mL

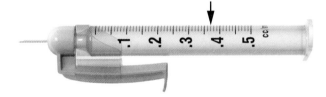

10. 100 unit insulin syringe; 51 units

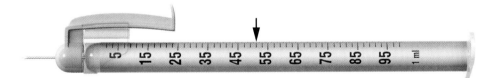

11. 12 mL syringe; 6.8 mL

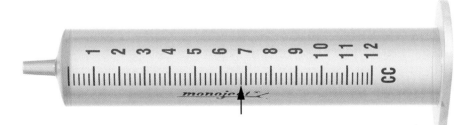

12. 1 mL tuberculin syringe; 0.72 mL

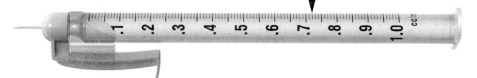

13. 12 mL syringe; 8.2 mL

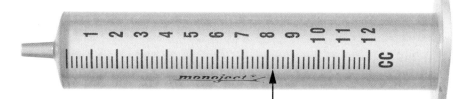

14. 35 mL syringe; 27 mL

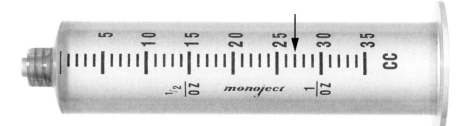

15. 26 units

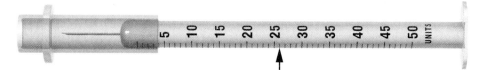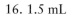

16. 1.5 mL

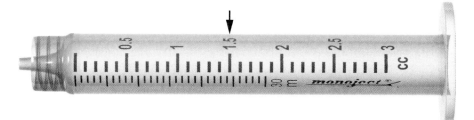

17. 14 units of regular insulin and 44 units of NPH insulin for a total of 58 units

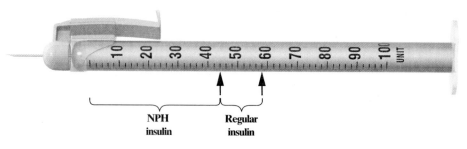

NPH
insulin

Regular
insulin

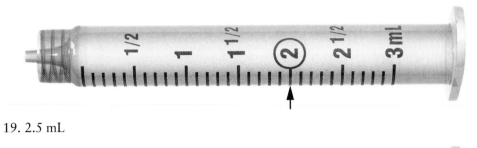

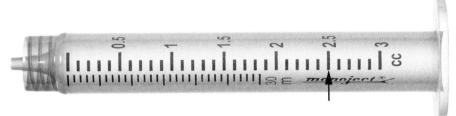

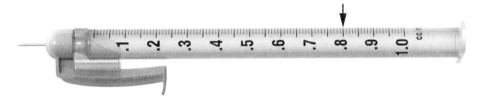

## Cumulative Review Exercises

1. (a) no insulin
   (b) 2 units
   (c) 8 units

2. 1.6 L          3. 28 capsules          4. 6 times per day

5. 0.8 mL          6. 8 tab          7. 4 oz

8. 240 mL          9. 3 mL          10. 0.3 mg

11. 3 cap          12. 3 tab          13. 1 cap

14. 1.5 mL          15. 0.025 mg

# Chapter 8

## Case Study 8.1

1. 0.5 mL—use 1 mL tuberculin syringe

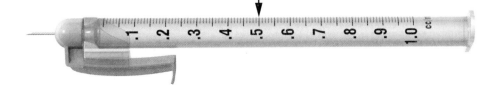

2. 180 mg = 120 mg + 60 mg

Use one 120 mg and one 60 mg tablet for each dose. Administer the two tablets daily.

3. 7.5 mL          4. Administer one 75 mg tablet.          5. 2 tab

6. Withdraw 10 units of Humulin R insulin, then into the same syringe withdraw 38 units of Humulin N insulin for a total of 48 units.

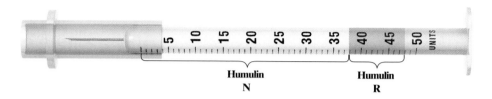

7. 9 g

## Try These for Practice

1. 0.025%

2. Take 20 tablets and dissolve with water, then add more water to the level of 1 L.

3. 80 mL

4. Use two 4-ounce cans of Sustacal and dilute with 16 ounces (4 cans) of water.

5. $\dfrac{0.25 \text{ mg}}{\text{mL}} = \dfrac{250 \text{ mcg}}{1 \text{ mL}} \times \dfrac{2}{2} = \dfrac{500 \text{ mcg}}{2 \text{ mL}}$

## Exercises

1. $\dfrac{\text{Solute}}{\text{Solution}} = \dfrac{15 \text{ mL}}{750 \text{ mL}} = \dfrac{15}{750} = \dfrac{1}{50}$

as a ratio 1:50, and as a percentage 2%

2. $\dfrac{\text{Solute}}{\text{Solution}} = \dfrac{60 \text{ g}}{2 \text{ L}} = \dfrac{60 \text{ g}}{2,000 \text{ mL}} = \dfrac{3 \text{ g}}{100 \text{ mL}}$

as a ratio 3:100, and as a percentage 3%

3. $\dfrac{0.9 \text{ g}}{100 \text{ mL}} = \dfrac{x \text{ g}}{300 \text{ mL}}$

$100x = 270$

$x = 2.7$

Take 2.7 g of sodium chloride crystals, dissolve with water, then add more water to the level of 300 mL.

4. $\dfrac{25 \text{ mg}}{5 \text{ mL}} = \dfrac{x \text{ mg}}{120 \text{ mL}}$

$5x = 3,000$

$x = 600 \text{ mg}$

5. $\dfrac{25 \text{ mg}}{5 \text{ mL}} = \dfrac{20 \text{ mg}}{x \text{ mL}}$

$100 = 25x$

$4 \text{ mL} = x$

6. $$\frac{50 \text{ mL (drug)}}{100 \text{ mL (solution)}} = \frac{x \text{ mL (drug)}}{400 \text{ mL (solution)}}$$

$$100x = 20{,}000$$

$$x = 200 \text{ mL}$$

Take 200 mL of the pure drug, and add water to the level of 400 mL.

7. $$\frac{6 \text{ g}}{100 \text{ mL}} = \frac{18 \text{ g}}{x \text{ mL}}$$

$$1800 = 6x$$

$$x = 300 \text{ mL}$$

8. $300 \text{ mg} = 0.3 \text{ g}$

$$\frac{4 \text{ g}}{100 \text{ mL}} = \frac{0.3 \text{ g}}{x \text{ mL}}$$

$$30 = 4x$$

$$x = 7.5 \text{ mL}$$

9. $2\% = \dfrac{2 \text{ g}}{100 \text{ mL}} = \dfrac{2000 \text{ mg}}{100 \text{ mL}} = 20 \text{ mg/mL}$

10. $$\frac{125 \text{ mg}}{\text{mL}} = \frac{0.125 \text{ g}}{1 \text{ mL}} = \frac{0.125 \times 1000}{1 \times 1000} = \frac{125}{1000} = \frac{1}{8}$$

$$\frac{1}{8} = 0.125 = 12.5\%$$

The strength is 1:8, $\frac{1}{8}$ strength, and 12.5%

11. $$\frac{3 \text{ mL (Sustacal)}}{4 \text{ mL (Solution)}} = \frac{x \text{ mL (Sustacal)}}{1600 \text{ mL (Solution)}}$$

$$4x = 4800$$

$$x = 1200 \text{ mL}$$

----

$$\frac{1 \text{ oz}}{30 \text{ mL}} = \frac{x \text{ oz}}{1200 \text{ mL}}$$

$$30x = 1200$$

$$x = 40 \text{ oz}$$

Use four 10-ounce cans of Sustacal and dilute with 400 mL of water.

12. $\dfrac{\text{Solute}}{\text{Solution}} = \dfrac{120 \text{ mL}}{600 \text{ mL}} = \dfrac{1}{5} = 20\%$

So the strength is 1:5 or 20%

13. $\dfrac{\text{Solute}}{\text{Solution}} = \dfrac{2000 \text{ mg}}{1 \text{ L}} = \dfrac{2 \text{ g}}{1000 \text{ mL}} = \dfrac{1}{500} = 0.2\%$

The strength is 1:500 or 0.2%

14. $$\frac{10 \text{ g}}{100 \text{ mL}} = \frac{x \text{ g}}{800 \text{ mL}}$$

$$100x = 8{,}000$$

$$x = 80 \text{ g}$$

----

$$\frac{20 \text{ g}}{1 \text{ tab}} = \frac{80 \text{ g}}{x \text{ tab}}$$

$$20x = 80$$

$$x = 4 \text{ tab}$$

Take 4 tablets, dissolve with water, then add more water to the level of 800 mL.

15. $\dfrac{5 \text{ mg}}{5 \text{ mL}} = \dfrac{x \text{ mg}}{12 \text{ mL}}$

$5x = 60$

$x = 12 \text{ mg}$

16. $\dfrac{5 \text{ mg}}{5 \text{ mL}} = \dfrac{35 \text{ mg}}{x \text{ mL}}$

$5x = (5)(35)$

$x = \dfrac{(\cancel{5})(35)}{\cancel{5}}$

$x = 35 \text{ mL}$

17. $\dfrac{25 \text{ g}}{100 \text{ mL}} = \dfrac{x \text{ g}}{1{,}200 \text{ mL}}$

$100x = (25)(1200)$

$x = \dfrac{(25)(12\cancel{00})}{1\cancel{00}}$

$x = 300 \text{ g}$

Take 300 g of the pure drug, dissolve with water, then add more water to the level of 1,200 mL.

18. $1\% = \dfrac{1 \text{ g}}{100 \text{ mL}} = \dfrac{10\cancel{00} \text{ mg}}{1\cancel{00} \text{ mL}} = 10 \text{ mg/mL}$

19. $\dfrac{25 \text{ mg}}{1 \text{ mL}} = \dfrac{0.025 \text{ g}}{1 \text{ mL}}$

$\dfrac{0.025 \times 1000}{1 \times 1000} = \dfrac{25}{1000} = \dfrac{1}{40} = 2.5\%$

The strength is 1:40, $\frac{1}{40}$ strength, or 2.5%.

20. 3

$\dfrac{2 \text{ oz (Isomil)}}{3 \text{ oz (Solution)}} = \dfrac{x \text{ oz (Isomil)}}{6 \text{ oz (Solution)}}$

$3x = 12$

$x = 4 \text{ oz of Isomil}$

Use one 4-ounce can and dilute with water to 6 ounces. No Isomil will be discarded.

## Cumulative Review Exercises

1. 12.5 g or 12,500 mg
2. Take 1.5 oz of hydrogen peroxide and dilute with NS to 6 oz.
3. 50 mL of $H_2O$ and 150 mL of Isocal
4. 16 oz
5. 0.6 mg
6. 66 in
7. 2.5 mL
8. 180 cm
9. 0.6 mL Use a 1 mL syringe.
10. 0.0004 g
11. 250 mcg
12. 0.2 mg
13. 3.6 g
14. 2 tab
15. 15 mL

# Chapter 9

## Case Study 9.1

1. (a) $\dfrac{2 \text{ mg}}{x \text{ mL}} = \dfrac{5 \text{ mg}}{1 \text{ mL}} \Rightarrow 5x = 2 \Rightarrow 0.4 \text{ mL}$

   (b) 0.5 mL or 1 mL tuberculin

2. (a) $\dfrac{5{,}000 \text{ units}}{x \text{ mL}} = \dfrac{20{,}000 \text{ units}}{1 \text{ mL}} \Rightarrow 20{,}000x = 5{,}000 \Rightarrow 0.25 \text{ mL}$

   (b) 0.5 mL or 1 mL tuberculin

3. Label reads 5 mg per 5 mL $\Rightarrow$ 5 mL

4. $\dfrac{150 \text{ lb}}{2.2} \approx 68.2 \text{ kg} \Rightarrow 68.2 \text{ kg} \times \dfrac{7.5 \text{ mg}}{\text{kg}} \approx 512 \text{ mg}$

5. Each dose is 1 mL, and four doses per 24 h means 4 mL in 24 hours.

6. 10 mg daily means 70 mg per week
   $0 . 0\ 7\ 0 .\ \text{mg} = 0.07\text{g}$

7. The strength is 0.5 mg/cap $\Rightarrow$ 1 cap

8. $\dfrac{10 \text{ mg}}{x \text{ tab}} = \dfrac{5 \text{ mg}}{1 \text{ tab}} \Rightarrow 5x = 10 \Rightarrow 2 \text{ tab}$

9. (a) 5 mg
   (b) 1 tab

10. $\dfrac{20 \text{ mg}}{x \text{ tab}} = \dfrac{10 \text{ mg}}{1 \text{ tab}} \Rightarrow 10x = 20 \Rightarrow 2 \text{ tab}$

## Try These for Practice

1. (a) 18 mL
   (b) 0.6 mL
   (c) 33 full doses
   (d) 5/5/2010, 0900 h, strength 250,000 units/mL, expires 5/12/2010, 0900 h, keep refrigerated, MJ

2. (a) Use 2 g IM vial
   (b) 5 mL
   (c) 6 mL
   (d) 330 mg/mL
   (e) 1.5 mL
   (f) 4 full doses

3. (a) 3.1 mg
   (b) 3.1 mL

4. (a) 0.8 mL

   (b) 1 mL tuberculin

5. (a) 2 tab

   (b) 5 mL

## Exercises

1. $\dfrac{750 \text{ mg}}{x \text{ mL}} = \dfrac{250 \text{ mg}}{1 \text{ mL}} \Rightarrow 250x = 750 \Rightarrow 3 \text{ mL}$

2. $1.5 \text{ g} = 1,500 \text{ mg}$

   $\dfrac{1,500 \text{ mg}}{x \text{ mL}} = \dfrac{375 \text{ mg}}{1 \text{ mL}} \Rightarrow 375x = 1,500 \Rightarrow 4 \text{ mL}$

3. (a) $\dfrac{155 \text{ lb}}{2.2} = 70.5 \text{ kg}$

   $70.5 \text{ kg} \times \dfrac{0.49 \text{ mcg}}{\text{kg}} = 34.5 \text{ mcg}$

   (b) $\dfrac{34.5 \text{ mcg}}{x \text{ mL}} = \dfrac{40 \text{ mcg}}{1 \text{ mL}} \Rightarrow 40x = 34.5 \Rightarrow 0.86 \text{ mL}$

4. (a) $1,200 \text{ mg} = 1.2 \text{ g}$. Use the 2 g vial

   (b) $\dfrac{1,200 \text{ mg}}{x \text{ mL}} = \dfrac{330 \text{ mg}}{1 \text{ mL}} \Rightarrow 330x = 1,200 \Rightarrow 3.6 \text{ mL}$

5. $\dfrac{500 \text{ mg}}{x \text{ mL}} = \dfrac{400 \text{ mg}}{1 \text{ mL}} \Rightarrow 400x = 500 \Rightarrow 1.3 \text{ mL}$

6. (a) $\dfrac{1.4 \text{ mg}}{x \text{ mL}} = \dfrac{2 \text{ mg}}{1 \text{ mL}} \Rightarrow 2x = 1.4 \Rightarrow 0.7 \text{ mL}$

   (b) $\dfrac{10 \text{ mL}}{0.7 \text{ mL}} \approx 14.3 \Rightarrow 14 \text{ full doses}$

7. $\dfrac{50 \text{ mg}}{25 \text{ mg}} = 2 \text{ vials}$

8. (a) $\dfrac{6,000 \text{ units}}{x \text{ mL}} = \dfrac{20,000 \text{ units}}{1 \text{ mL}} \Rightarrow 20,000x = 6,000 \Rightarrow 0.3 \text{ mL}$

   (b) 0.5 mL or 1 mL tuberculin

9. $\dfrac{60 \text{ mg}}{x \text{ mL}} = \dfrac{40 \text{ mg}}{1 \text{ mL}} \Rightarrow 40x = 60 \Rightarrow x = 1.5 \text{ mL}$

10. (a) $\dfrac{5 \text{ mg}}{x \text{ mL}} = \dfrac{15 \text{ mg}}{1 \text{ mL}} \Rightarrow 15x = 5 \Rightarrow 0.33 \text{ mL}$

   (b) 0.5 mL or 1 mL tuberculin

11. $\dfrac{30 \text{ mg}}{x \text{ mL}} = \dfrac{40 \text{ mg}}{1 \text{ mL}} \Rightarrow 40x = 30 \Rightarrow 0.75 \text{ mL}$

12. $\dfrac{3 \text{ mg}}{x \text{ mL}} = \dfrac{4 \text{ mg}}{1 \text{ mL}} \Rightarrow 4x = 3 \Rightarrow 0.75 \text{ mL}$

13. 320 is between 281 and 340. Give 6 units.

14. (a) $\dfrac{3,500 \text{ units}}{x \text{ mL}} = \dfrac{5,000 \text{ units}}{1 \text{ mL}} \Rightarrow 5,000x = 3,500 \Rightarrow 0.7 \text{ mL}$

    (b) 1 mL tuberculin

15. (a) 25 units

    (b) 30 unit Lo-Dose insulin

16. $\dfrac{650,000 \text{ units}}{x \text{ mL}} = \dfrac{1,000,000 \text{ units}}{1 \text{ mL}} \Rightarrow$

    $1,000,000x = 650,000 \Rightarrow 0.65 \text{ mL}$

17. (a) $\dfrac{0.2 \text{ mg}}{x \text{ mL}} = \dfrac{0.4 \text{ mg}}{1 \text{ mL}} \Rightarrow 0.4x = 0.2 \Rightarrow 0.5 \text{ mL}$

    (b) 1 mL tuberculin

18. (a) $\dfrac{110 \text{ lb}}{2.2} = 50 \text{ kg}$

    $50 \text{ kg} \times \dfrac{0.03 \text{ mg}}{\text{kg}} = 1.5 \text{ mg minimum}$

    (b) $50 \text{ kg} \times \dfrac{0.04 \text{ mg}}{\text{kg}} = 2 \text{ mg maximum}$

19. (a) $\dfrac{40 \text{ mg}}{x \text{ mL}} = \dfrac{25 \text{ mg}}{1 \text{ mL}} \Rightarrow 25x = 40 \Rightarrow 1.6 \text{ mL}$

    (b) 3 mL

20. (a) 18.2 mL

    (b) 8.2 mL

    (c) 5,000,000 units

    (d) $\dfrac{2,000,000 \text{ units}}{x \text{ mL}} = \dfrac{1,000,000 \text{ units}}{1 \text{ mL}} \Rightarrow$

    $1,000,000x = 2,000,000 \Rightarrow 2 \text{ mL}$

    Add 3.2 mL of diluent to the vial and administer 2 mL of the reconstituted solution to the patient.

## Cumulative Review Exercises

1. quinapril HCl

2. PO

3. Pfizer-Parke Davis

4. 8 tab

5. 2 tab

6. Celexa

7. 10 mg/5 mL

8. 10 mL

9. 12 doses

10. 2 cap

11. 0.4 mL

12. (a) 8 mL

    (b) 2 mL

    (c) 4 doses

13. 540 mL

14. (a) 1.8 mL

    (b) 250 mg/mL

    (c) 2 mL

    (d) 1 dose

15. (a) 0.25 mL

    (b) 40 doses

# Chapter 10

## Case Study 10.1

1. $\dfrac{1{,}000 \text{ mL}}{8 \text{ h}} = 125 \text{ mL/h}$

2. $FC = \dfrac{60}{15} = 4$

   $\dfrac{125}{4} = 31.25 \approx 31 \text{ gtt/min}$

3. $\begin{array}{l} 1900 \\ +0800 \\ \hline 2700 \end{array}$  $\begin{array}{l} 2700 \\ -2400 \\ \hline 0300 \end{array}$  0300 h the next day

4. $\dfrac{x \text{ g}}{1{,}000 \text{ mL}} = \dfrac{5 \text{ g}}{100 \text{ mL}}$

   $100x = 5{,}000$

   $x = 50 \text{ g dextrose}$

   $\dfrac{x \text{ g}}{1{,}000 \text{ mL}} = \dfrac{0.45 \text{ g}}{100 \text{ mL}}$

   $100x = 450$

   $x = 4.5 \text{ g NaCl}$

5. $\dfrac{100 \text{ mL}}{60 \text{ min}} = \dfrac{100 \text{ mL}}{1 \text{ h}} = 100 \text{ mL/h}$

6. (a) $\dfrac{3 \text{ mL}}{4 \text{ mL}} = \dfrac{x \text{ mL}}{800 \text{ mL}}$ $\qquad\qquad \dfrac{600 \text{ mL}}{x \text{ oz}} = \dfrac{30 \text{ mL}}{1 \text{ oz}}$

   $4x = 2400$ $\qquad\qquad\qquad\qquad\quad 30x = 600$

   $x = 600 \text{ mL (needed)}$ $\qquad\quad x = 20 \text{ ounces (needed)}$

   Use two 10-oz caus.

   (b) $\dfrac{800 \text{ mL}}{7 \text{ h}} = 114 \text{ mL/h}$

7. $\dfrac{1 \text{ mg}}{1 \text{ mL}} = \dfrac{0.5 \text{ mg}}{x \text{ mL}} \Rightarrow x = 0.5 \text{ mL}$

8. $\dfrac{10 \text{ mg}}{1 \text{ mL}} = \dfrac{200 \text{ mg}}{x \text{ mL}}$

   $200 = 10x$ $\qquad$ prepare 20 mL

   $20 = x$

9. $\dfrac{100 \text{ mg}}{x \text{ mL}} = \dfrac{60 \text{ mg}}{15 \text{ mL}}$

$60x = 1,500$

$x = 25 \text{ mL}$

## Try These for Practice

1. 10 gtt/min         2. 36 gtt/min         3. 375 mL

4. 108 mL/h         5. 67 mL/h

## Exercises

1. $\dfrac{750 \text{ mL}}{8 \text{ h}} = 93.8 \text{ mL/h};$    $\text{FC} = \dfrac{60}{10} = 6;$    $93.8 \div 6 \approx 16 \text{ gtt/min}$

2. $\dfrac{375 \text{ mL}}{3 \text{ h}} = 125 \text{ mL/h}$

3. $\dfrac{100}{30} = \dfrac{550}{x}$      $100x = 16,500$      $x = 165 \text{ mL}$

4. $\dfrac{1,000 \text{ mL}}{x \text{ h}} = \dfrac{125 \text{ mL}}{1 \text{ h}}$      $125x = 1,000$      $x = 8\text{h}$

5. $\dfrac{500 \text{ mL}}{3 \text{ h}} \approx 167 \text{ mL/h} = 167 \text{ mcgtt/min}$

6. (a) $\dfrac{1,500 \text{ mL}}{12 \text{ h}} = 125 \text{ mL/h}$     $\text{FC} = 3$     $\dfrac{125}{3} \approx 42 \text{ gtt/min}$

   (b) $\dfrac{1,200 \text{ mL}}{9 \text{ h}} = 133.3 \text{ mL/h}$     $\dfrac{133.3}{3} \approx 44 \text{ gtt/min}$

   (c) $25\%$ of $42 = 0.25 \times 42 = 10.5 \text{ gtt/min}$

       $44 - 42 = 2 \text{ gtt/min}$

       Because 2 is less than 10.5, the adjustment is within the guidelines.

7. $\dfrac{750 \text{ mL}}{8 \text{ h}} = 93.8 \text{ mL/h}$     $\text{FC} = \dfrac{60}{15} = 4$     $93.8 \div 4 \approx 23 \text{ gtt/min}$

8. $\dfrac{125 \text{ mL}}{1 \text{ h}} = \dfrac{750 \text{ mL}}{x \text{ h}}$     $125x = 750$     $x = 6\text{h}$

   It will finish at 6 P.M. the same day.

9. $\dfrac{1,000 \text{ mL}}{24 \text{ h}} \approx 42 \text{ mL/h}$

10. 90 mL/h     $\text{FC} = \dfrac{60}{20} = 3$     $90 \div 3 = 30 \text{ gtt/min}$

11. $\dfrac{1,000 \text{ mL}}{6 \text{ h}} \approx 167 \text{ mL/h}$

12. $\dfrac{40 \text{ mL}}{1 \text{ h}} = \dfrac{500 \text{ mL}}{x \text{ h}}$     $40x = 500$     $x = 12\frac{1}{2} \text{ hours}$

13. $\dfrac{750 \text{ mL}}{24 \text{ h}} \approx 31 \text{ mL/h}$

14. $\dfrac{500 \text{ mL}}{3.25 \text{ h}} \approx 153.8 \text{ mL/h}$     FC = 4     $\dfrac{153.8}{4} \approx 38 \text{ gtt/min}$

15. $\dfrac{90 \text{ mL}}{0.75 \text{ h}} = 120 \text{ mL/h}$

16. FC $= \dfrac{60}{15} = 4$     $35 \times 4 = 140 \dfrac{\text{mL}}{\text{h}}$

$\dfrac{140 \text{ mL}}{1 \text{ h}} = \dfrac{350 \text{ mL}}{x \text{ h}}$     $140x = 350$     $x = 2\frac{1}{2} \text{ hours}$

17. 32 mcgtt/min $= 32 \dfrac{\text{mL}}{\text{h}}$

$\dfrac{32 \text{ mL}}{1 \text{ h}} = \dfrac{x \text{ mL}}{6 \text{ h}}$     $x = 192 \text{ mL}$

18. $\dfrac{350 \text{ mL}}{5 \text{ h}} = 70 \text{ mL/h}$     FC = 4     $\dfrac{70}{4} \approx 18 \text{ gtt/min}$

19. FC $= \dfrac{60}{15} = 4$     $30 \times 4 = 120 \text{ mL/h}$

20. $\dfrac{50 \text{ mL}}{1 \text{ h}} = \dfrac{x \text{ mL}}{0.25 \text{ h}}$     $x = 12.5 \text{ mL}$

$500 \text{ mL} - 13 \text{ mL} = 487 \text{ mL}$

$\dfrac{487 \text{ mL}}{3.75 \text{ h}} \approx 130 \text{ mL/h}$

## Cumulative Review Exercises

| | | |
|---|---|---|
| 1. 4.5 mg | 2. 40 mL/h | 3. 156 mL/h |
| 4. 17 gtt/min | 5. 2.13 m$^2$ | 6. 1 cap |
| 7. 80 mL/h | 8. 3 mL | 9. 1 cap |
| 10. 63 mL/h | 11. 1.7 mL | 12. 2.11 m$^2$ |
| 13. 600 mcgtt | 14. 8 oz | 15. 30 mL |

# Chapter 11

## Case Study 11.1

1. $\dfrac{1{,}000 \text{ mL}}{8 \text{ h}} = 125 \text{ mL/h}$

2. $\dfrac{6 \text{ mg}}{x \text{ mL}} = \dfrac{8 \text{ mg}}{1 \text{ mL}} \Rightarrow 8x = 6 \Rightarrow x = 0.75 \text{ mL}$

3. $\dfrac{0.25 \text{ mg}}{x \text{ mL}} = \dfrac{1 \text{ mg}}{1 \text{ mL}} \Rightarrow x = 0.25 \text{ mL}$

4. $\dfrac{250 \text{ mg}}{x \text{ mL}} = \dfrac{350 \text{ mg}}{1 \text{ mL}} \Rightarrow 350x = 250 \Rightarrow x \approx 0.71 \text{ mL}$

5. FC $= \dfrac{60}{15} = 4$     $105 \text{ mL/h} \div 4 = 26 \text{ gtt/min}$

6. $\dfrac{255 \text{ mL}}{90 \text{ min}} = \dfrac{250 \text{ mL}}{1.5 \text{ h}} = 170 \text{ mL/h}$

7. (a) $\dfrac{4 \text{ g}}{x \text{ mL}} = \dfrac{40 \text{ g}}{1{,}000 \text{ mL}} \Rightarrow 40x = 4{,}000 \Rightarrow x = 100 \text{ mL}$

   $\dfrac{100 \text{ mL}}{20 \text{ min}} \times \dfrac{3}{3} = \dfrac{300 \text{ mL}}{\text{h}}$

   (b) $\dfrac{1 \text{ g}}{x \text{ mL}} = \dfrac{40 \text{ g}}{1{,}000 \text{ mL}} \Rightarrow 40x = 1{,}000 \Rightarrow x = 25 \text{ mL}$

   $\therefore \dfrac{1 \text{ g}}{\text{h}} = \dfrac{25 \text{ mL}}{\text{h}}$

8. $\dfrac{0.5 \text{ mU}}{\text{min}} \times \dfrac{60}{60} = \dfrac{30 \text{ mU}}{\text{h}} = \dfrac{0.03 \text{ units}}{\text{h}}$

   $\dfrac{.03 \text{ units}}{x \text{ mL}} = \dfrac{10 \text{ units}}{1{,}000 \text{ mL}} \Rightarrow 10x = 30 \Rightarrow x = 3 \text{ mL}$

   $\therefore \dfrac{0.03 \text{ units}}{\text{h}} = 3 \text{ mL/h}$

9. $\dfrac{9 \text{ mL}}{x \text{ units}} = \dfrac{1{,}000 \text{ mL}}{10 \text{ units}} \Rightarrow 1{,}000x = 90 \qquad x = 0.09 \text{ units}$

   $0.09 \text{ units} = 90 \text{ mU} \qquad \text{So,} \quad \dfrac{9 \text{ mL}}{\text{h}} = \dfrac{90 \text{ mU}}{\text{h}}$

10. $2 \text{ mg} = 1 \text{ mL} \qquad \therefore 1 \text{ mg} = 0.5 \text{ mL}$

## Try These for Practice

1. 25 gtt/min
2. 25 mL/h
3. 60 mg/h
4. 11 mcgtt/min
5. 12 mL/h

## Exercises

1. $\dfrac{20 \text{ mEq}}{100 \text{ mL}} = \dfrac{10 \text{ mEq}}{x \text{ mL}} \Rightarrow 20x = 1{,}000 \Rightarrow x = 50 \text{ mL}$

   $\dfrac{10 \text{ mEq}}{\text{h}} = \dfrac{50 \text{ mL}}{\text{h}} = 50 \text{ mcgtt/min}$

2. $\dfrac{2 \text{ mcg}}{\text{min}} \times \dfrac{60}{60} = \dfrac{120 \text{ mcg}}{\text{h}} = \dfrac{0.12 \text{ mg}}{\text{h}}$

   $\dfrac{0.12 \text{ mg}}{x \text{ mL}} = \dfrac{8 \text{ mg}}{250 \text{ mL}} \Rightarrow 8x = 30 \Rightarrow x = 3.75 \text{ mL}$

   $\dfrac{0.12 \text{ mg}}{\text{h}} = \dfrac{3.75 \text{ mL}}{\text{h}} \approx 4 \text{ mL/h}$

3. $\dfrac{40 \text{ mL}}{x \text{ mg}} = \dfrac{500 \text{ mL}}{1000 \text{ mg}} \Rightarrow 500x = 40{,}000 \Rightarrow x = 80 \text{ mg}$

   $\dfrac{40 \text{ mL}}{\text{h}} = \dfrac{80 \text{ mg}}{\text{h}} = \dfrac{80 \text{ mg}}{60 \text{ min}} \approx 1.3 \text{ mg/min}$

4. $91 \text{ kg} \times \dfrac{3 \text{ mcg}}{\text{kg} \cdot \text{min}} = \dfrac{273 \text{ mcg}}{\text{min}} = \dfrac{0.273 \text{ mg}}{\text{min}} \times \dfrac{60}{60} = \dfrac{16.38 \text{ mg}}{\text{h}}$

   $\dfrac{16.38 \text{ mg}}{x \text{ mL}} = \dfrac{400 \text{ mg}}{250 \text{ mL}} \Rightarrow 400x = 4095 \Rightarrow x = 10.2 \text{ mL}$

   $\dfrac{16.38 \text{ mg}}{\text{h}} = \dfrac{10.2 \text{ mL}}{\text{h}} \approx 10 \text{ mL/h}$

5. $\dfrac{500 \text{ mL}}{90 \text{ min}} = \dfrac{500 \text{ mL}}{1.5 \text{ h}} \approx 333 \text{ mL/h}$

6. $\dfrac{550 \text{ mL}}{x \text{ h}} = \dfrac{25 \text{ mL}}{\text{h}} \Rightarrow 25x = 550 \Rightarrow 22 \text{ h}$

7. $\dfrac{24{,}000 \text{ units}}{1{,}000 \text{ mL}} = \dfrac{1{,}000 \text{ units}}{x \text{ mL}} \Rightarrow 24{,}000x = 1{,}000{,}000$

   $x = 41.67 \text{ mL}$

   $\dfrac{1{,}000 \text{ units}}{\text{h}} = 42 \dfrac{\text{mL}}{\text{h}}$

8. $\dfrac{1 \text{ mL}}{\text{min}} \times \dfrac{60}{60} = \dfrac{60 \text{ mL}}{\text{h}}$

   $\dfrac{60 \text{ mL}}{x \text{ units}} = \dfrac{500 \text{ mL}}{50 \text{ units}} \Rightarrow 500x = 3{,}000 \Rightarrow x = 6 \text{ units}$

   $\dfrac{60 \text{ mL}}{\text{h}} = \dfrac{6 \text{ units}}{\text{h}}$

9. $\dfrac{40 \text{ mL}}{15 \text{ min}} = \dfrac{40 \text{ mL}}{\frac{1}{4} \text{ h}} = \dfrac{160 \text{ mL}}{\text{h}} \div 3 \Rightarrow 53 \text{ gtt/min}$

10. (a) $\dfrac{4 \text{ mcg}}{x \text{ mL}} = \dfrac{5 \text{ mcg}}{1 \text{ mL}} \Rightarrow 5x = 4 \Rightarrow x = 0.8 \text{ mL}$

    $\dfrac{4 \text{ mcg}}{\text{min}} = \dfrac{0.8 \text{ mL}}{\text{min}} \times \dfrac{60}{60} = \dfrac{48 \text{ mL}}{\text{h}}$

    (b) If $\dfrac{4 \text{ mcg}}{\text{min}} = \dfrac{48 \text{ mL}}{\text{h}}$ then $\dfrac{2 \text{ mcg}}{\text{min}} = \dfrac{24 \text{ mL}}{\text{h}}$

| Dosage Rate | Flow Rate |
|---|---|
| 4 mcg/min | 48 mL/h |
| 6 mcg/min | 72 mL/h |
| 8 mcg/min | 96 mL/h |
| 10 mcg/min | 120 mL/h |
| 12 mcg/min | 144 mL/h |

11. (a) $\dfrac{0.5 \text{ mg}}{x \text{ mL}} = \dfrac{0.1 \text{ mg}}{1 \text{ mL}} \Rightarrow 0.1x = 0.5 \Rightarrow x = 5 \text{ mL}$

    (b) $\dfrac{5 \text{ mL}}{5 \text{ min}} = \dfrac{5 \text{ mL}}{300 \text{ sec}} \div \dfrac{10}{10} = \dfrac{0.5 \text{ mL}}{30 \text{ sec}}$    Push 0.5 mL.

    (c) $\dfrac{5 \text{ mL}}{300 \text{ sec}} \div \dfrac{5}{5} = \dfrac{1 \text{ mL}}{60 \text{ sec}}$    So, 60 seconds are needed.

12. $\dfrac{100 \text{ mL}}{60 \text{ min}} = 100 \text{ mL/h} \div 4 = 25 \text{ gtt/min}$

13. $\dfrac{4 \text{ mcg}}{1 \text{ min}} \times \dfrac{60}{60} = \dfrac{240 \text{ mcg}}{1 \text{ h}} = \dfrac{0.24 \text{ mg}}{\text{h}}$

    $\dfrac{0.24 \text{ mg}}{x \text{ mL}} = \dfrac{2 \text{ mg}}{500 \text{ mL}} \Rightarrow 2x = 120 \Rightarrow x = 60 \text{ mL}$

    So $\dfrac{4 \text{ mcg}}{\text{min}} = 60 \text{ mL/h}$

14. $\dfrac{20 \text{ mL}}{x \text{ mg}} = \dfrac{1,000 \text{ mL}}{500 \text{ mg}} \Rightarrow 1,000x = 10,000 \Rightarrow x = 10 \text{ mg}$

$\dfrac{20 \text{ mL}}{\text{h}} = \dfrac{10 \text{ mg}}{\text{h}}$

15. $82 \text{ kg} \times \dfrac{3 \text{ mcg}}{\text{kg} \cdot \text{min}} = \dfrac{246 \text{ mcg}}{\text{min}} = \dfrac{0.246 \text{ mg}}{\text{min}} \times \dfrac{60}{60} = \dfrac{14.76 \text{ mg}}{\text{h}}$

$\dfrac{14.76 \text{ mg}}{x \text{ mL}} = \dfrac{50 \text{ mg}}{250 \text{ mL}} \Rightarrow 50x = 3,690 \Rightarrow x = 73.8 \text{ mL}$

$\dfrac{14.76 \text{ mg}}{\text{h}} = 74 \text{ mL/h}$

16. $2.33 \text{ m}^2 \times \dfrac{75 \text{ mg}}{\text{m}^2} = 174.75 \text{ mg}$

$\dfrac{174.75 \text{ mg}}{x \text{ mL}} = \dfrac{50 \text{ mg}}{1 \text{ mL}} \Rightarrow 50x = 174.75 \Rightarrow x = 3.495 \text{ mL} \approx 3.5 \text{ mL}$

17. $22 \text{ gtt/min} \times 3 = 66 \text{ mL/h}$

$\dfrac{1,000 \text{ mL}}{x \text{ h}} = \dfrac{66 \text{ mL}}{1 \text{ h}} \Rightarrow 66x = 1000 \Rightarrow x = 15.15 \text{ h}$

$\dfrac{0.15 \text{ h}}{x \text{ min}} = \dfrac{1 \text{ h}}{60 \text{ min}} \Rightarrow x = 9 \text{ min}$

It will take 15 h 9 min to finish.

It will finish at 1:04 A.M. the next day.

18. $\dfrac{70 \text{ mL}}{0.5 \text{ h}} = 140 \text{ mL/h}$

19. $\dfrac{1,200 \text{ units}}{x \text{ mL}} = \dfrac{40,000 \text{ units}}{500 \text{ mL}} \Rightarrow 40,000x = 600,000$

$x = 15 \text{ mL}$

$\dfrac{1,200 \text{ units}}{\text{h}} = \dfrac{15 \text{ mL}}{\text{h}}$

20. MIN $\dfrac{150 \text{ lb}}{2.2} = 68.18 \text{ kg}$

$68.18 \text{ kg} \times \dfrac{0.05 \text{ mg}}{\text{kg} \cdot \text{min}} = \dfrac{3.4 \text{ mg}}{\text{min}} \times \dfrac{60}{60} = \dfrac{204 \text{ mg}}{\text{h}}$

$\dfrac{204 \text{ mg}}{x \text{ mL}} = \dfrac{200 \text{ mg}}{50 \text{ mL}} \Rightarrow 200x = 10,200 \Rightarrow x = 51 \text{ mL}$

MIN is 51 mL/h

MAX $\dfrac{0.05 \text{ mg/kg/min}}{51 \text{ mL/h}} = \dfrac{0.1 \text{ mg/kg/min}}{x \text{ mL/h}}$

$5.1 = 0.05x \Rightarrow x = 102 \text{ mL/h}$

Yes.

## Cumulative Review Exercises

1. 4.4 mL

2. 2 tab

3. 3 mL

4. 1.7 mL

5. 10 mL

6. 10 mL

7. 2 tab

8. 20 mL

9. 0.4 mg/min

10. 36 mL/h          11. 1,091 mg          12. 1,091 mg/min
13. 1.83 m$^2$          14. 4 mL          15. 5 g

# Chapter 12

## Case Study 12.1

1. $\dfrac{30 \text{ lb}}{2.2} = 13.6 \text{ kg}$

$\left. \begin{array}{l} 10 \text{ kg} \times \dfrac{100 \text{ mL}}{\text{kg}} = 1,000 \text{ mL} \\[2.5ex] 3.6 \text{ kg} \times \dfrac{50 \text{ mL}}{\text{kg}} = 180 \text{ mL} \end{array} \right\} 1,180 \text{ mL}$

2. MAX daily dose is 400,000 units × 6 doses = 2,400,000 units/day

$\dfrac{600,000 \text{ units}}{\text{dose}} \times \dfrac{4 \text{ doses}}{\text{day}} = 2,400,000 \text{ units/day (ordered)}$

The ordered dose is safe.

3. 4.8 mL of diluent.

$\dfrac{600,000 \text{ units}}{x \text{ mL}} = \dfrac{750,000 \text{ units}}{1 \text{ mL}} \Rightarrow x = 0.8 \text{ mL}$

4. $\dfrac{50.8 \text{ mL}}{30 \text{ min}} \times \dfrac{2}{2} = \dfrac{101.6 \text{ mL}}{60 \text{ min}} \approx 102 \dfrac{\text{mL}}{\text{h}}$

5. $\dfrac{30 \text{ lb}}{2.2} = 13.6 \text{ kg}$

MIN:   $13.6 \text{ kg} \times \dfrac{0.1 \text{ mg}}{\text{kg}} = 1.4 \text{ mg}$

MAX:   $13.6 \text{ kg} \times \dfrac{0.15 \text{ mg}}{\text{kg}} = 2 \text{ mg}$

1 mg is too low; it is not safe.

6. $\dfrac{1}{2}$ of 2.5 mg = 1.25 mg

7. $\dfrac{1}{2}$ of 20 mg = 10 mg

8. VENTOLIN:   $\dfrac{3 \text{ mL}}{1.25 \text{ mg}} = \dfrac{x \text{ mL}}{1 \text{ mg}} \Rightarrow x = 2.4 \text{ mL}$

Intal:   $\dfrac{1}{2}$ of 2 mL = 1 mL

2.4 mL + 1 mL = 3.4 mL

9. $\dfrac{1}{2}$ of 1 mL = 0.5 mL

10. $\dfrac{1}{2}$ of 300 mg = 150 mg

## Try These for Practice

1. 9 units per day          2. It is safe.          3. 10 mL

4. 4 mL          5. 121 mL/h

# Exercises

1. $\dfrac{40 \text{ lb}}{2.2} = 18.18 \text{ kg}$

   $18.18 \cancel{\text{kg}} \times \dfrac{6 \text{ mg}}{\cancel{\text{kg}}} = 109 \text{ mg (min)}$

   $18.18 \cancel{\text{kg}} \times \dfrac{7.5 \text{ mg}}{\cancel{\text{kg}}} = 136 \text{ mg (max)}$

   $50 \text{ mg} \times 3 \text{ doses} = 150 \text{ mg daily}$
   No, the dose is not safe.

2. $4000 \text{ g} = 4 \text{ kg}$

   $4 \cancel{\text{kg}} \times \dfrac{10 \text{ mg}}{\cancel{\text{kg}}} = 40 \text{ mg}$

3. $\text{BSA} = \sqrt{\dfrac{42 \times 50}{3131}} = 0.81 \text{ m}^2$

   $0.81 \cancel{\text{m}^2} \times \dfrac{7.5 \text{ mg}}{\cancel{\text{m}^2}} = 6 \text{ mg (min)}$

   $0.81 \cancel{\text{m}^2} \times \dfrac{30 \text{ mg}}{\cancel{\text{m}^2}} = 24 \text{ mg (max)}$

   Since 2.9 mg is less than 6 mg, the ordered dose is not safe.

4. $32 \cancel{\text{kg}} \times \dfrac{10 \text{ mg}}{\cancel{\text{kg}}} = 320 \text{ mg}$

5. $1.2 \cancel{\text{m}^2} \times \dfrac{350 \text{ mg}}{\cancel{\text{m}^2} \cdot \text{day}} = 420 \text{ mg/day (min)}$

   $1.2 \cancel{\text{m}^2} \times \dfrac{450 \text{ mg}}{\cancel{\text{m}^2} \cdot \text{day}} = 540 \text{ mg/day (max)}$

   The safe dose range is 420–540 mg/day.

6. $\dfrac{77 \text{ lb}}{2.2} = 35 \text{ kg}$

   $35 \cancel{\text{kg}} \times \dfrac{30 \text{ mg}}{\cancel{\text{kg}} \cdot \text{d}} = 1{,}050 \text{ mg/d}$

   $\dfrac{1{,}050}{3} = 350 \text{ mg/dose}$

   $\dfrac{350 \text{ mg}}{x} = \dfrac{187 \text{ mg}}{1 \text{ mL}}$

   $x = 1.8 \text{ mL per dose}$

7. 65 mL/h = 65 mcgtt/min

8. $\dfrac{52 \text{ lb}}{2.2} = 23.6 \text{ kg}$

   $23.6 \cancel{\text{kg}} \times \dfrac{2 \text{ mg}}{\cancel{\text{kg}} \cdot \text{d}} = 47.2 \text{ mg/d (min)}$

   $23.6 \cancel{\text{kg}} \times \dfrac{4 \text{ mg}}{\cancel{\text{kg}} \cdot \text{d}} = 94.4 \text{ mg/d (max)}$

   $30 \text{ mg} \times 3 \text{ doses} = 90 \text{ mg}$
   90 is between 47.2 and 94.4
   and
   30 is less than 50
   So, the dose is safe.

9. (a) $\dfrac{55 \text{ lb}}{2.2} = 25 \text{ kg}$

$25 = 10 + 10 + 5$

$\left.\begin{aligned} 10 \text{ kg} \times \dfrac{100 \text{ mL}}{\text{kg}} &= 1000 \text{ mL} \\[6pt] 10 \text{ kg} \times \dfrac{50 \text{ mL}}{\text{kg}} &= 500 \text{ mL} \\[6pt] 5 \text{ kg} \times \dfrac{20 \text{ mL}}{\text{kg}} &= 100 \text{ mL} \end{aligned}\right\} \; 1{,}600 \text{ mL}$

(b) $\dfrac{1{,}600 \text{ mL}}{24 \text{ h}} = 66 \text{ mL/h}$

10. $0.82 \text{ m}^2 \times \dfrac{2{,}000{,}000 \text{ units}}{\text{m}^2} = 1{,}640{,}000 \text{ units}$

11. $1.2 \text{ g} = 1{,}200 \text{ mg}$

$\dfrac{1{,}200 \text{ mg}}{x \text{ mL}} = \dfrac{60 \text{ mg}}{1 \text{ mL}}$

$60x = 1{,}200$

$x = 20 \text{ mL}$

12. $\dfrac{7 \text{ lb}}{2.2} = 3.18 \text{ kg}$

$3.18 \text{ kg} \times \dfrac{100 \text{ mL}}{\text{kg}} = 318 \text{ mL}$

13. $1.1 \text{ m}^2 \times \dfrac{160 \text{ mg}}{\text{m}^2} = 176 \text{ mg}$

$\dfrac{176 \text{ mg}}{x \text{ mg}} = \dfrac{50 \text{ mg}}{5 \text{ mL}}$

$50x = 880$

$x = 17.6 \text{ mL}$

14. (a) $\dfrac{x \text{ mEq}}{500 \text{ mL}} = \dfrac{20 \text{ mEq}}{1{,}000 \text{ mL}} \Rightarrow x = 10 \text{ mEq}$

(b) $\dfrac{10 \text{ mEq}}{x \text{ mL}} = \dfrac{2 \text{ mEq}}{1 \text{ mL}} \Rightarrow x = 5 \text{ mL}$

(c) $\dfrac{30 \text{ mL}}{x \text{ mEq}} = \dfrac{500 \text{ mL}}{10 \text{ mEq}} \Rightarrow x = 0.6$

$\dfrac{30 \text{ mL}}{\text{h}} = \dfrac{0.6 \text{ mEq}}{\text{h}}$

15. (a) $\left.\begin{aligned} 14.5 \text{ kg} \times \dfrac{30 \text{ mg}}{\text{kg} \cdot \text{d}} &= 435 \text{ mg/d} \\[6pt] 14.5 \text{ kg} \times \dfrac{50 \text{ mg}}{\text{kg} \cdot \text{d}} &= 75 \text{ mg/d} \end{aligned}\right\} \; \text{recommended}$

$125 \text{ mg} \times 6 = 750 \text{ mg/d (ordered)}$

Since 750 is larger than 725, this dose is not safe.

(b) You would not administer any amount because the dose is unsafe.

16. $41 \ \cancel{kg} \times \dfrac{40 \ mg}{\cancel{kg} \cdot d} = 1{,}640 \ mg/d$

$\dfrac{1{,}640}{4} = 410 \ mg/dose$

$\dfrac{410 \ mg}{x \ mL} = \dfrac{50 \ mg}{1 \ mL} \Rightarrow x = 8.2 \ mL$

$\dfrac{200 \ mL}{90 \ min} = \dfrac{200 \ mL}{1.5 \ h} = 133 \ mL/h$

If 8.2 mL is included in the total volume, the answer is

$\dfrac{208.2 \ mL}{1.5 \ h} = 138 \ mL/h$

17. $\dfrac{100 \ mg}{20 \ min} = 5 \ mg/min$

18. $\dfrac{40 \ mL}{60 \ min} = \dfrac{40 \ mL}{h} = 40 \ mcgtt/min$

19. $\dfrac{35 \ lb}{2.2} = 15.9 \ kg$

$15.9 \ \cancel{kg} \times \dfrac{10 \ mg}{\cancel{kg} \cdot dose} = 159 \ mg/dose$

$\dfrac{159 \ mg}{x \ mL} = \dfrac{100 \ mg}{2.5 \ mL}$

$100x = 397.5$

$x = 3.975$

3.9 mL per dose

20. $\dfrac{22 \ lb}{2.2} = 10 \ kg$

$10 \ \cancel{kg} \times \dfrac{50 \ mg}{\cancel{kg} \cdot d} = 500 \ mg/d$ (recommended)

$125 \ mg \times 4 = 500 \ mg/d$ (ordered)

The prescribed dose is safe.

# Cumulative Review Exercises

1. 525 mg      2. 30 units

3. (a) 200 mg      4. 50 units
   (b) 0.2 g

5. 20 mL      6. (a) 2 cap
           (b) 0.3 g

7. 1 mg      8. 60 gtt/min      9. 2.5 mL/min

10. 83 mL/h      11. 3 tab      12. 1 tab

13. 5.2 mL      14. 2 tab      15. 10 mL

# Answers to the Comprehensive Self-Tests

## Comprehensive Self-Test 1

1. 735 mg
2. 2 cap
3. Take 40 mL of 100% Clorox solution and dilute to 400 mL
4. 0.1 g
5. 8 hours 20 min
6. 12.5 g
7.

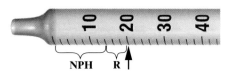

8. 2 tab
9. 100 mL/h, 1,000 mg
10.

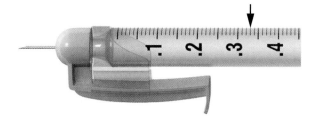

11. 0.75 mL
12. 3 mL/h
13. 6.8 units/h
14. 2.5 mL
15. 0.132 mg
16. 0.22 mg/d, 0.32 mg/d, yes
17. 160 mg, 63 mL/h
18. 25 gtt/min
19. 1 m²
20. 0.5 mL
21. 1.25 mL/min, 25 gtt/min, 13 hours 20 minutes
22. 2,000 mL
23. 30 mL
24. 10 mg, 60 mL
25. 21 mL/h

## Comprehensive Self-Test 2

1. 2,000 units per hour
2. 19.2 mg, 3.8 mL, 311 mL/h
3. 2 tab
4. 2 cap
5. 2.2 mL
6. Yes, 0.9 mL
7. 0900 h the next day
8. 4.1 mL
9. 2 mL, arrow at 2 mL
10. 218 mg/d, 681 mg/d
11. 2.25 g
12. 100 mL/h
13. 454 mL/d, 18.9 mL/h
14. No
15. 40 mL/h
16. 120 mL/h
17. 2.5 mL
18. 2 cap, 3.15 g
19. 30 mL
20. 21 mL/h

21. 45 mL, 2.75 mL/h          22. 0.7 mL

23. 1 mL, 1 mL tuberculin          24. Take 600 mL of Sustacal and dilute to 900 mL

25. 0400 h the next day

## Comprehensive Self-Test 3

1. 1,260 mL          2. 8 mL          3. 1.2 mL

4. 1,600 units/h, it is safe          5. 1,650 mg, 250 mL/h          6. 120 mL

7. 0.35 mL, 0.5 mL or 1 mL          8. No          9. 2.6 mL, 3 mL

10. 30 mL          11. 1,250 mL

12.

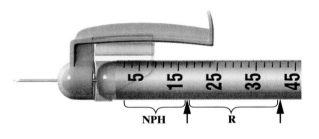

13. 32,600 units          14. 10 mL          15. 42 mL/h

16. 0500 h the next day          17. 3 tab          18. 0.3 g

19. 3 mL/h          20. 3 g          21. 1 mL tuberculin

22. 75 mcgtt/min          23. 2 tab          24. 0.52 m$^2$

25. 1,180 mL

## Comprehensive Self-Test 4

1. Yes          2. 2.7 mL          3. 2 tab

4. 8 h          5. 250 mL

6. 0.4 mL, 0.5 mL or 1 mL          7. 0.05 mg          8. 2 cap

9. 0.4 mL          10. 0.2 mL          11. 2 mL/min

12. 45 mL/h          13. 5 mL/min          14. 40 mL/h

15. 1.3 mL, 3 mL          16. 25 g

17. 6 hours 27 minutes          18. 32.4 mg          19. 1,090 mL

20. Yes          21. 20 units/h          22. 0.5 mL

23. 1.5 mL          24. 10 mL          25. Yes

# Appendix B

## The Apothecary System of Measurement

The apothecary system is one of the oldest systems of drug measurement. Although the apothecary system was used in the past to write prescriptions, it has largely been replaced by the metric system. Apothecary units are rarely used on drug labels, but when they are, the metric equivalents are also provided.

### Liquid Volume in the Apothecary System

The equivalents for the units of measurement for liquid volume in the apothecary system are shown in Table B.1 along with their abbreviations.

> **NOTE**
>
> In the apothecary system, the abbreviation or symbol for the unit is placed before the quantity (as in drams 8). Ounces are used for liquid volume in both the household and apothecary systems. To avoid errors, the abbreviations dr and oz are preferred over the formerly used abbreviations ℥ and ℨ.

| Table B.1 | Common Equivalents for Apothecary Liquid Volume Units |
|---|---|
| ounce (oz)1 | = drams (dr)8 |
| dram (dr)1 | = minims 60 |

> **NOTE**
>
> Decimal numbers are never used in the apothecary system.

### EXAMPLE B.1

How many minims would be equivalent to dr $\frac{1}{6}$?

Think:

$$dr\,\frac{1}{6} = minims\ ?$$

$$dr\ 1 = minims\ 60$$

Solve the proportion:

$$\frac{dr\,\frac{1}{6}}{minims\ x} = \frac{dr\ 1}{minims\ 60}$$

$$x = 10$$

So, minims 10 are equivalent to dr $\frac{1}{6}$.

### EXAMPLE B.2

How many ounces would be equivalent to dr 4?

Think:

$$dr\ 4 = ounces\ ?$$

$$dr\ 8 = ounce\ 1$$

Solve the proportion:

$$\frac{dr\ 4}{ounces\ x} = \frac{dr\ 8}{ounce\ 1}$$

$$8x = 4$$

$$x = \frac{1}{2}$$

So, dr 4 is equivalent to oz $\frac{1}{2}$.

## Weight in the Apothecary System

The grain (gr) is the only unit of weight in the apothecary system that is used in administering medications.

## Roman Numerals

Dosages in the apothecary system are sometimes written using Roman numerals. Table B.2 shows Roman numerals.

| Table B.2 Roman Numerals | | | | | |
|---|---|---|---|---|---|
| | Roman Numerals | | Roman Numerals | | Roman Numerals |
| 1 | I | 7 | VII | $\frac{1}{2}$ | ss |
| 2 | II | 8 | VIII | $1\frac{1}{2}$ | iss |
| 3 | III | 9 | IX | $7\frac{1}{2}$ | viiss |
| 4 | IV | 10 | X | | |
| 5 | V | 15 | XV | | |
| 6 | VI | 20 | XX | | |

## Equivalents of Common Units of Measurement

Tables B.3 and B.4 list some common equivalent values for weight, volume, and length in the metric, household, and apothecary systems of measurement. Although these equivalents are considered standards, many of them are approximations.

**NOTE**

Here are some useful equivalents:

1 t = 5 mL = dr 1

2 T = 30 mL = oz 1 = dr 8

| Table B.3 Equivalent Values for Units of Weight | | | |
|---|---|---|---|
| **Metric** | | **Apothecary** | **Household** |
| 60 milligrams (mg) | = | grain (gr) 1 | |
| 1 gram (g) | = | grains (gr) 15 | |
| 1 kilogram (kg) | | | = 2.2 pounds (lb) |

413

## Table B.4  Equivalent Values for Units of Volume

| Metric | | Apothecary | | Household |
|---|---|---|---|---|
| 1 milliliter (mL) | = | minims 15 | | |
| 5 milliliters (mL) | = | dram (dr) 1 | = | 1 teaspoon (t) |
| 15 milliliters (mL) | = | ounce (oz)$\frac{1}{2}$ | = | 1 tablespoon (T) |
| 30 milliliters (mL) | = | ounce (oz) 1 | = | 2 tablespoons (T) |
| 500 milliliters | = | ounces (oz) 16 | = | 1 pint (pt) |
| 1,000 milliliters | = | ounces (oz) 32 | = | 1 quart (qt) |

# Metric–Apothecary Conversions

### EXAMPLE B.3

**Convert 40 milligrams to grains.**

Think:

$$40 \; mg = gr \; ?$$
$$60 \; mg = gr \; 1$$

Solve the proportion:

$$\frac{40 \; mg}{gr \; x} = \frac{60 \; mg}{gr \; 1}$$
$$60x = 40$$
$$x = \frac{2}{3}$$

So, 40 milligrams are equivalent to grain $\frac{2}{3}$.

### EXAMPLE B.4

**Convert 0.12 milligrams to grains.**

Think:

$$0.12 \; mg = gr \; ?$$
$$60 \; mg = gr \; 1$$

Solve the proportion:

$$\frac{0.12 \; mg}{gr \; x} = \frac{60 \; mg}{gr \; 1}$$
$$60x = 0.12$$
$$x = 0.002$$

A decimal number cannot be used in the apothecary system. Therefore, 0.002 must be written in fractional form.

$$0.002 = \frac{2}{1,000} = \frac{1}{500}$$

So, 0.12 milligrams are equivalent to grain $\frac{1}{500}$.

## EXAMPLE B.5

**Convert 1.5 grams to an equivalent weight in grains.**

Think:

$$1.5\ g = gr\ ?$$
$$1\ g = gr\ 15$$

Solve the proportion:

$$\frac{1.5\ g}{gr\ x} = \frac{1\ g}{gr\ 15}$$
$$x = 22.5$$

A decimal number cannot be used in the apothecary system. Therefore, 22.5 must be written in fractional form as $22\frac{1}{2}$.

So, 1.5 grams are equivalent to grains $22\frac{1}{2}$.

**NOTE**

Grains are apothecary units and are expressed as fractions or whole numbers. Therefore, grains 22.5 should be expressed as grains $22\frac{1}{2}$.

## EXAMPLE B.6

**Convert grain $\frac{1}{300}$ to milligrams.**

Think:

$$gr\ \frac{1}{300} = ?\ mg$$
$$gr\ 1 = 60\ mg$$

Solve the proportion:

$$\frac{gr\ \frac{1}{300}}{x\ mg} = \frac{gr\ 1}{60\ mg}$$
$$x = 0.2$$

So, *grain* $\frac{1}{300}$ is equivalent to 0.2 milligrams.

## EXAMPLE B.7

**Convert grains $7\frac{1}{2}$ to grams.**

Think:

$$gr\ 7\frac{1}{2} = ?\ g$$
$$gr\ 15 = 1\ g$$

**NOTE**

Grams are metric units, so they are expressed as decimals or whole numbers. Therefore, $\frac{1}{2}$ gram is expressed as 0.5 gram.

Solve the proportion:

$$\frac{gr\ 7\frac{1}{2}}{x\ mg} = \frac{gr\ 15}{1\ g}$$

$$15x = 7\frac{1}{2}$$

$$x = \frac{1}{2}$$

So, *grains* $7\frac{1}{2}$ are equivalent to 0.5 gram.

# Household–Apothecary Conversions

### EXAMPLE B.8

**Convert ounces 2 to tablespoons.**

Think:

$$oz\ 2 = ?\ T$$
$$oz\ 1 = 2\ T$$

Solve the proportion:

$$\frac{oz\ 2}{x\ T} = \frac{oz\ 1}{2\ T}$$

$$x = 4$$

So, *ounces* 2 is equivalent to 4 tablespoons.

## Exercises

1. oz 1 = dr ?
2. dr 1 = minims ?
3. dr 12 = oz ?
4. dr $1\frac{1}{2}$ = minims ?
5. oz 64 = dr ?
6. dr 1 = ? t = minims ? = ? mL
7. oz 1 = ? T = dr ? = ? mL
8. 1 cup = ? glass = oz ? = ? pt
9. gr 1 = ? mg
10. 1 g = gr ?
11. 0.006 mg = gr ?
12. gr $3\frac{3}{4}$ = ? mg

## Answers

1. dr 8
2. minims 60
3. oz $1\frac{1}{2}$
4. minims 90
5. dr 512
6. dr 1  = 1 t = minims 60 = 5 mL
7. oz 1 = 2 T = dr 8 = 30 mL
8. 1 cup = 1 glass = oz 8 = $\frac{1}{2}$ pt
9. 60 mg
10. gr 15
11. gr $\frac{1}{10,000}$
12. 225 mg

# Appendix C

## Common Abbreviations Used in Medical Documentation

To someone unfamiliar with prescription abbreviations, medication orders may look like a foreign language. To interpret prescriptive orders accurately and to administer drugs safely, a qualified person must have a thorough knowledge of common abbreviations. For instance, when the prescriber writes, "**Dilaudid (hydromorphone) 1.5 mg IM q4h prn**" the health care professional knows how to interpret it as "hydromorphone, 1.5 milligrams, intramuscular, every four hours, whenever necessary." For measurement abbreviations, refer to Appendix D.

| Abbreviation | Meaning | Abbreviation | Meaning |
|---|---|---|---|
| ā | before (*abante*) | GT | gastrostomy tube |
| ac | before meals (*ante cibum*) | gtt | drop |
| ad lib | as desired (*ad libitum*) | h, hr | hour |
| A.M., am | morning | hs | hour of sleep; bedtime (*hora somni*) |
| amp | ampule | | |
| aq | aqueous water | IC | intracardiac |
| b.i.d. | two times a day | ID | intradermal |
| BP | blood pressure | IM | intramuscular |
| c̄ | with | IV | intravenous |
| C | Celsius; centigrade | USP | United States Pharmacopeia |
| cap | capsule | IVP | intravenous push |
| CBC | complete blood count | IVPB | intravenous piggyback |
| cc | cubic centimeter | IVSS | IV Soluset |
| CVP | central venous pressure | kg | kilogram |
| d | day | KVO | keep vein open |
| D/W | dextrose in water | L | liter |
| D5W or D5/W or D₅W | 5% dextrose in water | LA | long acting |
| daw | dispense as written | lb | pound |
| dr | dram | LIB | left in bag, left in bottle |
| Dx | diagnosis | LOS | length of stay |
| elix | elixir | MAR | medication administration record |
| ER | extended release | | |
| F | Fahrenheit | mcg | microgram |
| g | gram | mcgtt | microdrop |
| gr | grain | mEq | milliequivalent |

| Abbreviation | Meaning | Abbreviation | Meaning |
|---|---|---|---|
| mg | milligram | q2h | every two hours |
| min | minute | q3h | every three hours |
| mL | milliliter | q4h | every four hours |
| mU | milliunit | q6h | every six hours |
| n, noct | night | q8h | every eight hours |
| NDC | national drug code | q12h | every 12 hours |
| NGT | nasogastric tube | q.i.d. | four times a day *(quarter in die)* |
| NKA | no known allergies | | |
| NKDA | no known drug allergies | qn | every night *(quaque noct)* |
| NKFA | no known food allergies | qs | quantity sufficient or sufficient amount *(quantitas sufficiens)* |
| NPO | nothing by mouth *(per ora)* | | |
| NS | normal saline | R | respiration |
| NSAID | nonsteroidal anti-inflammatory drug | R/O | rule out |
| OTC | over the counter | Rx | prescription, treatment |
| oz | ounce | s̄ | without *(sine)* |
| p̄ | after | SIG | directions to the patient |
| PEG | percutaneous endoscopic gastrostomy tube | SL | sublingual |
| | | SR | sustained release |
| P | pulse | stat | immediately *(statum)* |
| pc | after meals *(post cibum)* | subcut | subcutaneous |
| PEJ | Percutaneous Endoscopic Jejunostomy | supp | suppository |
| PICC | peripherally inserted central catheter | susp | suspension |
| | | T or tbs | tablespoon |
| P.M., pm | afternoon, evening | t or tsp | teaspoon |
| PO | by mouth *(per os)* | T | temperature |
| POST-OP | after surgery | t.i.d. | three times a day *(ter in die)* |
| PR | by way of the rectum | | |
| PRE-OP | before surgery | tab | tablet |
| prn | when required or whenever necessary | TPN | total parenteral nutrition |
| Pt | patient | USP | United States Pharmacopeia |
| pt | pint | V/S | vital signs |
| q | every *(quaque)* | wt | weight |
| qh | every hour *(quaque hora)* | | |

# Appendix D

## Units of Measurement in Metric and Household Systems

| Abbreviations | | | |
|---|---|---|---|
| **Volume** | | | |
| **Metric** | | **Household** | |
| milliliter | mL | microdrop | mcgtt |
| liter | L | drop | gtt |
| cubic centimeter | cc | teaspoon | t or tsp |
| | | tablespoon | T or tbs |
| | | fluid ounce | oz |
| | | pint | pt |
| | | quart | qt |
| **Weight** | | | |
| **Metric** | | **Household** | |
| microgram | mcg | ounce | oz |
| milligram | mg | pound | lb |
| gram | g | | |
| kilogram | kg | | |
| **Length** | | | |
| **Metric** | | **Household** | |
| centimeter | cm | inch | in |
| meter | m | foot | ft |
| **Area** | | | |
| **Metric** | | | |
| square meter | $m^2$ | | |

# Appendix E

## Celsius and Fahrenheit Temperature Conversions

Reading and recording a temperature is a crucial step in assessing a patient's health. Temperatures can be measured using either the Fahrenheit (F) scale or the Celsius or centigrade (C) scale. Celsius/Fahrenheit equivalency tables make it easy to convert Celsius to Fahrenheit, or vice versa. Still, it is useful to be able to make this conversion yourself.

You can use the following formulas to convert from one temperature scale to the other

$$C = \frac{F - 32}{1.8} \quad \text{and} \quad F = 1.8\,C + 32$$

For those unfamiliar with algebra, the following rules are equivalent to the algebraic formulas.

> **First rule: To convert to Celsius.** Subtract 32 and then divide by 1.8.
> **Second rule: To convert to Fahrenheit.** Multiply by 1.8 and then add 32.

**NOTE**

Temperatures are rounded to the nearest tenth.

---

### EXAMPLE E.1

**Convert 102.5°F to Celsius.**

Using the first rule, you subtract 32.

$$\begin{array}{r} 102.5 \\ -32.0 \\ \hline 70.5 \end{array}$$

Then you divide by 1.8.

$$1.8\overline{)70.5000} \quad \Rightarrow \quad 39.17$$

So, 102.5°F equals 39.2°C.

---

### EXAMPLE E.2

**Convert 3°C to Fahrenheit.**

Using the second rule, you first multiply by 1.8.

$$\begin{array}{r} 1.8 \\ \times 3 \\ \hline 5.4 \end{array}$$

Then you add 32.

$$
\begin{array}{r}
5.4 \\
+32.0 \\
\hline
37.4
\end{array}
$$

So, 3°C equals 37.4°F

For those unfamiliar with the Celsius system, the following rhyme might be useful:

*Thirty is hot*
*Twenty is nice*
*Ten is chilly*
*Zero is ice*

# Appendix F

## Tables of Weight Conversions

Use the following tables to convert between the metric kilogram and the household pound.

| Table F.1 | Pounds to Kilograms | | | | |
|---|---|---|---|---|---|
| **lb** | **kg** | **lb** | **kg** | **lb** | **kg** |
| 2.2 | 1.0 | 120 | 54.5 | 240 | 109.1 |
| 5 | 2.3 | 125 | 56.8 | 245 | 111.4 |
| 10 | 4.5 | 130 | 59.1 | 250 | 113.6 |
| 15 | 6.8 | 135 | 61.4 | 255 | 115.9 |
| 20 | 9.1 | 140 | 63.6 | 260 | 118.2 |
| 25 | 11.4 | 145 | 65.9 | 265 | 120.5 |
| 30 | 13.6 | 150 | 68.2 | 270 | 122.7 |
| 35 | 15.9 | 155 | 70.5 | 275 | 125 |
| 40 | 18.2 | 160 | 72.7 | 280 | 127.3 |
| 45 | 20.5 | 165 | 75 | 285 | 129.5 |
| 50 | 22.7 | 170 | 77.3 | 290 | 131.8 |
| 55 | 25 | 175 | 79.5 | 295 | 134.1 |
| 60 | 27.3 | 180 | 81.8 | 300 | 136.4 |
| 65 | 29.5 | 185 | 84.1 | 305 | 138.6 |
| 70 | 31.8 | 190 | 86.4 | 310 | 140.9 |
| 75 | 34.1 | 195 | 88.6 | 315 | 143.2 |
| 80 | 36.4 | 200 | 90.9 | 320 | 145.5 |
| 85 | 38.6 | 205 | 93.2 | 325 | 147.7 |
| 90 | 40.9 | 210 | 95.5 | 330 | 150 |
| 95 | 43.2 | 215 | 97.7 | 335 | 152.3 |
| 100 | 45.5 | 220 | 100 | 340 | 154.5 |
| 105 | 47.7 | 225 | 102.3 | 345 | 156.8 |
| 110 | 50 | 230 | 104.5 | 350 | 159.1 |
| 115 | 52.3 | 235 | 106.8 | 355 | 161.4 |

## Table F.2 Kilograms to Pounds

| kg | lb | kg | lb | kg | lb |
|---|---|---|---|---|---|
| 2 | 4.4 | 56 | 123.2 | 110 | 242 |
| 4 | 8.8 | 58 | 127.6 | 112 | 246.4 |
| 6 | 13.2 | 60 | 132 | 114 | 250.8 |
| 8 | 17.6 | 62 | 136.4 | 116 | 255.2 |
| 10 | 22 | 64 | 140.8 | 118 | 259.6 |
| 12 | 26.4 | 66 | 145.2 | 120 | 264 |
| 14 | 30.8 | 68 | 149.6 | 122 | 268.4 |
| 16 | 35.2 | 70 | 154 | 124 | 272.8 |
| 18 | 39.6 | 72 | 158.4 | 126 | 277.2 |
| 20 | 44 | 74 | 162.8 | 128 | 281.6 |
| 22 | 48.4 | 76 | 167.2 | 130 | 286 |
| 24 | 52.8 | 78 | 171.6 | 132 | 290.4 |
| 26 | 57.2 | 80 | 176 | 134 | 294.8 |
| 28 | 61.6 | 82 | 180.4 | 136 | 299.2 |
| 30 | 66 | 84 | 184.8 | 138 | 303.6 |
| 32 | 70.4 | 86 | 189.2 | 140 | 308 |
| 34 | 74.8 | 88 | 193.6 | 142 | 312.4 |
| 36 | 79.2 | 90 | 198 | 144 | 316.8 |
| 38 | 83.6 | 92 | 202.4 | 146 | 321.2 |
| 40 | 88 | 94 | 206.8 | 148 | 325.6 |
| 42 | 92.4 | 96 | 211.2 | 150 | 330 |
| 44 | 96.8 | 98 | 215.6 | 152 | 334.4 |
| 46 | 101.2 | 100 | 220 | 154 | 338.8 |
| 48 | 105.6 | 102 | 224.4 | 156 | 343.2 |
| 50 | 110 | 104 | 228.8 | 158 | 347.6 |
| 52 | 114.4 | 106 | 233.2 | 160 | 352 |
| 54 | 118.8 | 108 | 237.6 | 162 | 356.4 |

# Index

Note: All registered drug names are referred to their generic names. Figures are indicated by an F. Tables are indicated by a T. Notes are indicated by an N.

Pearson Education, Inc.

**YOU SHOULD CAREFULLY READ THE TERMS AND CONDITIONS BEFORE USING THE CD-ROM PACKAGE. USING THIS CD-ROM PACKAGE INDICATES YOUR ACCEPTANCE OF THESE TERMS AND CONDITIONS.**

Pearson Education, Inc. provides this program and licenses its use. You assume responsibility for the selection of the program to achieve your intended results, and for the installation, use, and results obtained from the program. This license extends only to use of the program in the United States or countries in which the program is marketed by authorized distributors.

## LICENSE GRANT

You hereby accept a nonexclusive, nontransferable, permanent license to install and use the program ON A SINGLE COMPUTER at any given time. You may copy the program solely for backup or archival purposes in support of your use of the program on the single computer. You may not modify, translate, disassemble, decompile, or reverse engineer the program, in whole or in part.

## TERM

The License is effective until terminated. Pearson Education, Inc. reserves the right to terminate this License automatically if any provision of the License is violated. You may terminate the License at any time. To terminate this License, you must return the program, including documentation, along with a written warranty stating that all copies in your possession have been returned or destroyed.

## LIMITED WARRANTY

THE PROGRAM IS PROVIDED "AS IS" WITHOUT WARRANTY OF ANY KIND, EITHER EXPRESSED OR IMPLIED, INCLUDING, BUT NOT LIMITED TO, THE IMPLIED WARRANTIES OR MERCHANTABILITY AND FITNESS FOR A PARTICULAR PURPOSE. THE ENTIRE RISK AS TO THE QUALITY AND PERFORMANCE OF THE PROGRAM IS WITH YOU. SHOULD THE PROGRAM PROVE DEFECTIVE, YOU (AND NOT PRENTICE-HALL, INC. OR ANY AUTHORIZED DEALER) ASSUME THE ENTIRE COST OF ALL NECESSARY SERVICING, REPAIR, OR CORRECTION. NO ORAL OR WRITTEN INFORMATION OR ADVICE GIVEN BY PRENTICE-HALL, INC., ITS DEALERS, DISTRIBUTORS, OR AGENTS SHALL CREATE A WARRANTY OR INCREASE THE SCOPE OF THIS WARRANTY.

SOME STATES DO NOT ALLOW THE EXCLUSION OF IMPLIED WARRANTIES, SO THE ABOVE EXCLUSION MAY NOT APPLY TO YOU. THIS WARRANTY GIVES YOU SPECIFIC LEGAL RIGHTS AND YOU MAY ALSO HAVE OTHER LEGAL RIGHTS THAT VARY FROM STATE TO STATE.

Pearson Education, Inc. does not warrant that the functions contained in the program will meet your requirements or that the operation of the program will be uninterrupted or error-free.

However, Pearson Education, Inc. warrants the diskette(s) or CD-ROM(s) on which the program is furnished to be free from defects in material and workmanship under normal use for a period of ninety (90) days from the date of delivery to you as evidenced by a copy of your receipt.

The program should not be relied on as the sole basis to solve a problem whose incorrect solution could result in injury to person or property. If the program is employed in such a manner, it is at the user's own risk and Pearson Education, Inc. explicitly disclaims all liability for such misuse.

## LIMITATION OF REMEDIES

Pearson Education, Inc.'s entire liability and your exclusive remedy shall be:

1. the replacement of any diskette(s) or CD-ROM(s) not meeting Pearson Education, Inc.'s "LIMITED WARRANTY" and that is returned to Pearson Education, or

2. if Pearson Education is unable to deliver a replacement diskette(s) or CD-ROM(s) that is free of defects in materials or workmanship, you may terminate this agreement by returning the program.

IN NO EVENT WILL PRENTICE-HALL, INC. BE LIABLE TO YOU FOR ANY DAMAGES, INCLUDING ANY LOST PROFITS, LOST SAVINGS, OR OTHER INCIDENTAL OR CONSEQUENTIAL DAMAGES ARISING OUT OF THE USE OR INABILITY TO USE SUCH PROGRAM EVEN IF PRENTICE-HALL, INC. OR AN AUTHORIZED DISTRIBUTOR HAS BEEN ADVISED OF THE POSSIBILITY OF SUCH DAMAGES, OR FOR ANY CLAIM BY ANY OTHER PARTY.

SOME STATES DO NOT ALLOW FOR THE LIMITATION OR EXCLUSION OF LIABILITY FOR INCIDENTAL OR CONSEQUENTIAL DAMAGES, SO THE ABOVE LIMITATION OR EXCLUSION MAY NOT APPLY TO YOU.

## GENERAL

You may not sublicense, assign, or transfer the license of the program. Any attempt to sublicense, assign or transfer any of the rights, duties, or obligations hereunder is void.

This Agreement will be governed by the laws of the State of New York.

Should you have any questions concerning this Agreement, you may contact Pearson Education, Inc. by writing to:

Director of New Media
Higher Education Division
Pearson Education, Inc.
One Lake Street
Upper Saddle River, NJ 07458

**Should you have any questions concerning technical support, you may contact:**

**Product Support Department: Monday–Friday 8:00 A.M. –8:00 P.M. and Sunday 5:00 P.M.-12:00 A.M. (All times listed are Eastern). 1-800-677-6337**

**You can also get support by filling out the web form located at http://247.prenhall.com**

YOU ACKNOWLEDGE THAT YOU HAVE READ THIS AGREEMENT, UNDERSTAND IT, AND AGREE TO BE BOUND BY ITS TERMS AND CONDITIONS. YOU FURTHER AGREE THAT IT IS THE COMPLETE AND EXCLUSIVE STATEMENT OF THE AGREEMENT BETWEEN US THAT SUPERSEDES ANY PROPOSAL OR PRIOR AGREEMENT, ORAL OR WRITTEN, AND ANY OTHER COMMUNICATIONS BETWEEN US RELATING TO THE SUBJECT MATTER OF THIS AGREEMENT.